Robin L. West   Jan D. Sinnott
Editors

Everyday Memory and Aging

Current Research and Methodology

With 11 Illustrations

Springer-Verlag

New York Berlin Heidelberg London Paris
Tokyo Hong Kong Barcelona Budapest

Robin L. West
Department of Psychology
University of Florida
Gainsville, FL 32611-2065, USA

Jan D. Sinnott
Department of Psychology
Towson State University
Towson, MD 21204-7097, USA

Library of Congress Cataloging-in-Publication Data
Everyday memory and aging: current research and methodology/Robin
  Lea West, Jan D. Sinnott, editors.
      p. cm.
   Includes bibliographical references and index.
   ISBN 0-387-97624-8 (alk. paper)
      1. Memory—Age factors. 2. Memory—Research—Methodology.
I. West, Robin, 1951–   . II. Sinnott, Jan D.
BF378.A33E84 1991
155.67—dc20   91-21258

Printed on acid-free paper.

Typeset by Asco Trade Typesetting Ltd., Hong Kong.
Printed and bound by Book Mart, North Bergen, NJ.
Printed in the United States of America.

9 8 7 6 5 4 3 2 1

ISBN 0-387-97624-8 Springer-Verlag New York Berlin Heidelberg
ISBN 3-540-97624-8 Springer-Verlag Berlin Heidelberg New York

Preface: How This Book Came to Be and What You Can Expect to Find Here

JAN D. SINNOTT AND ROBIN L. WEST

It is certainly true that it has taken great effort to create this book on everyday memory! But routinely, even greater effort is expended by countless researchers because they are interested in everyday memory activities. In spite of recent attacks on "everyday memory" (e.g., Banaji & Crowder, 1989), researchers remain enthusiastic (e.g., Bruce, 1991; Klatzky, 1991; Loftus, 1991; Tulving, 1991), even though it is harder to study everyday thought than to study memory in the laboratory. The critical variables in practical memory research often prove difficult to conceptualize and operationalize reliably. It is hard to decide what is "naturalistic" or "everyday," even in a certain context. Investigators cannot create measures quickly because tasks, by their very nature, are valid only in specific contexts, not all contexts. Because everyday memory research represents a new paradigm, this field of inquiry lacks the track record laboratory measures have established in psychology. Everyday studies often meet opposition, in part because their creators do not use the generally accepted mechanistic models and theories of human behavior and, most frightening of all, because they implicitly challenge some of our most sacred world views as 20th century cognitive scientists. The list of difficulties could go on indefinitely. Yet few of us who do such research can easily say *why* it is that we bother. We seem sure that this work is important, perhaps even fundamental to understanding memory aging—but why?

It seems that one main reason for interest in these studies is that they ask better, richer, juicier, more meaningful questions (Sinnott, in press). That's why it's worth the trouble. The heart of the question and the uniqueness of everyday research is the often-neglected variable of choice: the investigator's choice of parameters to study; adaptive choice for the person or "subject"; choice within a theory among a larger number of questions and subtheories; our discovery within everyday cognition of the individual knower's very real choice about cognitive "truth"; and knowing that the knower's and the experimenter's creation of reality do matter immensely to the definitions of "reality" given by science. Choice creates cognitive filters. Everyday studies, finally, are about the knower as a creator of reality, working jointly with other creators, and therefore about the extension of the discipline of psychology.

What better questions does the study of everyday cognition allow us to ask? What agenda can everyday cognition give us? What are the benefits of taking this approach?

One immensely different set of questions *focuses on process*, on the dialogue rather than the monologue, on the melody rather than the chords, on the path rather than the destination. This is a benefit because an essential interest of psychology, after all, is in change from state to state, rather than on the states alone, although traditional studies usually focus on state. Some of the larger process questions are also: How do people change or develop? How should we train agents of change to do that effectively? How can we get people to change their knowledge state, that is, to learn? What form does it take when people move from "here" to "there"? How are experimental questions related to adaptive real-life behavior? In the everyday cognitive world, nothing lasts for long, and process is our most important product. Process may or may not be progress; but it is definitely different from state. The study of process can yield both basic and applied laws of psychology.

A second benefit of doing everyday memory research is that this field necessitates *a conscious choice about the level of research question to address*, making us acknowledge and work with the idea that any one paradigm or view of truth is not the only one. The fact that everyday cognitive research is so very complicated forces us to narrow that complexity to a meaningful but tolerable level, to choose a "truth." Few can help us decide how to narrow it; we must make our methodological choices alone. Methodology is an overriding theme for this text because the newness of this research area requires us to look inward and examine the logic and heuristic value of these choices. When we are forced to choose, and to examine our selection, we become better scientists because we can then recognize more clearly our own power in creating paradigms and reality. Acknowledging choice frees us creatively as scientists.

A third benefit is to question the *mechanisms of application* of a general principle to a specific, concrete, life experience. Notice that this approach differs in two ways from strictly laboratory research: (a) It broadens the search for basic cognitive processes by including overlooked aspects of the cognitive event, often those aspects that vary freely during in vivo experience; thus, it enlarges the problem space; and (b) it provides mechanisms for explaining the annoying, probabilistic, less-than-100% nature of occurrence of most basic cognitive processes. This is higher order basic research, involving top–down analysis, whatever critics might argue.

A fourth set of questions addresses *function and compensation*. Researchers have uncovered many processes that are a part of human thought but have not yet connected many of those processes to how well or how poorly humans get along in the world. Some cognitive processes inevitably fail at one time or another across the life span, but life goes on for the adaptive individual. We have yet to do many studies on how individuals use their skills to compensate for failure. Everyday cognitive studies are ideal for this task, on a basic and applied level.

Another set of questions that have been of interest for some time are questions about the dynamic interplay of *self-evaluation and performance.* No single chapter in this text addresses this issue. At the same time, few of these chapters fail to mention memory complaints, self-confidence, or memory self-report. This topic has played a vital role in the burgeoning field of practical cognition. We want, and need, to know whether self-evaluation affects performance in subtle or powerful ways, in a qualitative or quantitative fashion, in specific contexts or in a persistent interactive process.

Finally, development over the life span involves an individual's use of general, adaptive intelligence to his or her own unique life over time. Thus, a sixth benefit of studying mechanisms of everyday cognition can be to *create a better set of theories about life tasks, growth, and change in midlife and old age.* A number of midlife-development theories exist, but they do not make much use of cognitive variables, especially complex ones. The study of practical cognition affords the opportunity to remedy this.

Notice that the underlying theme in these special contributions or sets of questions is that of ongoing *process* and *choice* in a *complex context* embedded in *personal history.* The focus remains on quantitative and qualitative forces for change that influence the adapting individual. Pursuit of this research theme involves being analytical and scientific about cognition as a whole, nonfragmented process, connected to life experience.

Some Definitions

It may be worthwhile to clarify what we mean by three key terms in this book's title: *everyday, memory,* and *aging.* By *everyday,* we mean naturalistic or realistic, or related to everyday experience, not necessarily frequent or common. *Everyday* represents some point along a spectrum that ranges from elaborately controlled artificial to spontaneously occurring in nature. Various investigators and theorists in this book choose different points on that continuum, tending toward the everyday end of it. The term *aging* refers to differences or changes related to the passage of life time, beyond the early 20s, changes or differences that may potentially lead to adaptation or decline. In this definition of aging, more doors are left open for meaningful cognitive changes—not just losses—to occur. This definition makes it possible to take a different, broader tack in our research questions. *Memory* refers to a processing-storage-retrieval function of mind that must be seen as embedded in context. The nature and definition of context is left to the author of each chapter, but a key difference between basic researchers who tolerate everyday memory studies and those who do not is the belief that memory cannot float free of context. Even laboratory tests of memory measure memory in context, albeit an unusual one. Not all of these papers focus on memory. Authors with related interests in intelligence or perception contributed shorter "idea" papers to stimulate broader conceptions, considering factors that have an impact on everyday memory.

Overview of the Chapters

The chapters in this volume are organized into four parts, although in many cases, the subject matter of a chapter fits more than one part. Methodological issues are an overriding theme, which all authors were asked to address, and the first general part focuses specifically on methods. In Chapter 1, West uses the discussion of location-recall studies to demonstrate that methodological choices have real consequences for research outcome. The researcher who uses a broader set of methodologies from the research continuum, varying from naturalistic to laboratory studies, can use converging operations to address process in a specific memory domain. Cavanaugh and Hertzog, in Chapter 2, describe the major ways that daily diaries can be used in everyday memory research, key methodological issues, and potential abuses of such data. Of particular importance to everyday memory researchers is the potential for using diaries for insight into the emotions associated with remembering and forgetting, as well as the potential to use diary entries as material for long-term retention tests. Some newly collected data are summarized to illustrate these points. Ross and Berg (Chapter 3) report on individual differences in experience as the leading explanation for variations in scripted events. These experiential factors include frequency of occurrence, importance, and affectivity of an event. The authors convey how script methodology has influenced the data collected thus far and call for more flexibility in script paradigms. They outline proposed methodologies for exploring experiential factors in the study of aging and script. Next, Larrabee and Crook (Chapter 4) review the development and application of a computerized memory test battery, which employs laser disk technology, and an interactive touch-sensitive screen to simulate memory tasks of everyday life, including telephone number dialing, name–face memory, and object location recall. They describe the factor structure of the battery, the association of memory self-report with performance, and subject performance subtypes. They discuss the application of this test battery in a variety of research arenas, including memory training and clinical trials of potential memory-enhancing compounds. Last in Part 1, Sinnott and her colleagues (Chapter 5) outline several spatial memory aging studies that employ a paradigm useful for comparing memory performance across the spectrum from naturalistic to laboratory spatial layouts. The goals of their program are to bridge the dichotomy between everyday and laboratory research in an experimentally sound way. The authors present results from five studies.

Part 2 focuses on semantic memory and speech processing, a research domain that is growing in importance and influence, partly because it encompasses studies along the entire spectrum from laboratory (see Howard, 1988) to naturalistic investigation (e.g., Burke, Mackay, Worthley, & Wade, in press). In Chapter 6, Hess discusses the recent work in cognitive psychology that has emphasized the role of knowledge structures in organizing our experience and in determining developmental differences in memory performance. He reports on a detailed study of adult age differences in both the content and structure of scripts. Of primary concern is the extent to which age differences in memory for events might be predicted from variations in scripted knowledge. Wingfield and Stine (Chapter 7) then discuss the surprising lack of problems older adults have with conversation. Their fine-grained analysis of speech processing, working memory during conversations, and recall of discourse reveals deficits as well as compensatory mechanisms. They discuss alternative methodological approaches that yield germane data on elderly language processing. Next, Jepson and Labouvie-Vief (Chapter 8) examine adaptive change with age in symbolic thinking. While older adults are often said to be poorer processors of expository text, they actually may have a more complex style, switching from literal to symbolic meanings. An examination of recalled narrative summaries from adolescents, adults, and elderly adults demonstrates that older adults more often remember events in terms of complex, inner psychological processes. In the last chapter in Part 2, Kemper, Kynette, and Norman (Chapter 9) survey age differences in spoken language production. This review focuses on the role of working memory in the production of language and how age-related impairments of working memory may affect adults' production of complex narrative and syntactic structures. Age-group differences in spoken language are illustrated with data from multiyear samples of adults' spontaneous speech.

Part 3 focuses on intervention and instruction. Within geropsychology, this domain of study was one of the first to emphasize practical memory function (e.g., Treat, Poon, & Fozard, 1978). In the first chapter here, Camp and McKitrick (Chapter 10) consider the methodological and theoretical issues involved in the implementation of memory interventions for individuals with Alzheimer's-type Dementia (AD). A relatively new intervention—spaced retrieval—seems to overcome many of the difficulties associated with the use of traditional techniques for this population. Successful results from recent research using this technique with AD populations are reported. Recommendations for interventions conclude the chapter. Thompson's chapter (11) provides an overview of the applications of psychological research for the instruction of elderly adults. Content areas include mode and rate of presentation of material, reinforcement and feedback, organization of information, response time, and meaningfulness of material. In addition, attention is given to new areas of interest, such as computer-assisted instruction. Riley's chapter (12) emphasizes the importance of integrating empirical and laboratory research with clinically relevant issues, focusing on intervention methodologies that would be useful in both domains. Among other issues, she highlights those research design considerations that would make laboratory findings more useful for clinicians and illustrates her ideas with new clinical data. Last in Part 3, Hayslip and Maloy (Chapter 13) raise the issue of the ecological relevance of psychometric assessments. This chapter examines relationships between crystallized and fluid intelligence and measures of everyday intelligence. In addition, the authors explore the impact of cognitive training (targeting fluid skills) on everyday abilities and perceived cognitive failures. Such data will help us to more completely understand the interface between psychometric abilities and everyday cognitive function in the elderly.

Part 4 is devoted to specific issues in everyday memory research and illustrations of some useful paradigms for this research. Norris and Krauss, in Chapter 14, point out that memory skills are necessary for negotiating any environment. In a nursing home setting, two sets of nontraditional measures of memory and spatial ability predicted the use residents made of their surroundings. The authors address measurement issues and suggest interventions based on these relationships. Hoyer and Rybash (Chapter 15) provide a model for compensatory mechanisms and processes in everyday perception based on knowledge—in particular, knowledge of specific objects in context. They examine the decline in real-world perceptual processing that occurs as a result of capacity-demanding conditions. This work provides a methodological model for everyday memory research. In Chapter 16, Yoder and Elias describe the basic paradigms used to measure emotion and affect and point out their relevance for everyday memory. They analyze areas of memory research that could have affective components and suggest future research based on their recent studies. Plude and Murphy (Chapter 17) explore the role of attention in everyday memory, focusing on absentmindedness and the importance of selective attention. A primary thesis is that everyday memory complaints often may be due to deficient selective attention rather than faulty memory function. Adams-Price and Perlmutter (Chapter 18) note that research on eyewitness memory has focused on issues of importance to cognitive gerontologists, such as the relationship between accuracy and confidence, memory for details, and the suggestibility of witnesses. A review of the research on eyewitness memory reveals an interplay between practical issues and theory, which may serve as a model for other domains of everyday memory research. In a more speculative vein, Meacham (Chapter 19) examines ways in which autobiographical events are remembered in the course of everyday reminiscence. One's memory and interpretation of these events can give information about individual and social goals, as people construct a personal meaning for their life course. He explores the implicit social and constructive nature of autobiographical memory in the context of motivational issues in life-span memory development. Finally, Ventis (Chapter 20) discusses everyday memory and individual differences, focusing on theory, methodology, and intervention. She weaves her discussion around the issues of self-reported memory and age-related mental slowing. A focus on individual differences has implications for design, analysis, and interpretation of everyday memory studies. Taken together, these chapters offer a wide range of empirical evidence and considerable insight into everyday memory processes.

Thanks. Seeing this list of talented, creative thinkers is a reminder of the thanks we owe to our "fellow travelers" in our explorations of thought. We very much appreciate the creative sparks, emotional support, and concrete assistance of family, friends, institutions, colleagues, older adult subjects, and students! This book should be dedicated to all of them. The old models are incomplete; we do not think alone. The others who share our lives also help to create our good ideas.

In particular, a special thank you goes to the Brookdale Foundation in New York, whose research support made it possible for Robin to devote time and energy to this project. Thanks also to the Brookdale Institute of Gerontology and Adult Human Development in Israel for furnishing a "home away from home" for Robin during the last 6 months of writing and editing. Thanks to Cecile Chapman and Brigette Bellott at the University of Florida for their help in the production of this volume. Also, Ken, Dara, and Jaina are much appreciated for both the personal support and the lively distraction they provide.

Another special thank you from Jan to the staff and students of the Center for the Study of Adult Development and Aging and the staff of the Psychology Department at Towson State University Jan appreciates grants from the University, which made preparation of this book possible. Thanks also go to James and Gwenn for their patience and support.

Our hope is that this volume will contribute to broader conceptions of the science of memory and aging. New frontiers are open to us if we can only recognize that talents and approaches across a wide spectrum are valued and indeed essential. Science is not a "zero sum game." The more we exercise our thoughts and skills, the more fun the game of ideas gets to be for all of us. Thank you to all of you who made the game fun for us as we worked on this book, and welcome to newcomers whose fresh ideas, inventions, and insights will soon make the game even more fun.

References

Banaji, M.R., & Crowder, R.G. (1989). The bankruptcy of everyday memory. *American Psychologist, 44,* 1185–1193.

Bruce, D. (1991). Mechanistic and functional explanations of memory. *American Psychologist, 46,* 46–48.

Burke, D.M., Mackay, D.G., Worthley, J.S., & Wade, E. (in press). On the tip of the tongue: What causes word finding failures in young and older adults. *Journal of Memory and Language.*

Howard, D.V. (1988). Aging and memory activation: The priming of semantic and episodic memories. In L.L. Light & D.M. Burke (Eds.), *Language, memory, and aging* (pp. 77–99). New York: Cambridge University Press.

Klatzky, R.L. (1991). Let's be friends. *American Psychologist, 46,* 43–45.

Loftus, E.F. (1991). The glitter of everyday memory . . . and the gold. *American Psychologist, 46,* 41–42.

Sinnott, J.D. (in press). Yes, it's worth the trouble! Unique contributions from everyday cognitive studies. In H.W. Reese & J.M. Puckett (Eds.), *Mechanisms of everyday cognition.* Hillsdale, NJ: Erlbaum.

Treat, N.J., Poon, L.W., & Fozard, J.L. (1978). From clinical and research findings on memory to intervention programs. *Experimental Aging Research, 4,* 235–253.

Tulving, E. (1991). Memory research is not a zero sum game. *American Psychologist, 46,* 41–42.

Contents

Preface: How This Book Came to Be and What You Can Expect
to Find Here v
JAN D. SINNOTT AND ROBIN L. WEST

Contributors xv

Part 1.   Methodological Approaches

  1. Everyday Memory and Aging: A Diversity of Tests, Tasks,
      and Paradigms 3
      ROBIN L. WEST
  2. Uses of Diary Data in Cognitive and Developmental
      Research 22
      JOHN C. CAVANAUGH AND CHRISTOPHER HERTZOG
  3. Examining Idiosyncracies in Script Reports Across the Life
      Span: Distortions or Derivations of Experience 39
      BARBARA L. ROSS AND CYNTHIA A. BERG
  4. A Computerized Battery for Assessment of
      Everyday Memory 54
      GLENN J. LARRABEE AND THOMAS H. CROOK, III
  5. Age and Memory for Spatial Relations 66
      JAN D. SINNOTT, KEVIN BOCHENEK, MICHELLE KIM,
      LISA KLEIN, CHESTER ROBIE, KAREN DISHMAN, AND
      CAROLYN DUNMYER

Part 2.   Semantic Memory and Speech Processing

  6. Adult Age Differences in Script Content and Structure 87
      THOMAS M. HESS
  7. Age Differences in Perceptual Processing and Memory for
      Spoken Language 101
      ARTHUR WINGFIELD AND ELIZABETH A.L. STINE

8. Symbolic Processing of Youth and Elders 124
   KATHRYN L. JEPSON AND GISELA LABOUVIE-VIEF
9. Age Differences in Spoken Language 138
   SUSAN KEMPER, DONNA KYNETTE, AND SUZANNE NORMAN

Part 3. Intervention and Instruction

10. Memory Interventions in Alzheimer's-Type Dementia
    Populations: Methodological and Theoretical Issues 155
    CAMERON J. CAMP AND LESLIE A. MCKITRICK
11. Applications of Psychological Research for the Instruction
    of Elderly Adults 173
    DENNIS N. THOMPSON
12. Bridging the Gap Between Researchers and Clinicians:
    Methodological Perspectives and Choices 182
    KATHRYN PEREZ RILEY
13. The Interface Between Psychometric Abilities and
    Everyday Cognitive Functioning 190
    BERT HAYSLIP, JR., AND ROBIN M. MALOY

Part 4. Issues and Illustrations of Everyday Memory Research

14. Spatial Skills, Memory, and Environmental Use in a
    Nursing Home Setting 201
    KRISTEN K.A. NORRIS AND ISELI K. KRAUSS
15. Knowledge Factors in Everyday Visual Perception 215
    WILLIAM J. HOYER AND JOHN M. RYBASH
16. A Proposed Role for Affect in Everyday Memory 223
    CAROL Y. YODER AND JEFFREY W. ELIAS
17. Aging, Selective Attention, and Everyday Memory 235
    DANA J. PLUDE AND LISA J. MURPHY
18. Eyewitness Memory and Aging Research: A Case Study
    in Everyday Memory 246
    CAROLYN ADAMS-PRICE AND MARION PERLMUTTER
19. Cooperative Action and Reconstructing the Personal Past
    as Functions of Autobiographical Remembering 259
    JOHN A. MEACHAM
20. Individual Differences in Everyday Memory Aging:
    Implications for Theory and Research 270
    DEBORAH G. VENTIS

Author Index 281
Subject Index 291

Contributors

CAROLYN ADAMS-PRICE Department of Psychology, Mississippi State University, Mississippi State, MS 39762-6161, USA

CYNTHIA A. BERG Department of Psychology, University of Utah, Salt Lake City, UT 84112, USA

KEVIN BOCHENEK Department of Psychology, Towson State University, Baltimore, MD 21204, USA

CAMERON J. CAMP Department of Psychology, University of New Orleans, New Orleans, LA 70148, USA

JOHN C. CAVANAUGH Department of Psychology, Bowling Green State University, Bowling Green, OH 43403, USA

THOMAS H. CROOK, III Memory Assessment Clinics, Inc., 83-11 Wisconsin Avenue, Bethesda, MD 20814-3126, USA

KAREN DISHMAN Department of Psychology, Towson State University, Baltimore, MD 21204-7097, USA

CAROLYN DUNMYER Department of Psychology, Towson State University, Baltimore, MD 21204-7097, USA

JEFFREY W. ELIAS Department of Psychology, Texas Tech University, Lubbock, TX 79409-2051, USA

BERT HAYSLIP, JR. Department of Psychology, University of North Texas, Denton, TX 76203-3587, USA

CHRISTOPHER HERTZOG School of Psychology, Georgia Institute of Technology, Atlanta, GA 30332, USA

THOMAS M. HESS Department of Psychology, North Carolina State University, Raleigh, NC 27695-7801, USA

WILLIAM J. HOYER Department of Psychology, Syracuse University, Syracuse, NY 13244-2340, USA

KATHRYN L. JEPSON Department of Psychology, Wayne State University, Detroit, MI 48202, USA

SUSAN KEMPER Department of Psychology, University of Kansas, Lawrence, KS 66045-2160, USA

MICHELLE KIM Department of Psychology, Towson State University, Baltimore, MD 21204-7097, USA

LISA KLEIN   Department of Psychology, Towson State University, Baltimore, MD 21204-7097, USA

ISELI K. KRAUSS   Clarion University of Pennsylvania, Clarion, PA 16214, USA

DONNA KYNETTE   Department of Psychology, University of Kansas, Lawrence, KS 66045-2160, USA

GISELA LABOUVIE-VIEF   Department of Psychology, Wayne State University, Detroit, MI 48202, USA

GLENN J. LARRABEE   Memory Assessment Clinic, 1217 East Avenue South, Sarasota, FL 34239, USA

ROBIN M. MALOY   Department of Psychology, University of North Texas, Denton, TX 76203, USA

JOHN A. MEACHAM   Department of Psychology, State University of New York at Buffalo, Buffalo, NY 14260, USA

LESLIE A. MCKITRICK   Department of Psychology, University of New Orleans, New Orleans, LA 70148, USA

LISA J. MURPHY   Department of Psychology, University Maryland, College Park, MD 20742-4411, USA

SUZANNE NORMAN   Department of Psychology, University of Kansas, Lawrence, KS 66045-2160, USA

KRISTEN K.A. NORRIS   California State Polytechnic University, Pomona, CA 91768, USA

MARION PERLMUTTER   Department of Psychology, University of Michigan, Ann Arbor, MI 48109, USA

DANA J. PLUDE   Department of Psychology, University of Maryland, College Park, MD 20742-4411, USA

KATHRYN PEREZ RILEY   Department of Psychiatry, Marshall University, School of Medicine, Huntington, WV 25755-9460, USA

CHESTER ROBIE   Department of Psychology, Towson State University, Baltimore, MD 21204-7097, USA

BARBARA L. ROSS   Department of Psychology, University of Utah, Salt Lake City, UT 84112, USA

JOHN M. RYBASH   Department of Psychology, Hamilton College, Clinton, NY 13323, USA

JAN D. SINNOTT   Department of Psychology, Towson State University, Baltimore, MD 21204-7097, USA

ELIZABETH A.L. STINE   Department of Psychology, University of New Hampshire, Durham, NH 03824, USA

DENNIS N. THOMPSON   Department of Educational Foundations, Georgia State University, Atlanta, GA 30303-3083, USA

DEBORAH G. VENTIS   Department of Psychology, College of William and Mary, Williamsburg, VA 23185, USA

ROBIN L. WEST   Department of Psychology, University of Florida, Gainseville, FL 32611-2065, USA

ARTHUR WINGFIELD Department of Psychology, Brandeis University, Waltham, MA 02254-9110, USA

CAROL Y. YODER Department of Psychology, Indiana State University, Terre Haute, IN 47809, USA

Part 1
Methodological Approaches

1
Everyday Memory and Aging: A Diversity of Tests, Tasks, and Paradigms

Robin L. West

As a fledgling field, the study of everyday memory and aging is still searching for a definition and a methodology. The importance of this search is reflected by the number of presentations and articles since the mid-1980s that focused on this concern. These include conference papers (Neisser, 1988; Poon, Dudley, & Welke, 1990), journals (see Loftus, 1991), and books that define the field and its importance (Cohen, 1989; Gruneberg, Morris, & Sykes, 1988; Poon, Rubin, & Wilson, 1989). Articles and books have also explained applied cognition (Park, in press; Sinnott, 1989) and overviewed aging research on everyday memory (Cohen, 1988; West, 1986). Every one of these references includes an attempt to delineate the field of everyday memory or applied research and some guidelines for how practical memory should be studied. This chapter focuses on evidence gleaned from different types of practical memory investigations to show the rich data base that is being gathered in this research field. Examples from location-recall studies are used to illustrate the importance of maintaining diversity in our scientific tests, tasks, and paradigms, to provide more understanding of the effects of aging on memory.

Five Research Domains

Researchers must make many design decisions, and several decisions relevant to the study of everyday memory are highlighted here. Although some evidence on the impact of research design choices is examined here, more direct study of the effects of methodology, design, and/or paradigm selection is needed. As it is, the current research designs generally follow five patterns: (a) self-report measures, (b) naturalistic studies, (c) simulations, (d) laboratory component process experiments, and (e) test batteries. (Research on memory improvement is not included as a separate category here. The assessments employed for memory training studies have varied widely and, in fact, involve all five of the categories noted.)

Self-Report Measures

Self-reported everyday memory has been investigated extensively with questionnaires, and a number of studies have used diaries as well (see Chapter 2). Adults of all ages have reported their memory failures (Larrabee, West, & Crook, 1991), abilities (Dixon & Hultsch, 1983), strategies (Weinstein, Duffy, Underwood, McDonald, & Gott, 1981), attributions (Lachman, Steinberg, & Trotter, 1987), and their experiences with specific types of problems, like tip-of-the-tongue experiences (TOTs) (Burke, Worthley, & Martin, 1988).

These data have provided a framework for understanding memory self-evaluation and aging. The diary investigations have shown that age differences in everyday activities (e.g., Rice, 1986) and strategies (e.g., Burke et al., 1988) are often reflected in diary records. It has also been demonstrated repeatedly that depression can affect questionnaire responses concerning memory skills (Neiderehe, 1986). However, few principles about the relationship between actual memory performance and self-reported memory can be stated with any certainty. The findings regarding age differences in self-evaluated memory are mixed (Chaffin & Herrmann, 1983; Martin, 1986), but it is clear that older adults' "self-efficacy" is consistently lower than that of younger people (Berry, West, & Dennehy, 1989; Hertzog, Dixon, Schulenberg, & Hultsch, 1987). Performance–self-report correlations do not appear to vary systematically with age (cf. Berry et al., 1989; Zelinski, Gilewski, & Thompson, 1980), but such correlations have been stronger for everyday tests than for laboratory tests and stronger after testing than before (Berry et al., 1989; Gilewski & Zelinski, 1986; West & Dennehy, 1990). The extant data show that self-report measures cannot serve as a stand-in for performance. In fact, that may not be desirable. Instead, the study of memory self-report complements the study of performance, with the former research area focusing more on attitudinal, social, and affective factors influencing memory aging (Cavanaugh, Morton, & Tilse, 1989).

Naturalistic Studies

Naturalistic is defined: Learned in the context of ongoing activity in one's social or work environment (see Stevens, 1988). With this approach, there is a real-world motivation involved in the *encoding* of the material, although the motivation for retrieval is typically experimenter driven in the research setting. The best examples of this type of research are remote memory (see Erber, 1981) and autobiographical memory studies (see Rubin, 1986). In these studies, the encoding or learning of the to-be-remembered material occurs in real-world environments that are not controlled by experimenters, and in some remote memory studies, there is no guarantee that encoding even occurred for some items. Nevertheless, such studies have provided us with a valuable characterization of slow rates of forgetting and trends across long periods of time (e.g., Bahrick, 1984) and age-related patterns in forgetting of remote information (Rubin, Wetzler, & Nebes, 1986).

Also in this category are numerous studies of semantic memory. Semantic memory research is more likely to be conducted using an intelligence test (e.g., a vocabulary scale) or in a laboratory with tightly controlled priming stimuli, but in any case, it involves the examination of memory traces that were laid down in the real world. Like the studies of remote memory, this research has as one of its assumptions that all research subjects, at some point in time, were exposed to the relevant information (in this case, the meanings of the items used in the research) as part of their normal daily activities. This research domain has also contributed to our knowledge and understanding of aging, by showing that verbal intelligence measures and the organization of semantic networks show no dramatic changes as a function of aging (see Light & Burke, 1988).

Notice that this category of naturalistic studies is not limited to investigations in which both encoding and retrieval occur in naturalistic settings, that is, situations in which the motivation to remember is subject initiated in both cases. Studies that have used naturalistic encoding and retrieval include measures of appointment recall (Martin, 1986) or learning the way around a neighborhood (Walsh, Krauss, & Regnier, 1981). Naturalistic studies of this kind are extremely rare in the aging literature; most are studies of spatial memory. The impact of personal motivation to remember needs more study. In one particularly interesting study, Sinnott (1986) examined memory for information to which individual research subjects were exposed during a visit to a testing center. She found that motivation, that is, whether or not the information was needed later, was a critical determinant of performance. Thus, results may not be similar for conditions that only have naturalistic encoding (with recall that is motivated by a laboratory experimenter's needs) and other conditions that are naturalistic both for encoding and retrieval.

Simulation

An everyday task simulation is a laboratory memory test that bears some resemblance, at least in stimulus content, to an everyday memory experience. There is no requirement that the task exactly emulate in vivo memory activities. Simulated investigations of everyday memory lie along a continuum, with many "direct-simulation" tests closely resembling an everyday experience, such as hearing a phone number and then dialing it (West & Crook, 1990). Direct simulations tend to place the research participant into an everyday contextual framework in which stimulus familiarity and meaningfulness are important for memory because they enable the participant to access cues and strategies used in the real world (see Weinstein et al., 1981).

Other simulation studies use tests in which the stimuli are comparable to those that occur in everyday experience, but the testing situations differ markedly from everyday experience in terms of difficulty level (learning 12 name–face pairs in one setting, Yesavage, Rose, & Bower, 1983), and/or presentation format (putting 10 object pictures into a representative cross-section picture of a seven-room house, Crook, Ferris, & McCarthy, 1979). In spite of variations in difficulty level or presentation format, such studies clearly bear some resemblance to everyday experience, if only in the to-be-remembered content. For instance, recognition of faces is a common everyday event, but rarely do we see 50 faces presented for 8 s each (Smith & Winograd, 1978). I will refer to these as indirect simulations, but it is important to keep in mind that such studies are still characterized as simulations in this framework.

In some ways, simulation studies offer important advantages over both traditional laboratory work and naturalistic investigations. The stimuli resemble directly or indirectly (e.g., miniatures) information that people need to recall in the real world—names, phone numbers, maps, appointments, object locations, doctor's instructions, groceries. Poon and his colleagues (1990) refer to these types of stimuli as realistic (e.g., the street scenes used by Waddell & Rogoff, 1981) or actual (e.g., recall of a television program as in Cavanaugh, 1983). Thus, relative to the laboratory, simulation studies have the advantage of using stimuli that have more face validity for older adults. Although direct studies of the benefits of this face validity are rare, it is generally believed that older adults are more relaxed, more confident, and better able to understand a testing situation when the materials are familiar (Botwinick, 1984).

Simple manipulations of stimulus characteristics can affect patterns of age differences if the resulting display provides an everyday context for encoding. For instance, a recent study involving telephone number recall demonstrated that simply referring to a set of digits as *telephone numbers* rather than *number series* substantially improved the performance of the older adults but not the young (West & Crook, 1990). It has also been shown that older adults have higher confidence in their everyday memory abilities than their laboratory abilities and that this difference favoring everyday tasks is larger for the old than the young (Berry, West, & Scogin, 1983). The importance of placing to-be-remembered information into a familiar context more like everyday experience should not be underestimated.

Real-world environments are often highly complex, with many variables changing. Simulation studies can have advantages over naturalistic conditions in some cases because they provide the opportunity for the experimenter to design specific encoding and retrieval settings, to have some degree of control over these conditions, and to randomly assign individuals to conditions. Thus, in my view, these studies represent the "best situation" in terms of research (Banaji & Crowder, 1989), that is, research with high ecological validity and high generalizability. The ecological validity comes from using cues or stimuli that have potential utility in real-world environments (Petrinovich, 1989) whereas the generalizability, as defined by Banaji and Crowder (1989), comes from the laboratory control and potential for programmatic replicability. Among the aging research of this type, only the investigations of text processing have, thus far, fulfilled the potential of simulation work, that is, systematic and programmatic study of the effects of specific conditions and manipulations within an everyday domain (see Light & Burke, 1988).

Test Batteries

Two standardized batteries of everyday memory tests are now available for use by clinicians to assess the effects of head injury (Wilson, Cockburn, & Baddeley, 1985), to identify age-associated memory impairment (Cockburn & Collin, 1988; see also Chapter 4 of this text), and to test the impact of pharmaceutical (Crook, 1990) and memory-training interventions (West & Crook, in press). They are the Rivermead Behavioral Memory Test (RBMT), developed by Wilson and Baddeley, and the Memory Assessment Clinic (MAC) battery, developed by Crook. These batteries use (a) direct simulations of everyday memory experiences—learning of four faces presented in a realistic video format (Crook & West, 1990) or remembering to deliver a message (Cockburn & Collin, 1988); (b) naturalistic encoding—locating a personal belonging that is put away in a room (Wilson et al., 1985); and (c) laboratory memory tasks—a facial recognition test using a nonmatch to sample technique (Crook & West, 1990) or a story-recall test similar to the one in the Wechsler Memory Scale (Wilson et al., 1985).

The variety of tests used in these batteries encompasses the entire range of test types explored in this chapter, and data from these test batteries are cited throughout. Test batteries can be sensitive measures of decline. Using these batteries, investigators have obtained data on a wide range of tasks and have demonstrated large variation in age differences as a function of task characteristics (see Crook & West, 1990; West & Crook, 1990). Such findings reinforce the clinical and theoretical importance of continuing to investigate everyday memory and to maintain diversity in our research approaches, so as to better understand the conditions under which age differences occur and do not occur.

Laboratory Process-Oriented Research

Laboratory investigations of content domains that often need to be recalled in everyday experience, (e.g., spoken speech) are in the category of laboratory process-oriented research. These investigations focus on understanding component processes of a phenomenon. They do not look at overall performance (as most simulation studies do) as much as they examine subprocesses, such as rate of processing or decision accuracy. Purists might not include this type of research in a chapter on everyday memory, because with these investigations, there is no attempt to present the material in a way that is similar to everyday experience. Nevertheless, it is important in the early stages of this research not to be exclusive, for much of this work has clear implications for everyday memory experience.

Excellent examples of this type of work are the Wingfield and Stine studies of memory for spoken speech (see Chapter 7) and Charness's work on chess players (Charness, 1981a, 1981b). Tight control over both encoding and retrieval are maintained in this work so that components of encoding and retrieval—such as search patterns as opposed to reaction time, working memory as opposed to top–down organization—can be examined carefully.

The results of these studies have affected our understanding of memory and aging because they have often demonstrated that compensatory behavior with respect to one component process can help to reduce age differences. For example, Charness's work (1981a, 1981b) demonstrated that experienced older chess players use search processes that allow them to make effective decisions for moves in spite of poorer memory for exact chess piece locations. Other scientists demonstrated that older adults use prosodic knowledge to compensate for working memory deficits that might impair language processing in conversation (see Chapter 7). Thus, this particular paradigmatic approach can yield important information for understanding cognitive processing in everyday life, along with the other approaches noted previously.

Location-Recall Data as an Illustration

Selection of one of the previously mentioned paradigms can have consequences for research results and for the interpretation of these results. To illustrate the importance of research design decisions, I will discuss some location memory studies that use each of the methodological approaches outlined previously. Most research on location memory has used pre-arranged arrays of stimuli and has been concerned with issues such as automaticity (Puglisi, Park, Smith, & Hill, 1985) and distinctiveness (Park, Cherry, Smith, & Lafronza, 1990). Few studies have focused on the recall of object locations when the locations have been selected personally by the participants, in spite of the practical importance of such a task for normal functioning in the home. This discussion of location-recall research serves to illustrate the knowledge that can be gained by using converging operations to understand the relationship between aging and a specific type of skill.

Self-Report

Questions concerning memory for object locations and losing personal effects have often been included in memory self-evaluation questionnaires. Indeed, one study even focused on object-location recall as a central type of memory failure (Tenney, 1984). The results of these probes have consistently failed to find age differences in factors or individual items that assess self-reported ability to remember object locations (Chaffin & Herrmann, 1983; Crook & Larrabee, 1990; Rabbitt & Abson, 1990; Tenney, 1984). These self-report findings show no age differences in location recall of objects in the home.

Naturalistic Studies

A few reports of object-location memory fit the naturalistic category. One is an at-home interview study in which an object-location recall task was administered as part of a battery of everyday memory tasks (West & Walton, 1985). Participants were required to identify the current location of five common household items: telephone book, scissors, comb, address book (or calendar), and keys. This test assessed the ability of adolescents (M age = 16.3), community-dwelling younger subjects (M age = 32.4), and older adults (M age = 73.9) to remember object locations that were learned in a naturalistic environment, that is, in the home. Further, this test tapped semantic information, learned over a long period of exposure, for any object that was kept most of the time in the same location. Thus, to the extent that an individual household was well organized, and these common items were returned regularly to a designated place, the recall test assessed semantic rather than episodic memory. When there was no designated place for the item, the test was tapping episodic memory for the last location in which the object was placed. To ascertain the impact of such factors, subjects were asked to indicate if the object was always kept in the same place and when it was last used. All responses were checked by the experimenter, who went to find the household objects in the locations identified by the participants.

The results showed that most individuals remembered the location of 4/5 objects. The data were examined using chi-square analyses; the number of correct respondents for each object at each age group was entered into the analysis. The chi-square analyses showed an age difference in object-location recall for only one item, scissors, $\chi^2(2, N = 73) = 6.33$, $p < .05$, although the analysis approached significance for the location of one's address book, $\chi^2(2, N = 73) = 5.15$, $p < .10$. In both cases, the older adults were more often accurate than the young (see Table 1.1). For the other three items, the number of correct respondents was similar for all age groups.

An examination of responses to our questions concerning frequency of

TABLE 1.1. Percentage of respondents correctly recalling an item's location.

Item	Adolescents	Young adults	Older adults
Keys	.33	.30	.37
Address book	.27	.33	.40
Telephone book	1.00	.96	.92
Scissors	.30	.30	.41*
Comb	.30	.36	.34

*$p < .05$ in chi-square analyses.

use and regularity of placement of objects indicated that the older adults were more likely to recall a location because "I always keep it there." This may reflect an age-related life-style change (adolescents were least likely to indicate regularity of placement) that could be adaptive for memory problems in the home. Frequency or recency of object usage was not related to recall.

A second study similarly showed that older adults can perform very well in naturalistic settings. A group of 29 older adults ($M = 70.1$) and 29 younger adults ($M = 19.4$) were given a location-recall test as part of a large battery of everyday memory tests. All tests were administered either in the person's home or in a clinic room furnished like a sitting room. Ten common objects (e.g., a small note pad, a spoon) were placed, one by one, around the testing room. The subjects were permitted to select the locations, in a dialogue with the experimenter, and to place the objects at their own pace. However, the experimenter controlled the placement by offering recommendations about placement, so that 3 to 5 of the objects were in plain sight during a delay interval. Recall for the locations (with eyes closed) occurred approximately 30 min later. An analysis of variance showed no consistent age differences in performance ($M = 8.6$ and 8.8 correct out of 10, for the older and younger participants, respectively). The naturalistic studies, then, show no age differences in recall of small numbers of object locations. In both of these cases, however, performance was generally high, and ceiling effects obscured the meaning of the results.

Simulation

One of the earliest simulation studies was done by Crook and his colleagues, using a pictorial representation of rooms in a house (Crook et al., 1979). Ten object pictures were placed in seven "rooms" (no more than two objects per room) by subjects who had to recall these object locations 5 to 30 min later. The average score for the young-to-middle-aged group was 99%, significantly higher than the 89% average of the older adults (Crook et al., 1979). A replication of this task has been included in the MAC test battery (see following discussion).

Another simulation of location recall was carried out in a study of everyday memory and self-efficacy (Berry, West, & Powlishta, 1986). Adults (48 older and 20 younger adults) had to recall the placement of ten common items (e.g., eraser) put in various locations around the testing room. Although the placement was carried out by the subjects themselves, the object locations were preset by the experimenter and not chosen by the participants. In addition, the room was clearly arranged as a laboratory testing room. In this case, delayed recall performance (approximately 10 mins later) varied significantly as a function of age, $F(1, 66) = 13.64$, $p < .001$, with higher performance by the younger group ($M = 9.8/10$ correct) than the older group ($M = 7.9/10$ correct).

In a third simulation, conducted in my laboratory, systematic variations were introduced, to test the impact of familiarity on age differences. Jenkins's model (1979) was used to design the study. Jenkins suggested that memory studies can be distinguished according to their encoding and retrieval conditions, subject factors, and stimulus characteristics. In this particular investigation, the encoding and retrieval requirements, and the stimuli were varied in terms of their similarity to everyday situations. Our hypothesis was that the older adults' performance would be affected more than the young by increased task familiarity, and that age differences would not occur under conditions similar to everyday experience. The participants in this study were 300 college students (M age = 19, M education = 13 years) and community-dwelling older adults (M age = 68, M education = 14 years). All subjects were in good health. Anyone taking medications or with conditions known to affect cognitive performance (e.g., untreated high blood pressure) were excluded.

Six different location memory tasks were developed.[1] In the laboratory condition (L), 18 line drawings representing a variety of abstract shapes (e.g., sphere, cylinder) were placed by the subjects in a table-top array of 12 boxes of varying dimensions, using self-paced placement. The subjects were instructed to place the drawings in any box location they desired, and to name each drawing as it was placed, but they had to place at least one drawing in each box, and no box could contain more than two drawings. For retrieval, the experimenter held up a duplicate drawing and, using the name given by the subject, asked for its location. If the first response was incorrect, a second guess was permitted.

In a second condition, 18 pictures were again placed in 12 box locations in the same array. However, these pictures were not abstract. They were pictures of everyday objects having the same general shape as those used in

---

1. The location-recall task was presented in randomized order along with three other memory tasks (number recall, name–word recall, list recall). Order effects for these tests were not significant. Only the location-recall research is presented here because more location-recall data are available for the five design types outlined in this chapter.

condition L (e.g., ball [sphere], thread [cylinder]). This was called the everyday content–laboratory (ECL) condition, because the stimuli were pictures (common laboratory stimuli) of everyday objects. Encoding and retrieval procedures were identical to condition L.

In the everyday content (EC) condition, the array, and the encoding and retrieval requirements matched those of condition L, but the stimuli were those used in everyday experience. The subjects were given actual objects (e.g., a small ball and a spool of thread), and the subjects placed them in the 12 locations in the table-top array. Thus, this EC condition provided everyday content by using three-dimensional objects, with laboratory encoding and retrieval procedures like those of L and ECL.

In the condition with everyday content and encoding (ECE), the encoding situation changed to a more naturalistic one. The subjects were given the actual objects, as in EC, but they were asked to place them in 12 drawer or cabinet locations across the room. In all other respects, this ECE condition matched the others, for example, a duplicate object was used during retrieval and was given the name used by the subject during encoding. This condition added another element common to everyday experience—placement of objects in a *room* rather than an array.

In the last condition, using everyday content, encoding, and retrieval (ECER), the 18 objects were placed around the *room* by the subject as in ECE. Instead of pointing to the location during retrieval, however, subjects in ECER were asked to go to the location where they placed the items and show where the item had been placed. Both encoding and retrieval, then, involved locomotion, as in practical situations. Thus, there is an added component here—retrieval that simulates everyday conditions.

Across all conditions, the tasks were carefully matched along the following dimensions: self-paced presentation, number of stimuli, number of locations, stimuli shapes, placement rules and procedures, use of duplicate items for the retrieval test, number of retrieval trials, and self-paced retrieval. The dependent measure was the combined score of the two location attempts. At the same time, across the five conditions, the stimuli were varied, the locations for placing objects were varied, and subject movement was varied. These variations in conditions were introduced successively, in such a way that the impact of each variation could be studied independently. These changes, introduced to simulate an everyday experience, may have enhanced recall by adding more cues (e.g., a three-dimensional object may have more attributes than a picture, movement around a room may provide more kinesthetic cues than placement in a table-top array). On the other hand, the added cues could have made recall more difficult because individuals may have tried to process and remember these cues.

An overall analysis of variance was calculated for the effects of age and condition. There were main effects for age, $F(1,291) = 82.6$, $p < .001$, and condition, $F(4,291) = 13.6$, $p < .001$, and the interaction approached

TABLE 1.2. Correct object location recall (maximum score = 18) for two age groups.

Condition	Younger	Older	Overall
L (array)	13.9_{ab}	9.3_c	11.6
ECL (array)	14.9_{ab}	11.2_c	13.2
EC (array)	13.3_a	9.4_c	11.5
ECE (room)	15.4_b	13.1_b	14.6
ECER (room)	15.7_d	13.7_b	14.4
Overall	14.6	11.4	13.0
LEER (room)	16.1_b	13.3_b	14.7

L, laboratory; ECL, everyday content—laboratory; EC, everyday content; ECE, everyday content and encoding; ECER, everyday content, encoding, and retrieval; LEER, laboratory stimuli, everyday encoding and retrieval conditions.

Note. Means that are not significantly different have the same subscript letter.

significance, $F(4,291) = 2.0, p < .10$. More revealing were a priori comparisons between conditions for the two age groups. These showed that the young subjects, whose scores averaged between 13.3 (EC) and 15.7 (ECER) for all conditions, showed a significant difference only between the EC condition and the two *room* conditions (ECE and ECER) involving more naturalistic encoding. No other differences were significant. The younger adults' data, then, suggests that either the room cues or the familiarity effect (carrying out the task in a more naturalistic way) made a difference. It was a weak effect for the young, however, because performance in the room conditions did not exceed performance in all of the nonroom/ laboratory conditions. For the older adults, however, all laboratory conditions differed significantly from the two conditions that involved placement of real objects in locations around a room. Age differences were present in the laboratory nonroom conditions, but only approached significance in the two familiar room conditions (see Table 1.2).

These results suggested the value of examining another condition. The additional condition was designed to examine the differential impact of the specific cues provided in the room conditions as opposed to the impact of similarity to everyday experience. Individuals were drawn from the same population to participate in this new condition. The two room conditions, ECE and ECER, provided cues from locomotion in the room. They also were similar to everyday experience because real objects were employed rather than pictures. The new condition was designed to tease out the differential benefits of locomotion and use of real objects.

Subjects were asked to take the abstract drawings originally used in condition L and place them in the 12 *room* locations used in conditions ECE and ECER. This condition used laboratory stimuli, but everyday encoding and retrieval conditions (LEER). In the LEER condition, movement was

TABLE 1.3. Description of condition variations for three conditions.

ECER	LEER	L
Three-dimensional stimuli	Abstract stimuli	Abstract stimuli
Locomotion in a room	Locomotion in a room	Minimal locomotion
Everyday familiarity = realistic objects + movement cues	Movement cues only	No cues

L, laboratory; ECER, everday content, encoding, and retrieval; LEER, laboratory stimuli, everyday content and retrieval conditions.

provided but the abstract stimuli were not familiar, so this condition could not be seen as familiar or similar to everyday experience (see Table 1.3).

The logic for adding this condition was straightforward. This condition can be compared directly with the laboratory (L) condition that also used the abstract pictures (but no movement around the room to place items in actual drawers); it can also be compared with condition ECER, which was identical except for the stimuli. If older adults' LEER scores are comparable to scores in condition L (both use abstract pictures), but much worse than ECER performance (both conditions involve placing objects around a room), it would indicate that stimulus attributes had a significant impact on performance but that naturalistic encoding and retrieval (i.e., locomotion in a *room*) did not significantly aid performance. Alternatively, if LEER scores are comparable to ECER scores, and much better than scores in condition L, it would suggest that naturalistic encoding and retrieval (placement around a *room*) are the source for the improved scores in conditions ECE and ECER rather than familiarity (see Table 1.3). Finally, it is also possible that LEER, while better than condition L, could still result in lower performance than condition ECER, especially for the older adults. This would suggest that familiarity or similarity to everyday experience is the most critical factor because ECER provided both real objects and realistic procedures for remembering.

The results were fairly clear. In an analysis of variance using age and task (LEER vs. ECER), there were only main effects of age, $F(1,115) = 31.5$, $p < .001$, with no impact of condition, and no interaction of age and condition. A priori comparisons confirmed these findings. This reflects a high degree of similarity between LEER and ECER in performance. This similarity is probably due to the fact that these two conditions involved placement with locomotion and recall of items in a naturalistic *room* environment. In contrast, the analysis comparing LEER with L showed significant effects for age, $F(1,115) = 42.0$, $p < .001$, and condition, $F(1,115) = 29.8$, $p < .001$, and an interaction that approached significance, $F(1,115) = 2.7$, $p < .10$. A priori comparisons showed that the difference between L and

LEER was significant for both age groups and that age differences were larger for L than for LEER. These results confirm the work of Cherry and Park (1989) showing that age differences in recall of a prearranged array were not modified by object familiarity. Here, the critical factor affecting performance was not the nature of the objects so much as the conditions of encoding and retrieval.

With this evidence in hand, it cannot be concluded that familiarity, per se, led to higher performance and reduced age differences for conditions ECE and ECER. If overall familiarity had been the critical factor, that is, familiar objects *and* familiar encoding and retrieval, LEER performance should have been significantly worse than ECE and ECER. It was not. Thus, the appropriate conclusion is that locomotion around a room resulted in higher performance in the three conditions (ECE, ECER, and LEER) in which age differences were marginal. It is possible that this same factor accounts, at least in part, for the effects observed by Sharps and Gollin (cf. Park et al., 1990; Sharps & Gollin, 1987). Locomotion is undoubtedly part of a naturalistic setting. However, moving around a room to place abstract stimuli in drawers (LEER) cannot be considered as familiar. Without the LEER data, we could have erroneously concluded that familiarity accounted for the initial findings. Careful scrutiny in other cases may help to identify potential cues and factors, other than familiarity, per se, that could account for age–task interactions in everyday memory research.

Test Batteries

Both of the existing standardized test batteries include spatial memory items. The RBMT has a route memory test. The MAC battery has a misplaced objects test comparable to the study described earlier (Crook et al., 1979). The MAC version used 20 common items to be placed in 12 rooms using a simulation methodology. Recall of the self-selected locations occurred approximately 40 min later. Performance on this test was strongly affected by age, $r = -.40$. With age groups broken roughly into decades (age range = 18 to 88 years), individuals under age 50 consistently performed better than the older groups (Crook, Youngjohn, & Larrabee, 1990).

Laboratory Component-Process Studies

Quite a few laboratory studies of spatial memory have been conducted. Researchers have examined automaticity and aging (Puglisi et al., 1985), mental rotation (Bruce & Herman, 1983), and stimulus distinctiveness (Park et al., 1990), but to my knowledge, none of these studies has offered subjects the opportunity to place the stimuli themselves. Instead, adults are typically confronted with a prearranged array of 20 to 40 objects to memorize. The nature of this methodology precludes, at this time, any direct analogy to everyday experience. These studies have demonstrated that spatial location is not automatically encoded and that location recall does show age declines. But further study is needed to examine the differential benefits of self-placement versus experimenter placement of objects and to determine if the results from prearranged arrays will generalize to self-placement conditions.

Discussion

Several important points may be drawn from the location recall evidence. The results, using different approaches, tend to indicate that elderly adults, in their normal setting, do not have difficulty with intentional recall of fewer than 10 object locations even under delay conditions. At the same time, the simulation findings show clear age differences with 10 or more items, under many conditions, although the more naturalistic room conditions resulted in only marginal age differences. Looking across all five paradigms, generalizations cannot be made, that is, with any confidence, from self-report to performance, or from low-difficulty to high-difficulty tasks, or from laboratory to everyday contexts. It is clear from my findings, for example, that everyday familiarity, in particular, is not a straightforward phenomenon and can be very complex in its impact.

Familiarity needs more discussion and investigation, with greater sensitivity to the importance of analyzing the impact of specific cues provided by familiar conditions. With respect to location recall, the cues that require further study include locomotion, in particular, the effects of self-placement versus experimenter placement, and the effects of full locomotion (moving around a room) versus partial locomotion (placing objects in an array). In addition, "distinctiveness" has been considered to be a critical cue for location recall with prearranged arrays (Sharps & Gollin, 1987) and should be studied further, even though it does not appear to account for our findings or those of Park and her colleagues (Park et al., 1990).

Second, the number of items may be critical. If 10 or fewer items are used, the test bears more similarity to everyday experience, but ceiling effects are present. With larger numbers of items, ceiling effects are unlikely, but the test then no longer bears any resemblance, in its difficulty level, to most everyday experiences with object-location memory. Similarly, naturalistic location recall is often incidental; that is, the individual puts down one or two objects in the course of ongoing activity and later goes to find them. Intentionality does not appear to affect location recall with large, prearranged arrays (Puglisi et al., 1985) but it is not clear what its affect is on recall of self-placed, smaller arrays, because there are no incidental studies available.

Conclusions

This discussion of research designs, in general, and the results from location recall studies, in particular, reinforce the notion that researchers should take care in designing studies of everyday memory. The location-recall evidence shows that methodological choices have real consequences for outcome. The researcher who maintains a broader set of methodologies can use converging operations and can compare the findings gleaned from different approaches to gain more evidence for understanding aging in a specific memory domain.

The following list highlights many of the decisions that must be considered by investigators interested in everyday memory. Some, but not all, of these considerations were discussed in this chapter, but more research on the effects of test, task, and paradigm selection would be welcome. The researcher's decision process should be guided by both theory and empirical knowledge, and diverse scientific approaches should be embraced (see Ceci & Bronfenbrenner, 1991).

1. Measures: self-report or performance
2. Encoding: naturalistic or controlled by the experimenter (this is often equivalent to the choice between semantic and episodic memory tasks); self-paced or experimenter-paced
3. Motivation for remembering: individual and personal, or dictated by the experimenter
4. Content: realistic, actual, or laboratory stimuli
5. Context: simulated everyday, naturalistic, or laboratory
6. Retrieval: naturalistic or experimenter controlled
7. Performance: component processes examined, or overall score; strategies evaluated or not
8. Strategies: self-report, assessed directly (thinking out loud, measures of clustering, etc.), or inferred
9. Location: in home, in neighborhood, in laboratory
10. Task difficulty: comparable to everyday experience or laboratory tests

Whatever design and paradigm selections are made, it behooves us to validate any arguments about familiarity or meaningfulness of stimuli, encoding, and retrieval conditions by manipulation checks. Practical memory researchers (including myself) have been guilty of assuming that test conditions vary in meaningfulness to participants, but simple questions are not typically asked about familiarity that could easily be asked to validate our assumptions (Puckett, Reese, Cohen, & Pollina, 1991). This is particularly important for simulation investigations, in which subjects are brought into the laboratory for everyday memory studies. In addition to manipulation checks, another approach to confirmation of labels such as "everyday" or "familiar" is to do more exploration of the memory demands of adults. The life-styles of college students and retired elderly are clearly not the same, but there is little precise knowledge about these variations vis-à-vis memory. What is the most common kind of memory task done by younger adults? How do older adults typically use their memory skills? Investigation of these questions would be a fruitful area for further study.

It is important to support continued diversity in the study of aging and memory, with the recognition that laboratory and everyday research could very well lie on one continuum of variations in difficulty level, test format, stimulus familiarity, subject motivation, context effects, and other factors. Practical benefits are to be gained from tightly controlled laboratory studies (e.g., Richardson, 1989) as well as naturalistic studies (e.g., Neisser, 1988). Recognition of this possibility will widen the scope of investigation and strengthen our knowledge base about memory aging.

Acknowledgments. Special thanks are given to the Brookdale Foundation in New York for supporting this work and to the National Institute on Aging for its support of some location recall studies described here (AG06014).

References

Bahrick, H.P. (1984). Memory for people. In J.E. Harris & P.E. Morris (Eds.), *Everyday memory, actions, and absent-mindedness* (pp. 19–34). London: Academic.

Banaji, M.R., & Crowder, R.G. (1989). The bankruptcy of everyday memory. *American Psychologist, 44,* 1185–1193.

Berry, J.M., West, R.L., & Dennehy, D. (1989). Reliability and validity of the Memory Self-Efficacy Questionnaire (MSEQ). *Developmental Psychology, 25,* 701–713.

Berry, J.M., West, R.L., & Powlishta, K. (1986, November). *Self-efficacy and performance differences on laboratory and everyday memory tasks.* Paper presented at the meeting of the Gerontological Society of America, Chicago.

Berry, J.M., West, R.L., & Scogin, F. (1983, November). *Predicting everyday and laboratory memory skill.* Paper presented at the meeting of the Gerontological Society of America, San Francisco.

Botwinick, J. (1984). *Aging and behavior* (3rd ed.). New York: Springer.

Bruce, P.R., & Herman, J.F. (1983). Spatial knowledge of young and elderly adults: Scene recognition from familiar and novel perspectives. *Experimental Aging Research, 9,* 169–173.

Burke, D., Worthley, J., & Martin, J. (1988). I'll never forget what's-her-name: Aging and tip of the tongue experiences in everyday life. In M.M. Gruneberg, P.E. Morris, & R.N. Sykes (Eds.), *Practical aspects of memory: Current research and issues* (Vol. 2, pp. 113–118). Chichester, England: John Wiley & Sons.

Cavanaugh, J.C. (1983). Comprehension and retention of television programs by 20- and 60-year olds. *Journal of Gerontology, 38,* 190–196.

Cavanaugh, J.C., Morton, K.R., & Tilse, C.S. (1989). A self-evaluation framework for understanding everyday memory aging. In J.D. Sinnott (Ed.), *Everyday problem solving: Theory and application* (pp. 266–284). New York: Praeger.

Ceci, S.J., & Bronfenbrenner, U. (1991). On the demise of everyday memory. *American Psychologist, 46,* 27–31.

Chaffin, R., & Herrmann, D.J. (1983). Self reports of memory abilities by old and young adults. *Human Learning, 2,* 17–28.

Charness, N. (1981a). Aging and skilled problem solving. *Journal of Experimental Psychology: General, 110,* 21–38.

Charness, N. (1981b). Visual short-term memory and aging in chess players. *Journal of Gerontology, 36,* 615–619.

Cherry, K.E., & Park, D.C. (1989). Age-related differences in three-dimensional spatial memory. *Journal of Gerontology, 44,* P16–22.

Cockburn, J., & Collin, C. (1988). Measuring everyday memory in elderly people: A preliminary study. *Age and Ageing, 17,* 265–269.

Cohen, G. (1988). Memory and aging: Toward an explanation. In M.M. Gruneberg, P.E. Morris, & R.N. Sykes (Eds.), *Practical aspects of memory: Current research and issues* (Vol. 2, pp. 78–83). Chichester, England: John Wiley & Sons.

Cohen, G. (1989). *Memory in the real world.* London: Erlbaum.

Crook, T.H. (1990). Assessment of drug efficacy in Age-Associated Memory Impairment. In R. Wurtman, J.H. Growdon, S. Corkin, & E. Ritten-Walker (Eds.), *Advances in neurology, Vol. 51: Alzheimer's Disease* (pp. 211–216). New York: Raven Press.

Crook, T.H., Ferris, S.H., & McCarthy, M. (1979). The misplaced objects task: A brief test for memory dysfunction in the aged. *Journal of the American Geriatrics Society, 27,* 284–287.

Crook, T.H., & Larrabee, G.J. (1990). A self-rating scale for evaluating memory in everyday life. *Psychology and Aging, 5,* 48–57.

Crook, T.H., Youngjohn, J.R., & Larrabee, G.J. (1990). The misplaced objects test: A measure of everyday visual memory. *Journal of Clinical and Experimental Neuropsychology, 12,* 819–833.

Crook, T.H., & West, R.L. (1990). Name recall performance across the adult life span. *British Journal of Psychology, 81,* 335–349.

Dixon, R.A., & Hultsch, D.F. (1983). Metamemory and memory for text relationships in adulthood: A cross-validation study. *Journal of Gerontology, 38,* 689–694.

Erber, J.T. (1981). Remote memory and age: A review. *Experimental Aging Research, 7,* 189–199.

Gilewski, M.J., & Zelinski, E.M. (1986). Questionnaire assessment of memory complaints. In L.W. Poon (Ed.), *Handbook for clinical memory assessment of older adults* (pp. 93–107). Washington, DC: American Psychological Association.

Gruneberg, M.M., Morris, P.E., & Sykes, R.N. (1988). *Practical aspects of memory: Current research and issues* (Vols. 1 & 2). Chichester, England: John Wiley & Sons.

Hertzog, C., Dixon, R.A., Schulenberg, J.E., & Hultsch, D.F. (1987). On the differentiation of memory beliefs from memory knowledge: The factor structure of the Metamemory in Adulthood Scale. *Experimental Aging Research, 13,* 101–107.

Jenkins, J.J. (1979). Four points to remember: A tetrahedral model of memory experiments. In L.S. Cermak & F.I.M. Craik (Eds.), *Levels of processing in human memory* (pp. 429–446). Hillsdale, NJ: Erlbaum.

Larrabee, G.J., West, R.L., & Crook, T.H. (1991). The association of memory complaint with everyday memory performance. *Journal of Clinical and Experimental Neuropsychology, 13,* 484–496.

Light, L.L., & Burke, D.M. (Eds.) (1988). *Language, memory, and aging.* New York: Cambridge University Press.

Loftus, E.F. (1991). The glitter of everyday memory . . . and the gold. *American Psychologist, 46,* 16–18.

Martin, M. (1986). Ageing and patterns of change in everyday memory and cognition. *Human Learning, 5,* 63–74.

Neiderehe, G. (1986). Depression and memory impairment in the aged. In L.W. Poon (Ed.), *Handbook for clinical memory assessment of older adults* (pp. 226–237). Washington, DC: American Psychological Association.

Neisser, U. (1988). Time present and time past. In M.M. Gruneberg, P.E. Morris, & R.N. Sykes (Eds.), *Practical aspects of memory: Current research and issues* (Vol. 2, pp. 545–560). Chichester, England: John Wiley & Sons.

Park, D.C. (in press). Applied cognitive aging research. In F.I.M. Craik & T.A. Salthouse (Eds.), *Handbook of cognition and aging.* Hillsdale, NJ: Erlbaum.

Park, D.C., Cherry, K.E., Smith, A.D., & Lafronza, V.N. (1990). Effects of distinctive context on memory for objects and their locations in young and elderly adults. *Psychology and Aging, 5,* 250–255.

Petrinovich, L. (1989). Representative design and the quality of generalization. In L.W. Poon, D.C. Rubin, & B.A. Wilson (Eds.), *Everyday cognition in adulthood and late life* (pp. 11–24). Cambridge, England: Cambridge University Press.

Poon, L.W., Dudley, W.N., & Welke, D.J. (1990, April). *What is everyday cognition?* Paper presented at the West Virginia Conference on Life Span Developmental Psychology, Morgantown, WV.

Poon, L.W., Rubin, D.C., & Wilson, B.A. (1989). *Everyday cognition in adulthood and late life.* Cambridge, England: Cambridge University Press.

Puckett, J.M., Reese, H.W., Cohen, S.H., & Pollina, L.K. (1991). Age differences vs. age deficits in laboratory tasks: The role of research in everyday cognition. In J.D. Sinnott & J.C. Cavanaugh (Eds.), *Bridging paradigms: Positive development in adulthood and cognitive aging* (pp. 113–130). New York: Praeger.

Puglisi, J.T., Park, D.C., Smith, A.D., & Hill, G.W. (1985). Memory for two types of spatial information: Effects of instructions, age, and format. *American Journal of Psychology, 98,* 101–118.

Rabbitt, P., & Abson, V. (1990). "Lost and Found:" Some logical and methodological limitations of self-report questionnaires as tools to study cognitive ageing. *British Journal of Psychology, 81,* 1–16.

Rice, G.E. (1986). The everyday activities of adults: Implications for prose recall—Part II. *Educational Gerontology, 12,* 187–198.

Richardson, J.T.E. (1989). The practical benefits of cognitive psychology. *European Journal of Cognitive Psychology, 1,* 27–46.

Rubin, D.C. (Ed.) (1986). *Autobiographical memory.* Cambridge, England: Cambridge University Press.

Rubin, D.C., Wetzler, S.E., & Nebes, R.D. (1986). Autobiographical memory across the life span. In D.C. Rubin (Ed.), *Autobiographical memory* (pp. 202–221). Cambridge, England: Cambridge University Press.

Sharps, M.J., & Gollin, E.S. (1987). Memory for object locations in young and elderly adults. *Journal of Gerontology, 42,* 336–341.

Sinnott, J.D. (1986). Prospective/intentional and incidental everyday memory: Effects of age and passage of time. *Psychology and Aging, 1,* 110–116.

Sinnott, J.D. (Ed.) (1989). *Everyday problem solving: Theory and application.* New York: Praeger.

Smith, A.D., & Winograd, E. (1978). Adult age differences in remembering faces. *Developmental Psychology, 14,* 443–444.

Stevens, J. (1988). An activity theory approach to practical memory. In M.M. Gruneberg, P.E. Morris, & R.N. Sykes (Eds.), *Practical aspects of memory: Current research and issues* (Vol. 1, pp. 335–391). Chichester, England: John Wiley & Sons.

Tenney, Y.J. (1984). Ageing and the misplacing of objects. *British Journal of Developmental Psychology, 2,* 43–50.

Waddell, K.J., & Rogoff, B. (1981). Effect of contextual organization on spatial memory of middle-aged and older women. *Developmental Psychology, 17,* 878–885.

Walsh, D.A., Krauss, I.K, & Regnier, V.A. (1981). Spatial ability, environmental knowledge, and environmental use: The elderly. In L.S. Liben, A.H. Patterson, & N. Newcombe (Eds.), *Spatial representation and behavior across the life span* (pp. 321–357). New York: Academic.

Weinstein, C.E., Duffy, M., Underwood, V.L., MacDonald, J., & Gott, S.P. (1981). Memory strategies reported by older adults for experimental and everyday learning tasks. *Educational Gerontology, 7,* 205–213.

West, R.L. (1986). Everyday memory and aging. *Developmental Neuropsychology, 2,* 323–344.

West, R.L., & Crook, T.H. (1990). Age differences in everyday memory: Laboratory analogues of telephone number recall. *Psychology and Aging, 5,* 520–529.

West, R.L., & Crook, T.H. (in press). Video training of imagery for mature adults. *Applied Cognitive Psychology.*

West, R.L., & Dennehy, D. (1990, April). *Memory self-efficacy: The effects of age and experience.* Paper presented at the Cognitive Aging Conference, Atlanta.

West, R.L., & Walton, M. (1985, March). *Practical memory functioning in the elderly.* Paper presented at the meeting of the Second National Forum on Research in Aging, Lincoln, NE.

Wilson, B., Cockburn, J., & Baddeley, A. (1985). *The Rivermead Behavioural Memory Test.* Reading, England: Thames Valley Test Co.

Yesavage, J.A., Rose, T.L., & Bower, G.H. (1983). Interactive imagery and affective judgments improve face-name learning in the elderly. *Journal of Gerontology, 38,* 197–203.

Zelinski, E.M., Gilewski, M.J., & Thompson, L.W. (1980). Do laboratory tests relate to self assessment of memory ability in the young and old? In L.W. Poon, J.L. Fozard, L.S. Cermak, D. Arenberg, & L.W. Thompson (Eds.), *New directions in memory and aging: Proceedings of the George A. Talland Memorial Conference* (pp. 519–544). Hillsdale, NJ: Erlbaum.

2
Uses of Diary Data in Cognitive and Developmental Research

JOHN C. CAVANAUGH AND CHRISTOPHER HERTZOG

One of the most common written ways that people have kept track of their lives throughout history is by keeping a diary. Although the vast majority of diaries never see the light of day (and most people have preferred to keep it that way), a few have become classics in literature (e.g., Samuel Pepys's and Anne Frank's diaries). It is fair to say that many psychologists probably have kept a diary at some point during their lives and have read at least one of these classics. Perhaps a few have even marvelled at the richness of the entries or noticed examples of psychological constructs.

Given the ubiquitous nature of diary keeping and reading, it is somewhat surprising that psychologists have been loathe to use diaries as sources of data for testing theories of cognition. Because of this, we designed this chapter to make and to justify two arguments. First, psychologists' aversion to diaries, especially the labeling of diaries as unscientific, does not reflect the history of the discipline (Cavanaugh, 1981, 1985). Second, such attitudes preclude the uses and benefits of diary analyses for cognitive and developmental psychology.

For purposes of this chapter, we classify diaries into three groups. First, some diaries are primarily chronicles of personal and historical daily events. These diaries are mostly of literary or historical value and will not be considered here. A second type consists of systematic daily (or nearly daily) recording of other people's behaviors. Such diaries were widespread in the early days of psychology and are still commonly used in some areas of social science (e.g., anthropology). For example, the baby biographers of the 19th and early 20th centuries (e.g., Darwin, 1877; Taine, 1876/1877; see Cavanaugh, 1981, 1985, for more information) used extensive (and often nearly exhaustive) recording of infants' and children's behavior as the basis for theories of development. A third type, and the one we will focus on here, involves the systematic recording on a daily (or nearly daily) basis of one's own cognitive-emotional experiences. This type also has a long history in psychology. For example, Ebbinghaus (1913) used diary-like records of his memory performance as the basis for his keen observations and insights about memory that are still important today. The contents of this third type can be specific memory experiences (like Ebbinghaus's or other more autobiographical events) or self-reflections on one's experiences. We will describe research based on both.

We begin by addressing criticisms that diary methods are not psychometrically sound research tools. Next, we examine efforts to use diaries to investigate aspects of memory in everyday life. Finally, we summarize recent research using diaries to investigate various aspects of cognitive development. Our review is not exhaustive. Rather, we describe some typical studies in order to make our points. Throughout the chapter, we point out areas for future research and topics that need special attention.

Psychometric Issues and Diary Data

As interesting and rich as diary data may be, by modern standards their utility in scientific research will be limited if they are not reliable and valid. Strangely, despite the widespread modern criticism of the use of diaries in research, very few studies have examined the issue empirically in any area of psychology. Carp and Carp (1981) conducted one of the few investigations addressing these issues.

In a series of fairly extensive studies comparing diaries and interviews, Carp and Carp (1981) found diary data to be reliable and valid in some contexts and with some types of respondents. Concurrent and predictive validity were obtained over an 18-month period in one sample, and in general they noted considerable overlap between diary records and interviews. However, they found that reporting of negative events was, for some events, more likely in diary entries than in interviews and that higher frequencies of positive events were more likely in interviews. Carp and Carp also demonstrated that 1-day and retrospective diaries provide insufficient samples of behavior to be either reliable or valid.

Carp and Carp's (1981) findings also raise important issues about generalization and accuracy. Concerning generalization, Carp and Carp's findings show that diary data may have limited generalizability to the general population of elderly adults, given that cognitive ability and socioeconomic status were related to the completeness of diary entries. If one is only interested in healthy middle- or upper-class educated elderly, then generalization may be less problematic. Because Carp and Carp did not independently assess the validity of interview responses for those who did not complete diaries, it is possible that the greater representativeness of interviews is offset by lowered validity for their responses. Further comparisons between diary data and interviews are sorely needed, especially given Carp and Carp's hypothesis that affectively laden events may be more accurately reported in diaries rather than interviews.

The issue of accuracy of diary entries is extremely thorny. Some researchers claim that diary data cannot be considered valid unless they can be objectively verified; that is, unless there is independent evidence concerning the actual occurrence of a target event and some independent record of the actual attributes of the target event. Certainly, use of diary data for deriving measures of frequency of actual target events requires the assumption that diary entries reflect actual event frequency. The concern regarding objective characteristics of events is crucial if one wishes to use diary entries to distinguish subjective representations of events from their objective properties, including cognitive influences on processing event characteristics (e.g., selective attention) and the characteristics of memories for events (e.g., eyewitness testimony). Concern for the verisimilitude of diary entries, however, ignores the difficult philosophical question of whether, in principle, it is possible to obtain an objective account of personally experienced events and whether the factual quality of the diaries is the crucial issue, given the research question.

We argue that in at least two conditions the accuracy of diary entries is essentially moot. The first is when one treats the diary entries themselves as information to be remembered and asks how event representations manifested in the diary become altered during subsequent retrieval of event characteristics from memory. Second, diary entries may be very useful in documenting subjective reactions to events, even if and when the representations of the events and the reactions they cause are inconsistent with the "facts." For example, interpersonal conflict in everyday life (e.g., marital discord) might be traced to persons' discrepant event representations and attributions that are better measured by diary entries recording subjective event representations than by third-party recordings of the "facts" under dispute.

Ultimately, concerns about the construct validity of diary entries are no different than concerns regarding any self-report measure. Obtaining validity checks, in the form of independent evidence of the actual occurrence of the events and some of their properties is desirable but not always practically feasible. Often, a useful alternative is to obtain additional information that converges with the variables extracted from diary records or that can be used as indirect evidence for the construct validity of the recorded event (e.g., subsequent actions by the individual). In some cases, however, the spectre of invalid data that are due to the lack of an objective event record is simply irrelevant, relative to the research agenda.

Diaries as Tools in Memory Research

One of the most common uses of the diary method in contemporary research is to document people's use of various memory strategies in their everyday lives. In this section, we will consider three different approaches to this topic. First, we will consider studies that requested people to keep diary records of their remembering and forgetting experiences. Second, we will examine the use of diaries to document naturally occurring tip-of-the-tongue experiences. Finally, we will review research that examines the diary of a famous scientist (Michael Faraday) for evidence of a formal memory system that he used in his everyday life.

Self-Reports of Memory Strategies

Several researchers have adopted the diary method as a way to investigate people's use of memory strategies in everyday life. These investigators believe that having people record when, why, and how they use memory strategies as close to the actual event as possible and in the context of everyday life provides a more valid view of strategic activity than laboratory observation. Diary data can also be used to check self-reports of memory strategy use. Additionally, memory diaries provide an opportunity to investigate memory failures. Individuals can be asked to record episodes in which they realize that they have forgotten something, as well as their reactions to these events.

Most of the memory diary studies have been conducted on college students and young adults. For example, Shlechter and Herrmann (1981) examined whether diaries correlated with self-report measures (the Short Inventory of Memory Experiences; SIME) and with interviews. Their results showed that overall scores from diaries correlate with overall scores from the SIME but that specific scale (factor) scores from the SIME were unrelated to diary scores. Interview data correlated significantly with SIME scores. These findings corroborate the lack of strong correlations between diary records and interviews reported by Carp and Carp (1981) and reemphasize the point that multiple sources of data should be used in studying self-perceptions.

Cavanaugh, Grady, and Perlmutter (1983) were the first to use self-report diaries in research on everyday memory aging. They had 12 younger noncollege student adults and 12 middle-aged and elderly adults keep diary records of remembering and forgetting experiences 1 day per week for a month. Participants were asked to record strategy use and forgetting episodes and to note the time, content, context, subjective importance, and affective reaction for each episode. No age differences were found in the relative frequency of particular types of memory aids (the vast majority of which were external aids) or in the relative frequency of types of memory failures. Middle-aged and older adults, however, reported a higher absolute frequency of memory failures; were more upset at forgetting, independent of subjective importance of the content (see also Hulicka, 1982); and reported using memory aids more often than younger adults. Cavanaugh et al. (1983) concluded that middle-aged and older adults may be more sensitive to forgetting than younger adults in everyday life and may try to compensate for this problem by using more memory aids.

Other researchers have adapted the technique of Cavanaugh et al. (1983). For example, West (1984) provided her participants with a more structured diary-recording sheet that specifically requested certain information, with separate sheets used to record each memory experience. Her findings basically agree with those of Cavanaugh et al., but her method improves the quality of the data recorded. Overall, we recommend a compromise between the flexibility of the pocket notebook approach used by Cavanaugh et al. and West's more structured approach. Perhaps the two methods could be integrated so that pocket notebooks are pre-printed with the various types of information needed by the researcher.

Tip-of-the-Tongue Experiences

Reason and Lucas (1984) used a variation of diary recording of memory failures as a way to investigate naturally occurring tip-of-the-tongue (TOT) states. In a series of studies, they asked a total of 48 adult volunteers to keep track of their TOT experiences using a structured diary approach. For each TOT experience, respondents were asked to provide the sought-for memory item; the number of times the target item was searched for; the date, approximate time, and length of each search; the success or failure of each search; the aspects of the target information that were felt to be known before resolving the TOT state (e.g., first letter, other associations, etc.); any intermediate solutions; the strategies used to recover the target information; and the relative familiarity of the target information. Respondents were asked to carry the diaries with them for a 4-week period.

Reason and Lucas (1984) developed an extensive coding system that provided a thorough description of TOT experiences. They identified two main types of TOT states, blocked (where an incorrect solution keeps coming to mind) and nonblocked (where such intrusive thoughts did not occur). They discovered that nonblocked TOT experiences were resolved by using internal memory strategies, such as generation of similar words or names. Blocked TOT experiences, however, were resolved through external memory strategies, such as asking others. Additionally, nonblocked TOT states were more easily resolved (usually after just one search) and required less knowledge about the target information than blocked TOT states.

Reason and Lucas (1984) argue that this naturalistic approach to studying TOT experiences provides more insight into the process than do laboratory methods that induce TOT states. In particular, they argue that the differences between blocked and nonblocked TOT states are not adequately addressed in laboratory studies. Moreover, the need to use external memory strategies to resolve blocked TOT states is typically not met in laboratory studies; consequently, such experiences may be recorded as failures to resolve the TOT. Clearly, this is not representative of everyday experience.

Burke (e.g., Burke, Worthley, & Martin, 1988) has also used structured diaries to study age-related differences in TOT experiences. She found that TOT states increased with age, and that although young and old participants were equally successful in resolving them, they did so in different ways. Older adults were more likely to rely on spontaneous retrievals than to engage in strategic retrieval. Unlike Reason and Lucas (1984) however, Burke and colleagues did not find that blocked TOTs are more likely to involve external strategies for resolution.

These studies show that structured diaries are important tools in studying TOT states. More research is needed to resolve some issues (e.g., blocked TOTs and external strategies), but the method appears promising for systematic examination of spontaneous memory behaviors.

Memory Strategies in Michael Faraday's Diaries

Michael Faraday (1791–1867) was one of the most important scientific figures of the 19th century. His discoveries included electromagnetic induction, the quantitative laws of electrodeposition, benzene, diamagnetism, and the theoretical analysis of fields, which opened the way for Maxwell to integrate light, electricity, and magnetism (Nersessian, 1984). Tweney (e.g., 1989) has noted that Faraday left a much richer documentary legacy of his thinking than most other scientists. Records of roughly 30,000 successful and unsuccessful experiments, many books containing his speculative ideas, scrapbooks, bibliographies, indexes, and so forth still exist. These records provide an extraordinary opportunity to examine cognition in a variety of personal and professional settings.

In the present context, we focus on the data showing that Faraday relied a great deal on external memory aids (Tweney, 1989). Indeed, a major reason why so much of Faraday's records survive is that he did not trust his own memory. There is evidence that memory was a major problem for Faraday, certainly by age 40; he complained about the weakness of his memory at that time in correspondence and a bit later in his own diary. Records show that he repeated experiments that had been done earlier but apparently had been forgotten.

To combat this problem, Faraday created an elaborate system of memory storage, indexing, and retrieval devices (Tweney, 1989). Faraday's mnemonic system evolved over time. Initially, he developed a typical alphabetical index. Later, he incorporated John Locke's suggestions on constructing a real-time index. This system evolved into a chronological diary, which Faraday finally converted into a numbered chronological diary. Faraday also adapted the method of loci to an external format based on three overlapping orderings of locations. This elaborate mnemonic system allowed Faraday to develop two main types of retrieval devices: loose slips (small pieces of paper with short notes) and retrieval sheets (larger papers with 12 different types of more extensive cues). These retrieval devices were often constructed at roughly the same time as the diary entries (and often much later as well), indicating that Faraday intended the devices to help him organize information in a logical, easily retrievable way. Moreover, Tweney (1989) presents evidence that Faraday used these retrieval devices to keep track of and suggest important experiments, to assist him in writing manuscripts, and to impose order on his understanding of some physical process.

This extraordinary diary record allows great insight into how mnemonic systems come into being and evolve over time, processes about which we know very little. Moreover, the fact that Faraday developed the system at least in part because he did not trust his memory provides some interesting insights into the connection between self-perceptions of memory (e.g., metamemory) and actual strategy development and use. The diaries also provide insight into the ways in which Faraday dealt with a huge data base of (ultimately) 30,000 separate experiments. How he decided which retrieval cues to generate, among many other things, provides insight into his semantic and episodic memory structure. In short, Faraday's extensive records provide a unique opportunity to study cognitive processes in ways typically unavailable.

Diaries as Sources of Autobiographical Memory

As noted at the outset of this chapter, most people keep diaries as personal records. Consequently, diaries can be viewed as autobiographies, which for the cognitive researcher, provide data for potential use in studies of autobiographical memory. A distinct advantage of this approach is that, unlike the Galton method or a free-recall paradigm, there exists a record written at the time of the event that can be compared to a person's subsequent recollection of it. This advantage circumvents one of the most serious criticisms leveled at autobiographical memory research; namely, there is no way to gauge the accuracy of remembrances. That is, the question of interest is how well the diary record itself is retained over time.

Linton's 6-Year Study

One of the first, and still the most extensive, autobiographical diary investigations was Linton's (1975, 1978) 6-year investigation of her own memory. Every day during this period, she wrote at least two naturally occurring events in her life; these totaled roughly 5,500 through the course of the study. Linton also recorded salience ratings for each event. Each month, she tested herself on a semirandom subset of items; about 11,000 tests or retests of items occurred over the 6 years. Details of Linton's recording and scoring procedures are available (Linton, 1975).

Overall, Linton found forgetting occurred relatively slowly compared to the standard Ebbinghaus forgetting function. Interestingly, however, the shape of Linton's forgetting function was the same as Ebbinghaus's. Linton

(1978) speculates that the difference in rate was due to her use of cued recall as opposed to free recall and that events from a person's life are more easily and permanently encoded than are word lists or nonsense syllables. Linton also found that the rate of forgetting is independent of the opportunity of items to be tested; that is, frequency of retesting of items was unrelated to the rate of forgetting of these items.

Linton (1975) points out that one satisfying finding was that her data were quite orderly. That is, the criticism that diary data cannot be used in meaningful analyses of remembering and forgetting is clearly ill founded, at least when diary entries are made systematically. Moreover, data collected in this manner have the potential for addressing the question of how people form schemas in memory from discrete episodic events. That is, examination of how and what changes occur in the remembered episode over time provides information about the kinds of information extracted and incorporated into schemas.

BARCLAY'S APPROACH

Barclay (1986; 1988; Barclay & DeCooke, 1989) conducted some of the most carefully designed and interesting diary-based research on autobiographical memory. His approach is based on the notion that autobiographical memories are accurate in that they reflect people's *expectations* about what probably happened in their past lives, not necessarily what may have *actually* happened (see Barclay & Wellman, 1986). However, inaccuracies creep in at the level of details of the events, because most life events are not stored isomorphically with the way that the events really occurred. Barclay's creative solution to this issue was to test autobiographical memory through recognition tests, with foils constructed around certain rules (e.g., semantic similarity).

Barclay (e.g., 1988; see also Barclay & DeCooke, 1989) had three people complete a $2\frac{1}{2}$-year longitudinal study of events recorded in diaries over a period of 4 consecutive months. Each participant recorded at least three events per day, with recognition tests on them given at 3-, 6-, 9-, 12-, and 30-month delays. Each entry included a description of the event, its context, and personal reactions. Test format was as follows. Respondents were to decide first whether the test item was in their diary and then to rate on a 7-point scale how confident they were about this decision. Eighteen items on each test were original items, and 27 were foils. Like Linton (1975, 1978), Barclay (1988) found very high retention rates (94% correct after a 1-year delay and 76% after a 30-month delay). False recognition of foils, however, also increased to nearly .5 by the final test. These rates were comparable to other analyses (Barclay, 1986) that showed false-alarm rates of roughly .7 after a 1-year delay.

Hertzog conducted a small, unpublished pilot study in which three older adults were asked to record daily events and activities in a format similar to Barclay's. The goals of the pilot study were to determine whether relatively unstructured diaries could be used to generate measures of frequency of forgetting incidents and whether Barclay's procedures could be used to test older adults. Participants recorded at least five events per day which they nominated as memorable. One participant's diary was unusable due to failure to follow instructions. Entries in the remaining two diaries were analyzed for typological classes of events. Categorization of events was largely idiosyncratic to respondent but was reliably done by two independent raters.

Hertzog constructed a recognition test booklet, consisting of true events and foils, for each participant. The classified events were randomly assigned to be the basis for a true event description or for an event foil. Foils were created by taking an actual diary entry and changing it, either by significantly altering the nature of the event or the participant's evaluation of her own affective reaction and event evaluation. True event probes were rewritten by the experimenters. Participants were informed that test items might use different wordings than those actually recorded in the diaries. Recognition was tested approximately 3 months after the last diary entry. Both participants performed extremely well. False-alarm rates were low, and no significant relationship was found between date of diary entry and false-alarm rate.

However, these pilot data uncovered potential problems with Barclay's approach concerning the construction of recognition foils. Debriefing suggested that respondents often made choices based on self-schemas (cf. Markus, 1977), that is, complex, interrelated propositions about the self that are stored in long-term memory. Comments such as, "I know I didn't write it that way," or, "I know I didn't do that," were made when respondents were reviewing correctly rejected foils. This raises the issue that individuals may have insight into the way that they typically describe events and that tests involving rewriting or editing of diary entries may provide an unintended clue that the item is bogus. Indeed, James (1890) noted long ago that autobiographical memory involves a particular confluence of things, including one's personality and self, at one specific point in time. Thus, good performance on memory tests of diary entries may not necessarily imply good memory for past events. Rather, it may reflect the difficulty of writing good foils without elaborate knowledge about the individual diarist. This possibility needs to be carefully examined, as it could have potentially serious consequences for future research of this type. Certainly, it suggests that the use of cued recall may provide more valid indices of event memory than does recognition.

ADVANTAGES OF USING DIARIES IN AUTOBIOGRAPHICAL MEMORY RESEARCH

What can we conclude from diary-based research on autobiographical memory? Examination of Linton's as well as others' diary entries shows that most everyday events are routine and mundane. Yet, as Barclay and

DeCooke (1989) point out, such events form the "raw materials" for the construction and reconstruction of self-knowledge systems. People generally place great confidence in their memory of events from their past, perhaps because the only information that is available is the information that is retrieved. Consequently, Barclay and DeCooke (1989) argue, and we agree, that what is stored about autobiographical events is likely or probable occurrences that accumulate over many years and ultimately form self-schemas or ego (cf. Greenwald, 1980; Markus, 1977), a point made by James (1890) more than a century ago. An interesting hypothesis for future research, and one consistent with research on eyewitness testimony, is that episodic traces from events become less accessible over time, whereas inferences and other schematized representations of events are more easily accessed. For example, one may, over time, have difficulty reconstructing exactly which entrees were ordered during different visits to one's favorite restaurant, yet still be able to retrieve judgments about the relative quality of different entrees on the menu. Furthermore, people's reconstructions of autobiographical events over long time delays may be so heavily influenced by self-schemas that their remembrances are more akin to beliefs about their past than to what actually occurred.

The advantage of using diaries to investigate this process is that one gains insight into how this transformation occurs. Researchers can track the process by which recollections change over time and can document which aspects change and which remain constant. This allows greater insight into how self-schemas are formed and how they in turn affect subsequent construction and reconstruction of events.

Equally important, Linton (1975, 1978) and Barclay (1986, 1988; Barclay & DeCooke, 1989) have both demonstrated that it is possible to obtain detailed diary entries that can be used like any other kind of memory material. Diary entries can be reliably coded, can be used to track forgetting functions, and can be put into standard memory-testing paradigms. Such demonstrations remove many of the most serious claims against the use of diaries in research.

Future Directions in Diary-Based Memory Research

As has been demonstrated, diaries have most of the good qualities of traditional memory material but have the advantage of being more representative of everyday memory. For research on memory strategies, diaries offer the unique opportunity to measure the development and intentional use of strategies in natural settings. Considerably more information is needed on this issue, especially in view of the little data existing concerning older adults' memory experiences. The modified structured diary format described earlier appears to be the best alternative. Other possibilities include microcassette recorders, with which people could describe strategy use as it happens more easily than with pencil-and-paper methods.

In any case, we believe that carefully designed diary research on everyday use of memory strategies should focus on contextual factors, how strategies are selected, subjective feelings of importance, and reasons for using strategies. For example, one topic on which very little data are available concerns the rationale for using memory strategies. It would be valuable to establish whether individuals' reasons for using strategies vary with age in everyday settings and the extent to which these reasons are related to perceived rates and seriousness of forgetting.

We believe that diary-based methods for the study of autobiographical memory represent the approach of choice. We earlier described the various advantages of this method and believe that they will enable important advances to be made. We suggest, however, that more attention be paid to testing paradigms, with a special focus on the issue of constructing recognition foils. Additionally, we suggest that various testing approaches (e.g., free recall, cued recall, recognition) be included in a single study. This would allow additional insight into the construction and reconstruction of personal memories, as each retention test puts different demands on the system.

Because metamemory involves recollections of personal events (e.g., how well one performed on a particular memory task), improved diary research on autobiographical memory will advance metamemory theory as well. That is, how personal memories that are stored become transformed over time could provide insight into how one's self-evaluation of memory changes as well.

Diaries as Windows on Cognitive Development

Another interesting application of diary methods is in research on cognitive development. A long-standing debate in the field concerns whether the types of thinking that individuals demonstrate in the laboratory reflect their thinking in everyday life. Using diaries as indicators of everyday thought assists researchers in addressing this question. In this section, we will consider three different approaches to using diaries to study cognitive development. The first relies on published or widely available diaries, such as Anne Frank's, as the data. The second relies on participants recording their thoughts for a period of time. The third uses diaries to analyze the development of syntactic complexity.

Cognitive-Affective Development

Few developmental researchers have taken advantage of published diaries, despite the wide availability of such records. Kramer and Haviland (Haviland & Kramer, 1991; Kramer & Haviland, 1989) demonstrate the research potential of what they term *reflective diaries*, which are diaries that include lengthy discussions of the meaning of recorded events to the diarist. They conducted detailed analyses of two diaries: Anne Frank's and Vivienne's. In both cases, Kramer and Haviland looked for evidence of cognitive and affective development during adolescence. In particular, they examined diary entries and personal writings (e.g., letters) for evidence of formal and postformal thought, indications of affective involvement with current life experiences, and signs that affect and cognition were interrelated. Specifically, Kramer and Haviland focused on the hypothesis that affect and cognition are developmentally unrelated. The two sets of writings chosen for this research represent two very different individuals. Anne Frank was a well-adjusted mature girl, whereas Vivienne was a troubled adolescent who committed suicide.

Both diaries were coded as follows. Emotions and moods were categorized using Izard's (1971) dictionary list (interest-excitement, enjoyment-joy, surprise-startle, distress, anguish, disgust-contempt, anger-rage, shame-humiliation, fear-terror) plus a residual category of nonspecific terms (e.g., moody). Words in each category found in the text were tagged with the date of the entry, and with the person, object, or idea that is the referent of the emotion. Cognitions were categorized using a system based on Kramer and Woodruff (1986). Each sentence in the diaries was examined to see if it represented any of four categories of thought (absolutism, absolutism/relativism, relativism, or dialecticism). Reliability of codings was checked by having a second rater code 25% of all diary entries; very high levels of agreement were reported.

In the case of Anne Frank, Haviland and Kramer (1991) found three major cognitive shifts, each associated with specific types of affect. Absolutist thinking was most likely to occur during happy and angry moods and least likely during fearful moods. Relativistic thinking was most likely during fearful moods and least likely during angry moods. Finally, dialectical thinking was most likely during sad and angry moods and least likely during happy and fearful moods. Haviland and Kramer (1991) argue that these findings suggest that increases in affective activity may precede and perhaps facilitate the development of thinking during adolescence. New types of thinking never preceded emotional peaks, leading them to speculate that cognitive growth may not precede emotional periods. In their analysis, the divorcing of formal thought from emotionality occurred only after a prolonged pairing of affect and cognition. This may suggest that cognitive development is somehow interrelated to one's emotional life. Haviland and Kramer argue that certain types of emotion either facilitate or hinder cognitive activity, an interesting speculation that deserves greater attention. What is unclear from the examination of Anne's diary is whether it is emotionality in general as opposed to emotionality around certain kinds of themes that is important for cognitive development. It was the need to address this issue that led to the analysis of Vivienne's diary.

In the case of Vivienne, Kramer and Haviland (1989) found very different results. Happy word usage dropped considerably over time, whereas negative emotion words increased. Initially, there was considerable evidence of absolutist thinking, and some evidence of absolutist/relativistic and of relativistic thinking. By the end of the entries, these had all declined. No substantial evidence of dialectical thinking was identified. Although fairly closely linked at the beginning of the entries, cognition and affect became increasingly disconnected over time. Kramer and Haviland (1989) argue that these data help identify patterns of dysfunction in adolescence. Specifically, they point out that emotional dysfunction preceded cognitive dysfunction in Vivienne but that both were necessary for suicidal ideation. They also note that Vivienne's inability to understand or identify other people's emotions did not seem to interfere with cognitive growth up to adolescence, as evidenced by the relatively large number of codable cognitions at the outset. However, with the growing need to accommodate abstract reflections about interpersonal relationships, which develops during adolescence, the inability to understand others becomes problematic.

Everyday Thinking in College Women

Neimark and Stead (1981) conducted one of the only investigations of everyday thinking using diaries. They instructed 113 undergraduate women to keep a journal of their everyday thinking. Students were asked to describe some instance in which they were aware of their thinking and to provide as much detail about their thought process as possible. A detailed scoring system was devised that provided rankings within each category of analysis as to the complexity of thought.

Neimark and Stead reported three main results. First, the so-called average thinker concerns herself with commonplace events and impressions in a personal, concrete, and superficial manner. Personal thinking styles however, vary considerably. Second, five major dimensions of thinking emerged: creative thinking, assuming a broad perspective, intellectualizing, practical decision making, and preoccupation with the self. Third, blind sorting of randomly selected individuals was accomplished above chance. That is, randomly selected individuals' diary entries were scrambled and sorted into piles based on thinking styles; accuracy of these sorts, even though accomplished blindly, were above chance level. This finding supports the notion that individuals have identifiable, consistent, idiosyncratic thinking styles.

This research demonstrates that diaries produced by college women can be used to develop a typology of thinking, which in turn can be used to identify individual thinking styles. Neimark and Stead (1981) conclude their paper with a strong condemnation of what they term the "narrow focus of laboratory research on thinking" (p. 471) and a call for more direct investigation of everyday thought.

Development of Syntactic Complexity

Kemper (1987) also used existing diaries to conduct an interesting set of analyses on the development of syntactic complexity. In the longitudinal part of the study, she examined diaries of eight people born between 1856 and 1876 for seven or more decades. In the cohort-sequential part of the study, she analyzed diaries of 10 adults born between 1820 and 1829 and recorded during 1860 to 1869 and 10 adults born between 1986 and 1869 and recorded during 1900 and 1909 and again during 1940 and 1949. The data consisted of the two longest, usable entries from each half-decade (e.g., 20–24 years, 25–29 years). Kemper was particularly interested in the frequency of left- and right-branching embeddings and of coordinate and subordinate phrases and sentence fragments. She also analyzed the mean length of sentences in words and in clauses.

Kemper's (1987) results for both the longitudinal and the cohort-sequential analyses were consistent. Age-related declines were found for use of relative clauses, that-clauses, wh-clauses, infinitives, use of subordinates and coordinates, and double- and triple-embeddings. Sentence length in words did not change, but the mean number of clauses per sentence did decline. As Kemper notes, these findings corroborate similar evidence from oral speech and are consistent with processing based explanations of cognitive aging. Unlike most processing research, however, Kemper's use of diaries allowed her to examine such changes within individuals over very long periods of time.

Future Directions for Diary Research on Cognitive Development

Clearly, one must be cautious in interpreting the findings presented here. Kramer and Haviland (1989; Haviland & Kramer, 1991) examined only two diaries, written by two atypical adolescents. Likewise, Neimark and Stead (1981) studied adolescents and young adults. The problem here is that adolescence may not be representative of other life periods (e.g., old age). Kemper's (1987) analyses were based on a very small proportion of the diary records, leaving open the possibility that different selection criteria may have produced different results.

Despite these and other serious limitations (e.g., scoring systems tied to one specific theoretical orientation), these researchers have opened an extremely useful approach to studying everyday cognition. Rarely do developmental researchers have the luxury of collecting rich records of personal reflections recorded daily over extended periods of time in order to catch development as it happens naturally. Diaries offer such opportunities. As all of these researchers have shown, it is possible to code entries reliably for a variety of important developmental variables. Certainly, the choices of which behaviors to code were driven by theoretical reasons. One could have chosen other behaviors, such as social or moral cognition, interpersonal activities, love relationships, parent–child relationships, or a host of other experiences.

The important point is that, especially in cases when diaries have been kept for several decades, they could provide one of the few opportunities to test key developmental hypotheses of life-span theories (e.g., Erikson; postformal thought) that under normal circumstances is impossible. Additionally, diary records provide a way to develop taxonomies of thinking and feeling in everyday life that could be compared across age. Longitudinal records of the natural development of such taxonomies would be especially helpful.

In sum, as long as the limitations of multiple-case study methodology are kept in mind, diaries provide fertile ground for true developmental research. Hypotheses about personal change over time can be considered in ways unavailable to the average developmentalist. Results from such research would be extremely valuable in revising and extending existing theories as well as in opening new avenues of theory and research.

Summary and Conclusions

In this chapter, we have summarized several areas of research based on personal diaries. We have shown that diaries played an important part in the early history of psychology and that interest in them has increased over the past several years. Diaries present some unique opportunities to test psychological theories, as well as to provide insight into how people structure their everyday cognitive experiences. We believe that these opportunities will result in important theoretical advances, and we emphasize that cognitive and developmental research can be based on real-world experiences.

Acknowledgments. Preparation of this chapter was supported by a National Institute on Aging (NIA) RCDA award (K04 AG00335) to the second author. Collection of the memory event data was supported by an NIA research grant (R01 AG06162) to the second author. We thank Ryan Tweney for his comments on an earlier draft.

References

Barclay, C.R. (1986). Schematization of autobiographical memory. In D.C. Rubin (Ed.), *Autobiographical memory* (pp. 82–99). New York: Cambridge University Press.

Barclay, C.R. (1988). Truth and accuracy in autobiographical memory. In M.M. Gruneberg, P.E. Morris, & R.N. Sykes (Eds.), *Practical aspects of memory: Current research and issues: Vol. 1. Memory in everyday life* (pp. 289–294). Chichester, England: Wiley.

Barclay, C.R., & DeCooke, P.A. (1989). Ordinary everyday memories: some of the things of which selves are made. In U. Neisser & E. Winograd (Eds.), *Remembering reconsidered* (pp. 91–125). New York: Cambridge University Press.

Barclay, C.R., & Wellman, H.M. (1986). Accuracies and inaccuracies in autobiographical memories. *Journal of Memory and Language, 25,* 93–103.

Burke, D., Worthley, J., & Martin, J. (1988). I'll never forget what's-her-name: Aging and tip of the tongue experiences in everyday life. In M.M. Gruneberg, P.E. Morris, & R.N. Sykes (Eds.), *Practical aspects of memory: Current research and issues: Vol. 2. Clinical and educational implications* (pp. 113–118). Chichester, England: Wiley.

Carp, F.M., & Carp, A. (1981). The validity, reliability and generalizability of diary data. *Experimental Aging Research, 7,* 281–296.

Cavanaugh, J.C. (1981). Early developmental theories: A brief review of attempts to organize developmental data prior to 1925. *Journal of the History of the Behavioral Sciences, 17,* 38–47.

Cavanaugh, J.C. (1985). Cognitive developmental psychology before Preyer. Biographical and educational records. In G. Eckardt, W.G. Bringmann, & L. Sprung (Eds.), *Contributions to a history of developmental psychology* (pp. 187–207). Berlin: Mouton.

Cavanaugh, J.C., Grady, J.G., & Perlmutter, M. (1983). Forgetting and use of memory aids in 20 to 70 year olds' everyday life. *International Journal of Aging and Human Development, 17,* 113–122.

Darwin, C. (1877). A biographical sketch of an infant. *Mind, 2,* 285–294.

Ebbinghaus, H. (1913). *Memory: A contribution to experimental psychology.* New York: Teachers College, Columbia University. (Original work published 1885.)

Greenwald, A.G. (1980). The totalitarian ego: Fabrication and revision of personal history. *American Psychologist, 35,* 603–618.

Haviland, J.M., & Kramer, D.A. (1991). Affect-cognition relationships in an adolescent diary I: The case of Anne Frank. *Human Development, 34,* 143–159.

Hulicka, I.M. (1982). Memory functioning in late adulthood. In F.I.M. Craik & S. Trehub (Eds.), *Aging and cognitive processes* (pp. 331–351). New York: Plenum.

Izard, C. (1971). *The face of emotion.* New York: Appleton-Century-Crofts.

James, W. (1890). *The principles of psychology.* New York: Holt.

Kemper, S. (1987). Life-span changes in syntactic complexity. *Journal of Gerontology, 42,* 323–328.

Kramer, D.A., & Haviland, J.M. (1989). *Affect-cognition relationships in an adolescent diary II: The case of Vivienne.* Unpublished manuscript, Rutgers University, New Brunswick, NJ.

Kramer, D.A., & Woodruff, D.S. (1986). Relativistic and dialectical thought in three adult age groups. *Human Development, 29,* 280–290.

Linton, M. (1975). Memory for real-world events. In D.A. Norman & D.E. Rumelhart (Eds.), *Explorations in cognition* (pp. 376–404). San Francisco: Freeman.

Linton, M. (1978). Real world memory after six years: An in vivo study of very long term memory. In M.M. Gruneberg, P.E. Morris, & R.N. Sykes (Eds.), *Practical aspects of memory* (pp. 69–76). London: Academic Press.

Markus, H. (1977). Self-schemata and processing information about the self. *Journal of Personality and Social Psychology, 35,* 63–78.

Neimark, E.D., & Stead, C. (1981). Everyday thinking of college women: Analysis of journal entries. *Merrill-Palmer Quarterly, 27,* 471–488.

Nersessian, N. (1984). *Faraday to Einstein. Constructing meaning in scientific theories.* Dordrecht, Netherlands: Nijhoff.

Reason, J., & Lucas, D. (1984). Using cognitive diaries to investigate naturally occurring memory blocks. In J.E. Harris & P.E. Morris (Eds.), *Everyday memory, actions, and absent-mindedness* (pp. 53–70). London: Academic Press.

Shlechter, T.M., & Herrmann, D.J. (1981, April). *Multi-method approach to investigating everyday memory.* Paper presented at the annual meeting of the Eastern Psychological Association, New York.

Taine, H. (1877). M. Taine on the acquisition of language by children. *Mind, 2,* 252–257. (Original work published 1876.)

Tweney, R.D. (1989). *The use of external memory in science: A case study of Michael Faraday.* Unpublished manuscript.

West, R.L. (1984, August). *An analysis of prospective everyday memory.* Paper presented at the annual meeting of the American Psychological Association, Toronto.

3
Examining Idiosyncracies in Script Reports Across the Life Span: Distortions or Derivations of Experience

Barbara L. Ross and Cynthia A. Berg

When asked to describe "What happens when you go on an airplane trip starting with the decision to take the trip and ending when you are called to enter the plane?" an elderly woman in one of our studies (Ross & Berg, 1991) gave the following report:

Son sends the ticket
Get ticket
Become paralyzed with fear
Cut off appointments for 2 weeks
Tell people when I'll be gone
Look through my clothes to find the nicest
Put clothes on the davenport
Look at clothes
Pack by process of elimination
Take out what looks too shabby
Take out what looks too small
Take out suitcase
Take out the list of what I brought before
Judge by the list what I will need now
Put the list with the ticket
Wait for the day I go
Ask friend to take me
He takes me there 1 hour early
Get there
They assign seat
They put me in a wheelchair because the distance is long
They ask which seat I prefer
Get an aisle seat
They write the number of my seat
Sit
Read
They open the door to the plane

Although her report contained acts that other individuals generated for preparing for airplane travel (e.g., assign seat, read), many acts were different from those that other individuals, both young and old, generated when asked the same question. The idiosyncratic acts included in her script (e.g., son sends ticket, take out the list of what I brought before, they put me in a wheelchair) were related to her experience with airplane travel and reflected her personal habits and constraints. Our research suggests that such idiosyncratic acts are important as they guide her memory for new script-related events regarding airplane travel.

Script reports, such as the report here, have frequently been used to assess memory for everyday events, such as going on an airplane trip or going to a restaurant, in both children (Nelson, 1986; Schank & Abelson, 1977) and adults (see Chapter 6, this volume; Light & Anderson, 1983). Scripts have been defined as temporal-causal sequences of expectations that individuals have about common everyday events (Nelson, Fivush, Hudson, & Lucariello, 1983; Schank & Abelson, 1977). As individuals are thought to have similar knowledge of and experience with everyday events, the commonality of acts in script reports (i.e., similarity of acts) given by different individuals has been the primary focus of script research (Nelson, 1981). Idiosyncratic acts have been characterized as deviations and distortions in script reports (Nelson, 1981). Such idiosyncratic acts, however, may be based on an individual's experience with the event and may be integral to an individual's script (see also Chapter 6, this volume). As scripts are related to experience with routine events (Schank & Abelson, 1977) and as experience with routine events may become more heterogeneous during adult development (Baltes, Dittmann-Kohli, & Dixon, 1984; Charness & Bieman-Copland, in press), script reports may become more divergent.

The purpose of this chapter is to illustrate that individuals possess personalized scripts for routine events that relate to their specific experience and that personal scripts may become more idiosyncratic across adult development. The initial section briefly describes past script research that focuses on the common components of scripts in both children and adults. This is followed by a discussion of the methodological features of script research that may influence the degree of commonality in script reports. In the third section, we report results from a study examining individual differences in the script reports of young and older adults. Using a less directive methodology than has previously been used, these results support the notion that individuals possess personalized scripts for routine events that may become more idiosyncratic with development. This study also explores the importance of such personalized scripts for remembering new script-related information. In addition, the increased idiosyncracy of older adults' script reports has implications for age differences in memory for new script-related events. In the final section, we explore the role of experience in creating personalized scripts and suggest future research that may track the development of personalized scripts.

Commonality in Script Reports

Research on script development has focused on how common scripts are across individuals of the same age (e.g., Nelson, 1978) as well as across individuals of different ages (e.g., Light & Anderson, 1983; Nelson, 1986). Evidence for the high degree of similarity or "commonality" of scripts comes from both the child development (e.g., Nelson, 1986) and adult development literatures (e.g., Hess, 1985; Light & Anderson, 1983). We have included work on script reports with children here and throughout the chapter, as the child literature can inform the adult development literature regarding issues of commonality in scripts, methodological techniques in generating scripts, and the role of experience in script development.

A high level of commonality in script reports during childhood has been shown for a variety of different scripted events. Nelson and Gruendel (1986) examined commonality by describing the percentage of children who mentioned each act, referred to as "act consistency," for three different events. Commonality was high for all three events: an average of 63%, 75%, and 82% of 4- and 5-year-old children mentioned each act for eating lunch, eating dinner, and going to McDonald's, respectively. Similar act-consistency scores have been found among children's scripts for the event of going to school (Fivush, 1984) as well as for events such as getting dressed, going to a birthday party, making cookies, and grocery shopping (Nelson & Gruendel, 1986). Nelson and Gruendel (1986) reported that act-consistency scores increased during early childhood (4 to 6 years of age) for a variety of different scripted events and further suggested that scripts are well-established by early childhood (Nelson & Gruendel, 1986).

Scripts have also been found to be highly common during adulthood for a variety of events, using several different measures of commonality. For instance, Light and Anderson (1983) used the proportion of an individual's generated script acts that were uniquely reported by that individual as a measure of script idiosyncrasy. They found that the proportion of unique acts was relatively low, ranging from .16 to .26. Light and Anderson found that individuals more frequently generated items that were rated as typical in most people's experience.

Research also suggests that scripts are common across young and older adults. Light and Anderson (1983) reported no age differences in script reports using multiple sources of evidence: (a) no age differences in the proportion of unique acts, (b) similar ratings of the typicality of acts across young and older adults, and (c) high correlations between young and old act-consistency scores. Hess (1985) also found that ratings of act typicality were similar for young and old adults. Hess (Chapter 6, this volume), more recently, reports data that show more variability in script reports. Although the general picture that comes from the child and adult literatures is that scripts are common across individuals at a single age and across individuals of different ages, several methodological features of the way in which scripts were generated may have influenced the degree of commonality found in script reports.

Methodological Features That Influence Commonality in Script Reports

In their original theoretical work on scripts, Schank and Abelson (1977) posited that scripts consist of both common acts that are shared by individuals engaged in routine events as well as personalized acts that are specific to a particular individual's experience with the event. The majority of research on scripts has used methods, however, that highlight the common acts present in script reports. Scripts are typically elicited by asking individuals to generate acts related to routine events. Many variations on this basic method exist in the literature, including the manner in which the script is elicited and the nature of the scripted event being examined. Variations in the method and context in which scripts are elicited appear to differentially highlight common versus personalized acts in script reports. In this section, we discuss the ways in which methodology may influence script commonality across individuals.

INSTRUCTIONS

In much of script research, participants are given general instructions to "Tell me what happens when you . . ." (e.g., Nelson & Gruendel, 1986; Schank & Abelson, 1977). Some researchers, however, have been more specific regarding the kinds of acts (typical versus atypical) and number of acts to report. For example, Light and Anderson (1983) instructed their participants to "produce a list of common actions or events . . . that should not include idiosyncratic actions based on their own behavior but should list actions that would be typically performed by most people" (p. 437). Light and Anderson further provided participants with a detailed example of typical actions involved in the script of going to class, before participants elicited script reports of other events (e.g., going to a doctor's appointment, etc.). Such instructions were likely to restrict the reporting of idiosyncratic acts even if such acts were common in the participant's own experience with the event. Finally, participants in Light and Anderson's study (1983) were specifically instructed to produce approximately 20 actions, which may have led some individuals to shorten their reports and others to lengthen them. In contrast, Ross and Berg (1991) found that when individuals were not instructed as to the number or kinds of acts to report, individuals produced a larger number of total acts (young adults produced an average of 28.8 acts and older adults 24.1 acts) as well as a larger proportion of unique acts than reported by Light and Anderson (see following discussion).

PROMPTING

When scripts are generated orally, the types of prompts that are used to elicit more detail may affect the degree of commonality in script reports (Nelson, 1978, 1986). For example, in Nelson's studies, a series of prompts were used that became increasingly more specific (Nelson, 1978; Nelson & Gruendel, 1986). The general instructions to the child were "Can you tell me what happens when you . . . ?" (Nelson & Gruendel, p. 26, 1986). If the child paused, the child was asked "Can you tell me anything else about . . . ?" When the child answered no to this last prompt, the interviewer continued with a set of more specific prompts ("What happens next?" "What happens after . . . ?"). Such detailed prompting certainly made some features of scripts, such as temporal order and specific acts, evident in nearly all of the children's scripts. Furthermore, common acts were more extensively probed than less common acts (Nelson, 1978). Nelson (1978) has noted that such detailed prompting may lead to high commonality of script reports.

PROPS

In her work with children, Nelson (1978; Nelson & Gruendel, 1986) used props to elicit scripts and noted that such props affected script generation. For example, in one study, children were presented with a model of McDonald's and asked to act out the event of eating lunch at McDonald's. Nelson (1978) found that children generated more acts when they used the McDonald's prop than when they generated their script without the aid of a prop (although this was not true for other props). Props that are related to the scripted event provide individuals with cues to aid their recall of acts involved in the event and may lead to a higher degree of commonality for acts that are suggested from the prop.

In our pilot work with children, we found that the introduction of a relatively minor and *unrelated* prop such as asking children to give their script to a Mickey Mouse puppet greatly increased the length, detail, and idiosyncrasy of script reports. The idiosyncrasies in their reports were related to their experience with the event and not to their experience with Mickey Mouse. Thus, the use of certain types of props with young children, although necessary to engage the child in the task, may affect the level of individual differences found in script reports.

CONTEXT OF SCRIPT GENERATION

Several other features of the context in which a script is generated (e.g., where the script is generated and the participant's definition of the task) may affect the degree of commonality. Nelson and Gruendel (1986) examined whether the location in which scripts were generated impacted children's script reports. Children were asked to generate scripts for eating lunch at school and eating dinner at home, either at school or at home. The location of generation did not affect the number of acts children generated nor the consistency with which acts were generated. Although they did not find that location of generation affected act commonality, one can envision instances when location could increase act commonality. For example, when we asked young and older adults to describe what happens when they take an airplane trip, in a laboratory setting, only three individuals (two young and one old) mentioned the act of "going through the metal detector." This seems odd, as we hope that all individuals actually pass through the security metal detector before entering the plane. We suspect that had individuals generated their script at the airport many more individuals would have mentioned this act, thereby increasing commonality, because the metal detector itself would have provided a retrieval cue for this act.

One important contextual feature of script generation that has yet to be examined systematically is the participant's interpretation of what is meant by generating a script. That is, what kinds of acts does the participant believe should be mentioned: critically important acts, typical acts, or all acts involved in the event? The large range in the number of acts mentioned for events in our study (12–78), may reflect, in part, participants' different interpretations of the task of generating a script. In fact, many of the participants in our study asked specific questions regarding what types of acts they should mention. If participants vary greatly in their definition of the task, such different definitions may result in less commonality in script reports than if such definitions were similar. Some researchers (Light & Anderson, 1983; Ross & Berg, 1991) have addressed this issue by presenting individuals with beginning and end points of the script in order to help define the task for the participants.

CONTENT OF SCRIPTED EVENT

Commonality also appears to be affected by the nature of the scripted event (see also Chapter 6). For instance, Nelson and Gruendel (1986) found that act-consistency scores for children were low for the event of a fire drill. They posited that children's limited experience with fire drills may have produced less commonality than expected. However, in our work with young and older adults, we have found that script reports differ in commonality using events for which individuals are very experienced. We found less commonality in script reports for the event of going to a doctor's appointment than for the event of going on an airplane trip. We expect that the diversity in people's experience with different types of doctors may have led to less commonality.

In sum, several methodological features of existing script research may be related to the extent of commonality found in the script reports of both children and adults. The bulk of the extant script literature has involved methods that emphasize the common acts in script reports. Idiosyncratic or personalized script acts may not be anomalous in script reports but have yet to be highlighted by existing methodologies. As a result, caution should be exercised in making conclusions about the prevalence of individual differences in script reports and the lack of age differences in script reports (see also Chapter 6). To examine whether a less directive methodology might highlight personalized information in script reports, we asked individuals to relate their script without specifying the number or kinds of acts they should report.

Individual Differences in Script Reports

To examine individual differences in script reports, we asked 30 young adults (mean age 22.9) and 30 older adults (mean age 66.7 years) to relate their scripts for two events using a methodology that did not direct individuals to report acts of a particular type (e.g., highly common acts). Each individual was asked "What happens when you go on an airplane trip, beginning when you decide to take the airplane trip and ending when you leave the airport at your destination?" and "What happens when you go for a doctor's appointment, beginning when you decide to make the appointment and ending when you leave the doctor's office?" Participants were asked to report each event in two parts to ensure that all of the participants had a similar understanding of the dimensions of the task. For example, for the airplane script, individuals were first asked to describe events between the time "You decide to take an airplane trip" and "You are called to enter the plane" and second, to describe events between the time "You are called to enter the plane" and "You leave the airport at your destination." Individuals were asked to give these reports in enough detail so that another person would know exactly what they did. In addition, they were prompted with "Does anything else happen?" until they reported that nothing else happened.

To assess the prevalence of individual differences in script reports, two different measures were examined: act-consistency scores (Nelson, 1986) and proportion of unique acts (Light & Anderson, 1983). Act-consistency scores, or the percentage of individuals mentioning each act, revealed that the overwhelming number of acts generated for both events were mentioned by very few individuals. Acts were mentioned by an average of 7% of the young adults and 6% of the older adults. It should be noted, however, that a few acts were mentioned by a majority of the young participants (pack, make an appointment to see the doctor, and wait to see the doctor); whereas, no acts were mentioned by the majority of older participants. The proportion of unique acts also revealed that individual differences were prevalent in script reports. The proportion of unique acts ranged from 0 to .88 with an average of .31 for the young adults and .40 for the older adults, indicating that the scripts of older adults in this study contained significantly more idiosyncratic acts than the scripts of younger adults.

In sum, measures of act consistency and proportion of unique acts, the same individual difference measures used in past script research (e.g., Light & Anderson, 1983; Nelson & Gruendel, 1986), indicated that individual differences were more prevalent in the script reports obtained in this study than in past research, particularly in the reports of older adults. Because several researchers have suggested that individuals use their scripts to remember script-related events (e.g., Bower, Black, & Turner, 1979; McCartney & Nelson, 1981; Schank & Abelson, 1977), we were interested in assessing the impact of individual differences in script reports and the increased idiosyncracy of older adults' script reports on memory for new script-related events.

Rather than asserting that individuals use a common script to remember new script-related events, we hypothesized that individuals use their own personal scripts to aid in their memory of new events. In our study of individual differences in adults' scripts (Ross & Berg, 1991), we tested this hypothesis by tailoring script-related stories to be either similar to or different from each individual's personal script. Each participant was told a story that was similar to their script report (contained 12 out of 16 acts that were included in their personal script) and another that was different from their script report (contained 4 out of 16 acts that were included in their personal script) for two different events, going on an airplane trip and going to a doctor's appointment. These stories contained acts that were equated in their rated general typicality, such that high- and low-similarity stories contained approximately equal numbers of high-, moderate-, and low-typical acts as rated by pilot subjects. Therefore, any differences in the recall of these two stories could be attributed to the similarity of the story to the individuals' personal script, not to differences in general typicality.

We found that individuals in both age groups recalled significantly more acts from stories that were similar to their personal scripts than from stories that were different from their personal scripts (recalled 46% of the acts from high-similarity stories and 32% of the acts from low similarity stories). In addition, individuals made more errors in recalling stories that were less similar to their personal scripts. We interpret these results as suggestive that adults use their personal scripts to guide their memory of new script-related events. Additional support for this claim comes from participants' reports of their strategies for remembering the stories. Sixty-seven percent of the participants reported that they were using their own personal script to remember the new script-related stories. No age differences existed in the strategies used to remember the new script-related stories.

Young adults appeared to be more reliant than older adults on their personal scripts in remembering the stories. The difference in recall of high- versus low-similarity stories was greatest for young adults. Further, young adults intruded more acts from their own personal script in their recall than older adults.

Our results suggest that individual differences are more prevalent in script reports using a methodology that is less directive than used in past research (see also Chapter 6). The prevalence of individual differences found in this study may suggest that scripts consist of not only the common information typically associated with scripts but also more personal, idiosyncratic information. The extent to which idiosyncratic information is actually present in scripts is important in terms of gaining a better understanding of how scripts guide memory for script-related events. These results have implications for research indicating age differences in memory for script-related events (Hess, 1985; Hess, Donley, & Vandermaas, 1989; Light & Anderson, 1983). For instance, Hess (1985) found that older adults are more reliant on script structure than young adults, whereas Light and Anderson (1983) found no age differences between young and older adults on script reliance. Our results indicate that older adults may be less reliant on script structure than young adults, because they benefited less in their recall from the similarity between their own personal script and script-related stories than young adults. Given the extent of individual differences found in this study, further research regarding adults' reliance on scripts in their memory for new events apparently must take into account both the common and personalized components of scripts.

Because individual differences appear to be prevalent in script reports and impact memory for new script-related stories, we were interested in examining the nature of these individual differences. Because scripts are considered to be based on experience with events (e.g., Fivush, 1984; Nelson, 1986; Schank & Abelson, 1977), we began by examining the role of different components of experience on script representation and development.

The Impact of Experience on Script Representation

Amount of Experience

Researchers examining the impact of amount of experience on script representation have found that differences between the script reports of young and older children are related to quantitative differences in experience with routine events (Hudson & Nelson, 1986; Nelson & Gruendel, 1986). The relation between experience and the quality of scripts (e.g., elaboration, conditionals, idiosyncrasies), however, is not clear. Fivush (1984) found that with increasing experience, children produced longer, more elaborate scripts (e.g., temporally complex, more conditionals). Hudson and Nelson (1986), however, reported that with increasing experience, children produced more generic and less detailed scripts of events. Taylor and Winkler

(1980) also suggested that with increasing experience, individuals may develop more succinct and automatized schemas of events.

In our study of individual differences in adults' scripts (Ross & Berg, 1991), we examined the relationship between many experiential factors (number of experiences, types of experiences, attitude toward the experiences) and individual difference measures of script reports. There were great ranges in the amount of experience individuals had with the events, both in terms of recent and distant past experience (e.g., in the 5 years before the study, participants' experience with airplane travel ranged from 2 to 98 trips). However, no strong relationships were found between amount of experience and our individual difference measures. We must point out, however, that the role of amount of experience should be further examined as it may be difficult for individuals to assess accurately the amount of experience they have had with frequently occurring events.

Kind of Experience

In our work (Ross & Berg, 1991), we found that the specific content of participants' experience appeared more critical in producing individual differences in script reports than individuals' amount of experience with an event. Participants included acts in their scripts that were consistent with their own specific experience, even when the acts were nonconventional in terms of most people's experience. For example, the elderly woman's report at the beginning of the paper included "Take out the list of what I brought before," an act that no other individual generated, but which she rated as very typical in her experience with airplane travel.

Several other researchers have noted that the content of individuals' experience may have a stronger impact on memory performance than the quantity of their experience (Chi & Ceci, 1987; Thorndyke & Stasz, 1979). The impact of qualitative differences in individuals' experience on scripted events has been given less attention than quantitative differences in terms of script development. One exception is the early work of Schank and Abelson (1977), in which they described many different kinds of experiential factors that may characterize how specific experience impacts scripts. These factors can be divided into those that are a function of differences in personal perspective and those that are a function of differences in actual experience.

One element of perspective that Schank and Abelson (1977) offered to account for individual differences in scripts was the individual's role in the event. For example, a pilot and a passenger, because of their different roles in participating in airplane travel, are likely to have different perspectives of the event, which may lead to differences in their script for the event. For example, a pilot might mention acts such as "Establish communication with the air traffic controllers," whereas a passenger would be unlikely to include such acts in the script report. Another element of personal perspective that might produce individual differences in script reports involves differences in goals. Individuals who travel by airplane for business may mention acts such as "You prepare for the presentation," whereas individuals who travel for pleasure would not mention such acts. Other elements of perspective that may impact script reports involve motivation, habits, and affectivity.

A second set of factors that Schank and Abelson (1977) discuss involve variations in the objective experience individuals have with script-related events. Frequent exposure to obstacles or exceptions with an event may lead to the inclusion of idiosyncratic acts in a script report. For example, an individual who is consistently late for flights may include acts in the airplane travel script that may not be present for other individuals (e.g., "Reschedule the flight").

We found that the factors suggested by Schank and Abelson (1977) did account for some of the individual differences in script reports of airplane travel and doctor's appointments. These categories, however, did not account for all of the differences in script reports. One category that accounted for a large proportion of the differences in script reports of airplane travel and doctor's appointments was thoughts and opinions (e.g., "Wonder if the plane will crash" "Think that I should charge the doctor for his time"). Other categories that accounted for differences in script reports included differences in religion (e.g., "Find out who another Christian Science friend uses" [for a doctor during pregnancy]"); ethnic background (e.g., "Know some words [in English] about the illness for the doctor"); salience of particular experiences (e.g., "Know what your chances are [in preparation for heart surgery]); associates (e.g., "Call my father to see if he has any questions for the doctor"); health (e.g., "They put me in a wheelchair because she distance is long" [at the airport]); and responsibilities (e.g., "Cut off all appointments for 2 weeks" [before traveling]). Although similar categories were represented in the reports of young and older adults, the frequency with which some of the categories were included in script reports differed as a function of age. For example, acts that related to the categories of responsibilities and health were more prevalent in the reports of older adults than young adults.

Although many of the acts generated for our events seemed quite specific (e.g., son sends the ticket), such acts were rated as very typical in the individual's overall experience with the event. The idiosyncratic acts that participants mentioned in our study did not appear to be slot fillers (Lucariello & Nelson, 1985; Schank & Abelson, 1977), that is, specific, incidental details regarding a particular instantiation of an event (e.g., flying with a specific airline). Subsequent research will need to establish whether such idiosyncratic acts are consistently generated over time and guide people's actions as well as their memory for everyday events.

To summarize, the relationship between experience and individual differences in script reports appears to derive more from the kind of experience an individual has with an event rather than the amount of experience. As individuals differ in the kinds of experience they have with everyday events, it is important to examine the role of experience on script development and the process by which specific experiences with events become incorporated in script reports.

The Role of Specific Experience in Script Development

Several researchers have suggested that scripts are defined by an individual's first experience with an event and that with increasing experience the initial scripts become more detailed (Fivush, 1984). Schank and Abelson (1977) suggested, however, that the first experience with an event remains as a foundation for a script only to the extent that there is continuity between early and later experiences. Therefore, it is only when individuals' experience remains the same over time that their script for an event is defined by their first experience with the event. Because many researchers have suggested that individuals' experience with routine events is very common across individuals (Nelson, 1981), few have considered how changes in experience may alter the content of established scripts for particular events.

The results of our work indicate that specific experiences with events may be critical in the initial construction of scripts and in further development of existing scripts. When examining the script reports of the participants in our study, we noted that several individuals' scripts seemed to be influenced by a few particularly salient experiences (e.g., preparation for open heart surgery). Research following script structure over time is needed to determine if changes in specific experiences produce only minor changes in script structure (e.g., such acts become optional acts in the script) or produce more major long-term changes in overall script structure.

The consistency of such specific experiences over time will be a crucial factor in whether specific experience produces long-term changes in script structure. Across adult development, adults' experience with everyday events may change in a consistent and long-term fashion as a result of developmental life changes (e.g., Havighurst, 1972; Neugarten, Moore, & Lowe, 1968). That is, changes in life-style during adulthood may be so profound that they impact individuals' perceptions and experiences relating to routine events. Life events such as having an occupation, marriage, having children, retirement, and loss of a spouse impact an adult's participation in and perspective of routine events. For example, the older woman's report given at the beginning of this chapter contained acts related to diminished health in that she needed to arrange for a wheelchair at the airport. Other individuals mentioned acts that corresponded with adult responsibilities related to owning a home, having an occupation, and increased opportunities for leisure as a result of retirement. The extent to which life changes affect one's experience for everyday events and the process by which such experiences alter existing scripts are questions for future research.

Research examining developmental life changes and their impact on scripts must take into account that as a group, older adults are more heterogeneous than other age groups with regard to nearly every facet of adult life: health, intelligence, and personality (Baltes & Reese, 1984; Birren & Schaie, 1990). This diversity of older adults may relate to our findings that the script reports of older participants were more idiosyncratic than the reports of younger adults. The diversity and increased specialization of older adults' experience with routine events (Baltes et al., 1984) may be responsible for their increased idiosyncracy in script reports. However, as a result of the cross-sectional nature of this study, age differences in the extent to which different types of idiosyncratic acts were present in script reports may reflect cohort differences. Subsequent research will need to address whether the increased idiosyncracy in the script reports of older adults extends to routine events other than the ones examined in our work.

Summary

Past research on script development has indicated that scripts are highly consistent across individuals and over time (Nelson, 1981). However, several methodological features of the research have discouraged children and adults from reporting idiosyncratic information in their script reports (Light & Anderson, 1983; Nelson, 1978). In our work (Ross & Berg, 1991), we found that individual differences were prevalent in the script reports of both young and older adults and that the script reports of older adults were more idiosyncratic than those of younger adults. The results of our work suggest that individual differences in script reports appear to be based on the specific experiences and perspective of the individual generating the script rather than on the amount of experience with the event.

We found that individual differences in script reports are important because they impact memory for new script-related information. For instance, the increased idiosyncracy of older adults' script reports limits comparisons that can be made between the memory performance of young and older adults regarding script-related information. Future research should address how individual differences become incorporated into script reports, why young and old adults differ in the idiosyncracy of their script reports, and whether other groups of individuals also may differ in the idiosyncracy of their script reports (e.g., young children).

The view of scripts that we have presented in this chapter reflects a perspective of scripts that differs slightly from the traditional view. We have suggested that scripts include not only the highly common information that is traditionally associated with scripts but also more personalized information that may be closely associated with individuals' personal experiences. This modified view of scripts is consistent with the traditional view (Schank & Abelson, 1977) in that, from both perspectives, scripts are derived from individuals' experiences with routine events and function as a guide for remembering routine events (see also Chapter 6).

Such work on the development of scripts will be important because scripts organize much of our experience with everyday events. Examining the role of specific experience for each individual as the determinant of differences in script reports will significantly increase the complexity of script research. Such complexity, however, seems necessary to better understand individuals' experience with and memories of everyday events.

Acknowledgments. Preparation of this chapter was supported, in part, by grant HD 25728 from the National Institute of Child and Human Development and the National Institute of Aging and a University of Utah Research Committee Faculty Grant awarded to Cynthia A. Berg.

References

Baltes, P.B., Dittmann-Kohli, F., & Dixon, R.A. (1984). New perspectives on the development of intelligence in adulthood: Toward a dual-process conception and a model selective optimization with compensation. In P.B. Baltes & O.G. Brim, Jr. (Eds.), *Life-span development and behavior* (Vol. 6, pp. 33–76). New York: Academic Press.

Baltes, P.B., & Reese, H.W. (1984). The life-span perspective in developmental psychology. In M.H. Bornstein & M.E. Lamb (Eds.), *Developmental psychology: An advanced textbook* (pp. 493–531). Hillsdale, NJ: Erlbaum.

Birren, J.E., & Schaie, K.W. (Eds.). (1990). *Handbook of the psychology of aging* (Vol. 2). New York: Van Nostrand.

Bower, G.H., Black, J.B., & Turner, T.J. (1979). Scripts in memory for text. *Cognitive Psychology, 11,* 177–220.

Charness, N., & Bieman-Copland, S. (in press). The learning perspective: Adulthood. In R.J. Sternberg & C.A. Berg (Eds.), *Intellectual development.* New York: Cambridge University Press.

Chi, M., & Ceci, S. (1987). Content knowledge: Its role, representation, and restructuring in memory development. In H.W. Reese & L.P. Lipsitt (Eds.), *Advances in child development and behavior* (Vol. 20, pp. 91–142). New York: Academic Press

Fivush, R. (1984). Learning about school: The development of kindergartners' school scripts. *Child Development, 55,* 1697–1709.

Havighurst, R. (1972). *Developmental tasks and education.* New York: Van Nostrand.

Hess, T. (1985). Aging and context influences on recognition memory for typical and atypical script actions. *Developmental Psychology, 21*(6), 1139–1151.

Hess, T., Donley, J., & Vandermaas, M. (1989). Aging-related changes in the processing and retention of script retention. *Experimental Aging Research, 15,* 89–96.

Hudson, J., & Nelson, K. (1986). Repeated encounters of a similar kind: Effects of familiarity on children's autobiographical memory. *Cognitive Development, 1,* 253–271.

Light, L., & Anderson, P. (1983). Memory for scripts in young and older adults. *Memory and Cognition, 11*(5), 435–444.

Lucariello, J., & Nelson, K. (1985). Slot-filler categories as memory organizers for young children. *Developmental Psychology, 21,* 272–282.

McCartney, K.A., & Nelson, K. (1981). Children's use of scripts in story recall. *Discourse Processes, 4,* 59–70.

Nelson, K. (1978). How young children represent knowledge in their world in and out of language. In R.S. Seigler (Ed.), *Children's thinking: What develops?* (pp. 255–273). Hillsdale, NJ: Erlbaum.

Nelson, K. (1981). Social cognition in a script framework. In J.H. Flavell & L. Ross (Eds.), *Social cognitive development: Frontier and possible futures* (pp. 97–118). New York: Cambridge University Press.

Nelson, K. (Ed.). (1986). *Event knowledge: Structure and function in development.* Hillsdale, NJ: Erlbaum.

Nelson, K., Fivush, R., Hudson, J., & Lucariello, J. (1983). Scripts and the development of memory. In M.T.H. Chi (Ed.), *Contributions to human development: Trends in memory development research* (Vol. 9, pp. 52–70). New York: Karger.

Nelson, K., & Gruendel, J. (1986). Children's scripts. In K. Nelson (Ed.), *Event knowledge: Structure and function in development* (pp. 21–46). Hillsdale, NJ: Erlbaum.

Neugarten, B.L., Moore, J.W., & Lower, J.C. (1968). Age norms, age constraints, and adult socialization. In B.L. Neugarten (Ed.), *Middle age and aging* (pp. 22–28). Chicago, IL: University of Chicago Press.

Ross, B.L., & Berg, C.A. (1991). *The impact of individual differences in scripts on memory for script-related stories in young and older adults.* Manuscript submitted for publication.

Schank, R.C., & Abelson, R. (1977). *Scripts, plans, goals, and understanding.* Hillsdale, NJ: Erlbaum.

Taylor, S., & Winkler, J. (1980, August). *The development of schemas.* Paper presented at the meeting of the American Psychological Association, Montreal, Canada.

Thorndyke, P., & Stasz, C. (1979). Individual differences in procedures for knowledge acquisition from maps. *Cognitive Psychology, 12,* 137–175.

4
A Computerized Battery for Assessment of Everyday Memory

GLENN J. LARRABEE AND THOMAS H. CROOK, III

The field of clinical psychology in general, and neuropsychology in particular, has witnessed a rapid increase in the development of memory-testing procedures. During the 1980s, several memory tests and batteries have been published, including the Denman Neuropsychology Memory Scale (Denman, 1984), the New York University Memory Test (Randt, Brown, & Osborne, 1980), the California Verbal Learning Test (Delis, Kramer, Kaplan, & Ober, 1987), the Continuous Visual Memory Test (Trahan & Larrabee, 1988), and the Wechsler Memory Scale—Revised (Wechsler, 1987).

The increased availability of memory-testing procedures is directly related to the central importance of memory functioning in such common clinical conditions as closed head trauma, stroke, and Alzheimer's-type dementia (AD) (Kapur, 1988; Larrabee & Crook, 1988). The cognitive changes attendant to these clinical disorders frequently produce memory problems in everyday life.

Memory testing is also important in a variety of different research settings. Research may be conducted to differentiate clinical conditions associated with memory disorders of aging, for example, determining which memory tests differentiate AD from Age-Associated Memory Impairment (AAMI; Crook, Bartus, Ferris, Whitehouse, Cohen, & Gershon, 1986). Memory testing may also be conducted to evaluate change in a variable of interest such as drug treatment or fatigue.

In both clinical and research applications, the questions of fundamental interest in memory testing are questions of behavioral capacities in everyday functioning. In this vein, several recent reviews of memory testing have recommended an increased focus on prediction of everyday function, with face-valid procedures that have memory demands similar to those encountered in everyday settings (Cunningham, 1986; Erickson & Howieson, 1986; Ferris, Crook, Flicker, Reisberg, & Bartus, 1986).

In the present chapter, we describe a computer-simulated everyday memory battery. The battery is based on previous research by Crook and colleagues, who have been addressing the measurement of everyday mem-

54

ory for names, faces, object location, telephone numbers, and grocery list learning over the past 10 years (Crook, Ferris, & McCarthy, 1979; Crook, Ferris, McCarthy, & Rae, 1980; Ferris, Crook, Clark, McCarthy, & Rae, 1980; Flicker, Ferris, Crook, & Bartus, 1987). In its current form, the test battery is fully computerized (Crook, Salama, & Gobert, 1986). Laser disk technology, advanced computer graphics, and a touch-sensitive screen are employed for realistic simulation of everyday memory tasks with the added precision of measurement afforded by computerized stimulus presentation, response storage, and scoring. Although the battery is computerized, persons being tested do not come in contact with a keyboard, joystick, or other manipulanda that may be unfamiliar. Rather, subjects being tested respond either verbally (with the verbal response recorded on the computer by the tester), by pressing the video touchscreen, or by operating familiar manipulanda such as a telephone.

The design of the current battery was based on previous research on everyday memory tasks, knowledge of the psychometric properties of standard memory batteries, and standard memory measurement paradigms. Five of the tests are technologically advanced modifications of tasks developed previously and found to be of particular utility in studies of aging and dementia. These include a telephone dialing task (Crook et al., 1980); a facial recognition task employing a signal detection paradigm (Ferris et al., 1980); a facial recognition task employing a delayed nonmatching to sample paradigm (Flicker et al., 1987); a name–face learning and delayed recall task (Ferris et al., 1986); and a misplaced objects task requiring subjects to place computer-generated pictures of common objects within the representation of a house and later recall the locations chosen (Crook et al., 1979). Additional measures in the battery include narrative recall for factual information from an abbreviated television news broadcast, reaction time based on a simulated automobile driving task, recall of a radio broadcast occurring during a divided attention part of the driving task, grocery list learning, and learning of first and last name pairs.

Reviews of standard memory tests and batteries have highlighted several basic psychometric features (Cunningham, 1986; Erickson & Scott, 1977; Larrabee & Crook, 1988; Loring & Papanicolaou, 1987). Modality and material-specific stimuli are needed, including auditory and visual modalities and verbal and nonverbal material. Testing also should include learning trial performance, as well as delayed recall. Factor analysis should reflect, at minimum, verbal and visual factors, as well as dimensions for attention and psychomotor speed (Larrabee, Kane, & Schuck, 1983; Larrabee, Kane, Schuck, & Francis, 1985; Wechsler, 1987).

These psychometric considerations guided the development of the computer-simulated everyday memory battery, including initial evaluation of the factorial validity of the battery. We will present factorial validity data following description of the tests making up the battery.

Last, we incorporated standard memory measurement paradigms with the everyday memory simulations (Larrabee & Crook, 1988). These paradigms include paired associate learning for first and last names, name–face memory, and object location recall; verbal selective reminding (Buschke, 1973) for grocery list learning; text recall for television news broadcast and divided attention radio broadcast; signal detection methodology, for facial recognition memory; delayed nonmatching to sample, for a second test of facial recognition memory; digit recall for telephone dialing; and reaction time for psychomotor speed.

In summary, we attempted to enhance the everyday validity of the battery through realistic computer-graphic simulations, while we incorporated standard memory measurement paradigms to enhance the psychometric and clinical validity of our tests. Next we will present a detailed description of the computer-simulated everyday memory battery, followed by presentation of recent research on these procedures. In the concluding section, we will discuss future applications of the simulated everyday memory battery.

Equipment and Specific Everyday Memory Tasks

The computerized tests are administered in a standardized manner in a controlled clinical setting. The subject is seated in front of a large color monitor and the other manipulanda required for testing while the tester, who is present throughout the session, operates the computerized equipment behind, and generally out of view of, the subject. Tests are administered using a computer equipped with a 20-megabyte hard-disk drive and customized computer graphic hardware, a laser-disk player, a color monitor with a Personal Touch touchscreen, and various customized peripheral hardware and manipulanda. Subject responses are recorded and stored for later data analysis during the actual testing session. Responses involving a motor component (e.g., touching the screen for object placement, dialing the telephone) are automatically scored and stored. Subject verbal responses (e.g., to verbal selective reminding) are entered by the tester. Description of the various tasks follows.

A variety of tasks evaluate associate learning. The standard paired associate learning format is used for Name–Face Association and First–last Names tests. In the Name–Face Association test (Crook & West, 1990), a variety of scores are obtained. The test presents live video recordings (stored on laser disk) of individuals (actors) who introduce themselves by common first names. Recall is assessed by showing the same individuals in a different order and asking the subject to remember the person's name. Span testing (two, four or six name–face pairs, presented for a single trial) as well as supraspan learning (14 name–face pairs presented over three trials) and 40-minute delayed recall (of the 14 individuals) are evaluated. In the First–Last Names test (Youngjohn, Larrabee, & Crook, in press), subjects are presented, on each of five trials, with a series of six paired first and last names, followed by a presentation of the last names only. The subject has to recall the first name that was paired with each last name.

A different type of associative learning is evaluated with the Misplaced Objects test (Crook, Youngjohn, & Larrabee, 1990a). This test presents subjects with computer-generated images of 20 common objects (e.g., eyeglasses) that are frequently misplaced. This is followed by a computer-generated detailed interior of a 12-room house. This image remains on the screen while the subject "places" the 20 objects (by touching the screen) in the 12-room house, with the limitation of no more than two objects per room. Forty minutes later, the 12-room interior is presented, and the subject is asked to recall the room in which each object was placed. Two attempts are allowed for recall of the location of each object.

Two measures of memory for narrative material are included in the battery. The Narrative Recall test (Crook, Youngjohn, & Larrabee, 1990b) presents the subject with a 6-min television news broadcast. Then, the subject is given a series of 25 factual, multiple-choice questions on the touch-screen and asked to select the correct answer by touching a corresponding box on the screen. The second narrative memory task, Divided Attention (Crook, West, & Larrabee, 1991) is conducted as part of a divided attention procedure in which the subject is performing a simulated driving task (touching a simulated gas or brake pedal in response to a red or green traffic signal) while listening to a radio broadcast of weather and traffic conditions. Subjects are asked to recall as much information as possible in a free-recall format.

Supraspan list learning is evaluated with the Selective Reminding test (Youngjohn, Larrabee, & Crook, in press). This follows a standard selective reminding format for presentation of 15 common grocery items (the names are printed individually on the video screen), over five trials. Following each recall attempt, the words that subjects have not recalled reappear on the screen, and the subjects must then attempt to recall the entire list, having been selectively reminded of the words they omitted on the previous trial. Traditional selective reminding scores are calculated (e.g., consistent long-term retrieval; long-term storage; cf., Buschke, 1973), and half-hour delayed free recall is assessed.

Memory span is evaluated with the Telephone Dialing test (West & Crook, 1990). This is a variation on the standard digit-recall test, which is intended to provide greater ecologic validity. Subjects are shown a series of 7- or 10-digit numbers (as in local or long-distance numbers) on the monitor screen and asked to read the series aloud. Immediately after the final digit is read and the number disappears from the screen, subjects must dial the total number on a touchtone phone interfaced with the computer. Credit is given for each digit dialed in the correct position, regardless of errors made elsewhere in the sequence. This task can be presented without interference (as just described) or with interference, in which the number dialed by the subject is followed by either a ringing telephone or by a busy signal; if busy, the subject must redial the number.

Facial recognition memory is evaluated with two procedures (Crook & Larrabee, 1991). The first, Recognition of Faces—Delayed Nonmatching to Sample, employs a delayed nonmatch-to-sample paradigm (Mishkin, 1978), in which the subject must identify the new facial photograph on each of 24 successive trials (starting with one face, the task increments by a new face each trial). The second, Recognition of Faces–Signal Detection, employs signal-detection procedures for evaluation of recognition memory employing 156 facial photographs, with scores based on acquisition, as well as on 40-min delayed recognition memory.

A psychomotor-speed measure considered to be a memory-related variable is the Reaction Time test (Crook et al., 1991). This can be administered in one of two formats. First, reaction time can be measured under a single task condition such that the subject must lift his or her finger off a computer-simulated (on the touchscreen) image of a gas pedal or brake pedal in response to a red or green traffic light. Both lift and travel (from gas to brake pedal or vice-versa) reaction times are computed. Second, this task can be administered as a simultaneous processing task (divided attention condition) such that the subject must perform the gas pedal/brake pedal maneuvers while listening to a radio broadcast of road and weather conditions.

Alzheimer's Battery

The computer-simulated everyday memory battery is also available, with modifications, for use in research on early stage AD. Name–Face Association is modified, with single-trial presentations of two, three and four name–face pairs, followed by six pairs over three learning trials, and 40-min delayed recall. First–Last Names consists of four pairs over five trials. Telephone Dialing is conducted without interference, measuring recall of 3, 7, and 10 digits. Selective Reminding includes 10 items over five trials with 30-min delayed recall. Reaction Time is conducted without the Divided Attention condition. Misplaced Objects is presented unmodified. Recognition of Faces—Delayed Nonmatching to Sample is presented with one modification, termination of the test after three consecutive misses. Recognition of Faces—Signal Detection is not administered.

Current Status of the Computer-Simulated Everyday Memory Battery

In the 1980s, the computer-simulated everyday memory battery was employed as the major set of dependent variables in numerous clinical trials of potential cognition-enhancing compounds for memory disorders of aging

TABLE 4.1. Varimax-rotated principal components analysis: immediate-recall raw scores.*

	Factors			
Variables	1	2	3	4
Name–face association, sum	.77			
Name–face association, 6 faces	.50			−.59
Narrative recall	.58	.34		
Telephone dialing, 3 digits				.81
Telephone dialing, 10 digits	.55			
Misplaced objects, first try	.61	−.54	−.32	
Misplaced objects, second try		.88		
Recognition of faces—signal detection	.61			
Reaction time, lift component		−.49	.52	
Reaction time, travel component			.85	
Recognition of faces—Delayed nonmatching	.41		−.40	

*Loadings of .30 or greater are reported.

Note. From "Interrelationships among everyday memory tests: Stability of factor structure with age," by T.H. Crook and G.J. Larrabee, 1988, *Neuropsychology, 2,* p. 6. Copyright 1988 by Taylor & Francis, NY.
Reprinted by permission.

in the United States and Europe. The battery is available in at least six alternate forms in English, French, Italian, Dutch, Spanish, Danish, Finnish, and Swedish. Normative data have been collected on approximately 1,300 to 1,600 subjects for each test procedure, covering the range of 18 to 90 years of age. Consistent with expectation, there are significant associations of age and performance (Crook & Larrabee, 1988b; Crook et al., 1986). Additional data are available on more than 2,000 persons manifesting AAMI (Crook et al., 1986; Crook & Larrabee, 1988a), and on over 200 subjects with presumed AD.

We have recently reported on the factorial validity of the computer-simulated everyday memory battery (Crook & Larrabee, 1988b; Larrabee & Crook, 1989a). Table 4.1 displays the orthogonal four-factor principal components solution obtained on 158 normal adults, ages 18 to 77 (Crook & Larrabee, 1988b). The first factor is a general (verbal and visual) memory factor, the second factor represents a dimension of attention/vigilance, the third factor represents psychomotor speed, and the fourth factor represents simple attention span. This same basic factor pattern was obtained when performance measures were residualized (statistically adjusted) for the effects of age, indicating that while the tests are sensitive to level of performance differences associated with age, they measure the same basic abilities irrespective of the age of the adult subject.

As can be seen in Table 4.1, a general memory factor was obtained rather than separate verbal and visual factors. This was attributed to the lack of more purely verbal tasks in the analysis reported in Table 4.1. This, in fact, was true, because in a subsequent analysis with additional measures

TABLE 4.2. Varimax-rotated principal components analysis: everyday and standard memory tests.

Variables	Factors 1	2	3	4	5	6
Name–face association, sum	.75				.34	
Name–face association, 6 faces	.45				.36	
Recognition of faces—Delayed nonmatching-to-sample				.38	.75	
Recognition of faces—Signal detection					.55	
Reaction time, lift component			.75			
Reaction time, travel component			.76			
Telephone dialing, 7 digits				.83		
Telephone dialing, 10 digits				.68		
Incidental memory for radio broadcast		.60				
First–last names	.75					
Selective reminding, total consistent long-term retrieval	.69	.84				
WMS logical memory						.82
WMS easy paired associates	.65					
WMS hard paired associates			.50			.42
Benton Visual Retention Test, errors					−.53	
WAIS Vocabulary		.82				

Note. Loadings of .30 or greater are reported. $N = 110$.
WAIS, Wechsler Adult Intelligence Scale; WMS, Wechsler Memory Scale.
Note. From "Dimensions of everyday memory in Age-Associated Memory Impairment," by G.J. Larrabee and T.H. Crook, 1989, Psychological Assessment: A Journal of Consulting and Clinical Psychology, 1, p. 96. Copyright 1989 by The American Psychological Association. Reprinted by permission.

of everyday verbal memory, separate verbal and visual memory factors were demonstrated (Larrabee & Crook, 1989a). The results of this analysis, based on 110 persons suffering AAMI (Crook et al., 1986) are depicted in Table 4.2.

Tables 4.1 and 4.2 demonstrate that the computer-simulated everyday memory battery contains performance dimensions of verbal and visual memory and attention/concentration/psychomotor speed similar to those found in standard memory batteries (Larrabee et al., 1985; Wechsler, 1987). Indeed, in Table 4.2, standard and everyday measures converge on the appropriate factors (e.g., Wechsler Memory Scale (WMS) Hard Paired Associates with everyday verbal measures; WMS Logical Memory with Incidental Recall of the Radio News Broadcast; Benton Visual Retention with everyday facial memory measures). Moreover, the primary association of name–face memory appears to be with other everyday verbal memory measures with only a weak secondary association with everyday visual-facial memory (factor 5).

In continuing the analysis of the validity of the everyday battery, the relationship of performance on the battery to self-rated everyday memory skills was investigated. This analysis involved a subset of the 158 subjects from Crook and Larrabee (1988b). One hundred twenty-five subjects, who had also completed a rating scale of everyday memory abilities (Memory Assessment Clinic Self-Report Scale, MAC-S; Crook & Larrabee, 1990, Winterling, Crook, Salama, & Gobert, 1986), were studied (Larrabee, West, & Crook, 1991). Larrabee et al. found a significant canonical correlation of .528 between the computerized everyday general factor reported in Table 4.1 and a number of MAC-S factors including self-rated ability scale factors for remote, everyday, and semantic memory and self-rated frequency factors for concentration and forgetfulness. The Geriatric Depression Scale (GDS; Yesavage et al., 1983), included as a control variable, was not associated with this complaint-performance dimension.

Hence, the Crook and Larrabee (1988b) and Larrabee and Crook (1989a) investigations support the factorial validity of the computer-simulated everyday memory battery, whereas the Larrabee et al. (1991) analysis of self-ratings and computer-simulated everyday performance supports the concurrent validity of the everyday battery. Additional research has been conducted on performance subtypes (Larrabee & Crook, 1989b) and on memory training (West & Crook, in press).

Larrabee and Crook (1989b) performed cluster analysis of the 158 normal subjects reported in Crook and Larrabee (1988b). Cluster analysis was conducted on the computerized everyday raw scores, as well as on scores that had been residualized for the effects of age. In each set of cluster analyses, a variety of patterns of everyday strengths and weaknesses were demonstrated. Table 4.3 depicts the discriminant function results for the nine-cluster raw score solution. Subgroup 5 had the poorest overall performance in this and the age-residualized analysis. In both the raw and

TABLE 4.3. Canonical discriminant functions at group centroids for computerized everyday memory performance, nine cluster raw score solution.

	Discriminant functions			
Groups (size)	Everyday verbal-visual 1	Everyday visual-facial 2	Everyday visual object location 3	Everyday attentional 4
1 (13)	5.686	1.294	− .354	− .067
2 (18)	.709	1.331	1.051	.442
3 (25)	−1.789	−1.219	.091	− .422
4 (14)	3.137	−2.750	.227	.391
5 (25)	−5.338	− .096	− .106	− .233
6 (11)	1.878	3.221	− .610	−1.141
7 (19)	2.287	−1.029	.647	− .462
8 (15)	−2.087	2.133	.097	1.029
9 (18)	.821	− .960	−1.343	.540

Note. From "Performance subtypes of everyday memory function," by G.J. Larrabee and T.H. Crook, 1989, *Developmental Neuropsychology, 5*, p. 277. Copyright 1989 by L. Erlbaum. Reprinted by permission.

age-residualized solutions, subgroup 5 also had the poorest overall memory self-ratings and comprised older subjects, particularly in the raw score solution. These data, based on normal adult subjects, provide empirical support for the construct of AAMI.

West and Crook (in press) employed Misplaced Objects, Name–Face Association, Recognition of Faces, Grocery List Selective Reminding, and First–Last Names tests from the computer-simulated everyday memory battery in an imagery-based memory training study for mature adults. Because the computer-simulated everyday memory battery displays the test stimuli on a color monitor screen, West and Crook (in press) were able to produce a memory-training videotape that the subjects could take home for further study and practice. West and Crook employed interactive imagery training for object location recall and grocery list learning, and the image–name match method for name–face learning. Significant training effects were found for performance on Misplaced Objects, Name–Face Association, and Grocery List Selective Reminding. Additional evidence was reported for generalization of the imagery training to performance on the nontrained tasks.

Future Research with the Computer-Simulated Everyday Memory Battery

The computer-simulated everyday memory battery is employed in ongoing clinical drug trials of potential cognition-enhancing compounds for AAMI and AD. Future projects will include analysis of performance subtypes of

AAMI and AD, and comparisons of self-rated memory (MAC-S) and family-rated memory using a relative-rating version of the MAC-S, with performance on standard memory tests and computer-simulated everyday memory performance. Research will also focus on the everyday memory performance dimensions that are the most sensitive to discriminating AAMI from AD's.

Data collection is ongoing in other clinical populations, including persons suffering closed head trauma, stroke, and human immunodeficiency virus (HIV) dementia. Additionally, the computer-simulated battery is being employed in the investigation of memory functioning of patients undergoing temporal lobectomy for seizure control. Last, we are preparing analyses of cross-cultural patterns of performance in normal populations tested in the United States and Western Europe.

Summary

In closing, we have presented descriptive and validity data on a computer-simulated everyday memory battery, which combines enhanced computer graphic capabilities for realistic everyday memory simulation with current clinical and experimental memory measurement paradigms. Our evidence supports the factorial and concurrent validity of the battery, and we discuss current and future clinical and research applications. The computer technology described need not be constrained to the assessment of everyday memory but can also be extended to the evaluation of other everyday cognitive functions. This is an intended direction of future research and development.

Note: Address reprint requests to Glenn J. Larrabee, Ph.D., Memory Assessment Clinics, Inc., 1217 East Avenue South, Suite 209, Sarasota, FL 34239.

References

Buschke, H. (1973). Selective reminding for analysis of memory and learning. *Journal of Verbal Learning and Verbal Behavior, 12*, 543–549.

Crook, T.H., Bartus, R.T., Ferris, S.H., Whitehouse, P., Cohen, G.D., & Gershon, S. (1986). Age-Associated Memory Impairment: Proposed diagnostic criteria and measures of clinical change. Report of a National Institute of Mental Health work group. *Developmental Neuropsychology, 2*, 261–276.

Crook, T.H., Ferris, S., & McCarthy, M. (1979). The misplaced objects task: A brief test for memory dysfunction in the aged. *Journal of the American Geriatric Society, 27*, 284–287.

Crook, T.H., Ferris, S.H., McCarthy, & Rae, D. (1980). The utility of digit recall tasks for assessing memory in the aged. *Journal of Consulting and Clinical Psychology, 48*, 228–233.

Crook, T.H., & Larrabee, G.J. (1988a). Age-Associated Memory Impairment:

Diagnostic criteria and treatment strategies. *Psychopharmacology Bulletin, 24,* 509–514.

Crook, T.H., & Larrabee, G.J. (1988b). Interrelationships among everyday memory tests: Stability of factor structure with age. *Neuropsychology, 2,* 1–12.

Crook, T.H., & Larrabee, G.J. (1990). A self-rating scale for evaluating memory in everyday life. *Psychology and Aging, 5,* 48–57.

Crook, T.H., & Larrabee, G.J. (1991). *Changes in facial recognition memory across the adult age span.* Manuscript submitted for publication.

Crook, T.H., Salama, M., & Gobert, J. (1986). A computerized test battery for detecting and assessing memory disorders. In A. Bes, J. Cohn, S. Hoyer, J.P. Marc-Vergenes, & H.M. Wisniewski (Eds.), *Senile dementias: Early detection* (pp. 79–85). London-Paris: John Libbey Eurotext.

Crook, T.H., & West, R.L. (1990). Name recall performance across the adult life span. *British Journal of Psychology, 81,* 335–349.

Crook, T.H., West, R.L., & Larrabee, G.J. (1991). *The Driving-Reaction Time Test: Assessing age declines in dual-task performance.* Manuscript submitted for publication.

Crook, T.H., Youngjohn, J.R., & Larrabee, G.J. (1990a). The Misplaced Objects Test: A measure of everyday visual memory. *Journal of Clinical and Experimental Neuropsychology, 12,* 819–833.

Crook, T.H., Youngjohn, J.R., & Larrabee, G.J. (1990b). The TV News Test: A new measure of everyday memory for prose. *Neuropsychology, 4,* 135–145.

Cunningham, W.R. (1986). Psychometric perspectives: Validity and reliability. In L.W. Poon, T. Crook, K.L. Davis, C. Eisdorfer, B.J. Gurland, A.W. Kaszniak, & L.W. Thompson (Eds.), *Handbook for clinical memory assessment of older adults* (pp. 27–31). Washington, DC: American Psychological Association.

Delis, D.C., Kramer, J.H., Kaplan, E., & Ober, B.A. (1987). *California Verbal Learning Test, research edition: Manual.* San Antonio: The Psychological Corporation: Harcourt, Brace, Jovanovich.

Denman, S.B. (1984). *Denman Neuropsychology Memory Scale.* Charleston, SC: Sidney B. Denman.

Erickson, R.C., & Howieson, D. (1986). The clinician's perspective: Measuring change and treatment effectiveness. In L.W. Poon, T. Crook, K.L. Davis, C. Eisdorfer, B.J. Gurland, A.W. Kaszniak, & L.W. Thompson (Eds.), *Handbook for clinical memory assessment of older adults* (pp. 69–80). Washington, DC: American Psychological Association.

Erickson, R.C., & Scott, M.L. (1977). Clinical memory testing: A review. *Psychological Bulletin, 84,* 1130–1149.

Ferris, S.H., Crook, T. Clark, E., McCarthy, M., & Rae, D. (1980). Facial recognition memory deficits in normal aging and senile dementia. *Journal of Gerontology, 35,* 707–714.

Ferris, S.H., Crook, T., Flicker, C., Reisberg, B., & Bartus, R.T. (1986). Assessing cognitive impairment and evaluating treatment effects: Psychometric performance tests. In L.W. Poon, T. Crook, K.L. Davis, C. Eisdorfer, B.J. Gurland, A.W. Kaszniak, & L.W. Thompson (Eds.), *Handbook for clinical memory assessment of older adults* (pp. 139–148). Washington, DC: American Psychological Association.

Flicker, C., Ferris, S.H., Crook, T., and Bartus, R.T. (1987). A visual recognition memory test for the assessment of cognitive function in aging and dementia. *Experimental Aging Research, 13,* 127–132.

Kapur, N. (1988). *Memory disorders in clinical practice.* London: Butterworths.

Larrabee, G.J., & Crook, T. (1988). Assessment of drug effects in age-related memory disorders: Clinical, theoretical, and psychometric considerations. *Psychopharmacology Bulletin, 24,* 515–522.

Larrabee, G.J., & Crook, T.H. (1989a). Dimensions of everyday memory in Age-Associated Memory Impairment. *Psychological Assessment: A Journal of Consulting and Clinical Psychology, 1,* 92–97.

Larrabee, G.J., & Crook, T.H. (1989b). Performance subtypes of everyday memory function. *Developmental Neuropsychology, 5,* 267–283.

Larrabee, G.J., Kane, R.L., & Schuck, J.R. (1983). Factor analysis of the WAIS and Wechsler Memory Scale: An analysis of the construct validity of the Wechsler Memory Scale. *Journal of Clinical Neuropsychology, 5,* 159–168.

Larrabee, G.J., Kane, R.L., Schuck, J.R., & Francis, D.E. (1985). The construct validity of various memory testing procedures. *Journal of Clinical and Experimental Neuropsychology, 7,* 239–250.

Larrabee, G.J., West, R.L., and Crook, T.H. (1991). The association of memory complaint with computer-simulated everyday memory performance. *Journal of Clinical and Experimental Neuropsychology, 13,* 484–496.

Loring, D.W., & Papanicolaou, A.C. (1987). Memory assessment in neuropsychology: Theoretical considerations and practical utility. *Journal of Clinical and Experimental Neuropsychology, 9,* 340–358.

Mishkin, M. (1978). Memory in monkeys severely impaired by combined but not by separate removal of amygdala and hippocampus. *Nature, 273,* 297–298.

Randt, C.T., Brown, E.R., & Osborne, D.P., Jr. (1980). A memory test for longitudinal measurement of mild to moderate deficits. *Clinical Neuropsychology, 2,* 184–194.

Trahan, D.E., & Larrabee, G.J. (1988). *Professional manual: Continuous Visual Memory Test.* Odessa, FL: Psychological Assessment Resources.

Wechsler, D.A. (1987). *Wechsler Memory Scale-Revised: Manual.* San Antonio: The Psychological Corporation: Harcourt, Brace Jovanovich.

West, R.L., & Crook, T.H. (1990). Age differences in everyday memory: Laboratory analogues of telephone number recall. *Psychology and Aging, 5,* 520–529.

West, R.L., & Crook, T.H. (in press). Video training of imagery for mature adults. *Applied Cognitive Psychology.*

Winterling, D., Crook, T., Salama, M., & Gobert, J. (1986). A self-rating scale for assessing memory loss. In A. Beg, J. Cohn, S. Hoyer, J.F. Marc-Vergenes, & H.M. Wisniewski (Eds.), *Senile dementias: Early detection* (pp. 482–486). London-Paris: John Libbey Eurotext.

Yesavage, J., Brink, T., Rose, T., Lum, O., Huang, O., Adey, V., & Leirer, V. (1983). Development and validation of a geriatric depression scale: A preliminary report. *Journal of Psychiatric Research, 17,* 37–49.

Youngjohn, J.R., Larrabee, G.J., & Crook, T.H. (in press). First–Last Names and the Grocery List Selective Reminding Tests: Two computerized measures of everyday verbal learning. *Archives of Clinical Neuropsychology.*

5
Age and Memory for Spatial Relations

JAN D. SINNOTT, KEVIN BOCHENEK, MICHELLE KIM, LISA KLEIN, CHESTER ROBIE, KAREN DISHMAN, AND CAROLYN DUNMYER

Two foci of memory aging studies are spatial relations and modes of spatial representation. Within these areas are studies based on animal and human models, the latter conducted in both laboratory and naturalistic settings. Each model and setting can give single-faceted information on basic or applied questions related to aging; a combination of models and settings give many points of view to yield a multifaceted picture.

This chapter focuses on the development and testing of a model and a measure that is flexible enough to cross the boundaries between animal and human, laboratory and naturalistic studies of spatial memory aging. Five studies using this model are described as part of a research program. Goals of the program are to relate human, animal, laboratory, and "everyday" models, to link these results to other memory processes and other cognitive processes, to look at individual differences or styles, and to describe this memory performance in the context of the adaptive behavior of the physical, psychological, social human who is an active agent in his or her adult development. The chapter contains a brief overview of selected spatial memory aging literature, a description of the paradigm or model used in this program, reports on the five studies and suggestions for further work and measures.

Background

Some Key Factors in Memory Aging Models

Researchers and lay people alike agree that there is a negative correlation between age and performance on memory tasks. The decline is not uniform, however, across different types of memory tasks (Zacks, 1982). On examining experimental studies, it is clear that memory, as tested in laboratory situations, declines with age. We know much less from experimental studies about everyday memory. Only a handful of experimental studies used naturalistic materials or situations, however restricted in scope, and most of these related to spatial memory (e.g., Allen & Kirasic, 1985; Baroni, Job, Peron & Salmaso, 1980; Evans & Pezdek, 1980; Kirasic, 1983; Light & Zelinski, 1983; Perlmutter, Metzger, Nezworksi, & Miller, 1981; Pezdek, 1983a; Pezdek & Evans, 1979; Salmaso, Baroni, Job, & Peron, 1983; Sherman, Oliver, & Titus, 1980; Waddell & Rogoff, 1981).

This chapter will focus specifically on age-related abilities on spatial memory tasks. Several theoretical issues related to age-related memory deficits of this type are worth noting. Memory studies involving older adults have typically been conducted in laboratory settings and usually have employed experimental tasks. Most results have supported the notion of cognitive decline (Kausler, 1982). Memory failure and its consequences are concerns of both professionals and older adults, but as Hartley, Harker, and Walsh (1980) have stated, it is not known how ecologically valid some of the tasks may be on which older adults show decline. This is true for spatial tasks also. If tasks directly represented the cognitive demands that adults typically face, or could be validated with everyday memory performance, concerns about decline would be on clearer ground. Even more important gains in knowledge about memory processes might be made in the context of more naturalistic studies. Neisser (1982a, 1982b) has argued that orthodox memory research has shown us too little. He noted that, for example, in animal research, great progress was made when more naturalistic ethological studies were combined with traditional approaches. This argument for everyday tasks also was made by Cavanaugh (1982) and Sinnott (1986, 1989a, 1989b) in regard to memory.

A researcher's model of memory processes also seems to influence and limit research results by limiting questions posed by the memory reseacher. Some models are created in laboratory environments and may pertain only to such environments (McNamara, 1986). The earlier associative model was based on a mechanistic metamodel and led to an irreversible decrement view of aging with biological antecedents. The next approach historically was the information processing approach, based on an organismic metamodel and leading to a view of age-related decrement balanced by an individual's compensation. A contextual approach, suggesting that only relevant material in a context is remembered, led to a nondecremental view of aging (Hultsch, 1977). Proponents of the contextual view use a living systems metamodel (Miller, 1978) in that what is remembered at any age is a function of all intra- and extraorganismic system parameters like biology and the social environment. The contextual view would suggest that salient memories do not decline.

The decline in spatial ability over the life span has been observed in a wide range of cognitive tasks and also has been attributed to an overall slowing of central nervous system processing, although this applies mainly when reaction time is considered as a factor (Ohta, Walsh, & Krauss, 1981). These authors state that storage and retrieval systems for spatial information appear to decline more rapidly across the adult life span than do systems for constructing spatial information. Ohta et al. (1981) also state that because of these deficiencies, the elderly tend to form less organized representations of large-scale environments, which may cause older people to avoid exposure to new environments, thus reducing their geographical experience.

Georgemiller and Hassan (1986) argue that, to more accurately test the spatial ability of older people, we must do so in settings that are more familiar to older people and use tasks that hold more meaning for them. Seemingly simple acquisition, organization, and storage of an everyday spatial layout involves complex mental processes that may help us understand basic memory processes.

One perspective that is useful in discussing spatial memory tasks, as in the present study, is the automatic versus effortful memory distinction. Several researchers have proposed that spatial memory is automatically encoded (Hasher & Zacks, 1979; Moore, Richards,& Hood, 1984; Perlmuter, Metzger, Nezworski, & Miller, 1981). More importantly, some have held the view that spatial abilities do not decline with age (Moore et al., 1984; Permutter et al., 1981). In three studies, however (Light & Zelinski, 1983; Perlmutter et al., 1981; Pezdek, 1983a), using maps and household objects as stimuli, the old performed more poorly than the young. Waddell and Rogoff (1981) and Kirasic (1983) each found that the young outperformed the old only in unfamiliar settings (object arrays and model towns) that demanded additional learning. None of the studies appeared to support the view (Hasher & Zacks, 1979) that spatial memory is automatic in everyday settings but rather supported the view that energy is involved in remembering.

The present studies ranged from naturalistic to laboratory contexts using the same basic paradigm in each phase.

Variables Influencing Spatial Memory

There has been general agreement that subject motivation is an important variable. Naturalistic, familiar materials have been thought to be more motivating than laboratory tasks, but few investigators have been certain that memory for a city layout, for example, is much more salient than memory for a string of numbers. How can we be sure that respondents care? Perhaps motivation is even more important for the old, who have less energy to encode numerous items into memory (Hasher & Zacks, 1979). The present study predicted that age differences in spatial memory would occur such that older subjects would do less well than younger subjects when laboratory-like stimuli were used.

Age-related memory deficits may also be due to problematic encoding. Charness (1981) found age-related differences for the recall of chess positions that were possibly due to an encoding inaccuracy and not to a storage or retrieval problem. Participants in Charness's study seemed to encode less accurate information per unit of time.

The cues people use to encode spatial memory vary in many ways. People seem to use cues idiosyncratically to facilitate the encoding process. The comparison and the analysis of such idiosyncratic cues might reveal a pattern in mental representation for spatial memory. It has been reported that real-world schema play an important role in encoding and memory for spatial information (Mandler & Parker, 1976). Encoding thus may be a factor in spatial tasks. The present studies manipulated encoding.

Context also seems to influence the success of older subjects on memory tasks (Hultsch, 1977). Waddell and Rogoff (1981) found that older women did as well as middle-aged women when a spatial memory task was contextually organized, though context was not as important for middle-aged women (Waddell & Rogoff, 1981). Older individuals often needed more time to complete unstructured tasks and had difficulty developing organizational strategies (Waddell & Rogoff, 1981). It seems that older people become overwhelmed by the complex demands of tasks not put into a clear context. In the present set of studies, we gave an organizing context for every experimental condition. We predicted that older subjects would be more successful in mazes having a naturalistic context, and that the elderly would perform more poorly as the maze layout became less similar to a naturalistic context.

Georgemiller and Hassan (1986) describe "defective route-finding ability" as being partially caused by age. This defect, these authors explain, can cause inaccuracy in path-tracing mazes of both paper-and-pencil and locomotor type. Elderly people with this disorder may neglect turns in one specific direction, become confused at points where a directional decision must be made, reverse left and right turns, or reproduce relative route lengths inaccurately (Georgemiller & Hassan, 1986). In the present studies, we gave subjects a chance to make these errors.

Another factor that seems to affect subject performance on spatial tasks is the intentionality of the memory process. Light and Zelinski (1983) tested young and old subjects in intentional (remember object and location) and incidental (remember the object name) conditions. These experimenters concluded that both age and test expectations affect spatial memory, because older subjects and those in the incidental condition did not perform as well as other groups. A similar study by Pezdek (1983b) supports these results, and the experimenter explains these age differences in terms of differing encoding and rehearsal strategies used by the two age groups (Pedzek, 1983b). In the present studies, one phase varied intentionality.

Pezdek's results are supported by those of Bruce and Herman (1986) in their study of spatial memory in young and older women. The latter investigators used two trials and found that on the second trial older women performed comparably to younger women. The researchers believe this implies that the elderly require more practice than do the young, which possibly is due to their having more difficulty using encoding strategies (Bruce & Herman, 1986). In the present studies, we controlled practice.

Spatial Orientation

Spatial memory can be characterized as the extent to which one can accurately represent physical space using primarily mental faculties. One of the components in this process is the ability to interact with space (spatial orientation) to interpret and then remember what one has sensed. Considerable research has been conducted on how people orient themselves to facilitate their spatial memory processes, and this research has identified several important qualitative criteria for evaluating and predicting one's orientation performance potential. These criteria include one's ability to estimate distance and time as well as one's sense of direction (Kozlowski & Bryant, 1977). Other factors that are conducive to spatially orienting oneself are the establishment of reference points and (especially in a non-laboratory setting) the presence of hierarchical and "clustered" organization of these reference points (landmarks) as well as semantic information concerning the landmarks (Hirtle & Jonides, 1985).

Research also elucidates the relationship between orientation and the interpretations of a particular spatial phenomenon. Levine, Jankovic, and Palij (1982) argue that spatial information is generally interpreted and stored in a specific way and must be recalled in the same specific orientation as initially learned (much the same as state-dependent memory). This then suggests that spatial judgments are easy when the layout is presented as learned initially, but the spatial judgments become more difficult when the layout is presented in a different orientation (Presson, DeLange, & Hazelrigg, 1987). Presson et al. concur with previous research that certain types of spatial information (maps) consistently show orientation-specific effects; however, other types of spatial information (navigation of large-scale environments and nonsighted navigation of simple routes) can be coded and recalled more flexibly in an orientation-free manner that employs multiple orientations. These multiple frames of reference, which facilitate more flexible learning and recall of spatial information, are specific to real-world complex environments and are difficult to replicate or observe in a simple, sterile laboratory situation (Smyth & Kennedy, 1982).

Spatial Memory Paradigm Used in the Present Studies

Our model for testing spatial memory is based on the real but maze-like floor plan of a research center where volunteers from the Baltimore Longitudinal Study of Aging (Shock et al., 1985) are tested. Many variations of

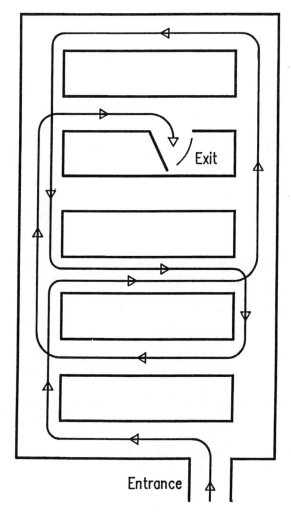

FIGURE 5.1. Maze layout including the actual route used.

this same floor-plan model can be created (Sinnott, 1987). The general layout is shown in Figure 5.1. Respondents at the research center move through this real environment to get to their various tests. Movement though the real environment can also be simulated using videotape. The same layout can be created in a simple way using styrofoam panels as walls, and movement through this "mock-up" can also be real or be presented on videotape. The environment in its general form can also be presented in a paper-and-pencil format on which a respondent sees a path drawn or has his or her hand guided through the path. The layout and path also can be described verbally for the respondent to remember. These are just a few of the possible experimental manipulations that can be done with the same spatial layout to test for age effects, mode of encoding effects, cognitive style effects, and the like, in a maze that represents any point on a continuum from life-like to laboratory-like.

Following are reports of five experiments using the model, arrayed along this realism–abstraction continuum, addressing various aspects of memory for special relations. Additional details, precluded here by space considerations, are available on request and will be published elsewhere in their entirety.

Experiment 1

Experiment 1 was conducted in the real building to test the effects of age and attention on memory for spatial relations. Our hypothesis was that while age would not be a factor in this real environmental task, attention would influence performance.

Method

SUBJECTS

52 members of the Baltimore Longitudinal Study of Aging (Shock et al., 1985) took part in experiment 1. Participants consisted of 26 men and 26 women; their ages ranged from 26 to 85, with a mean age of 55.44; they were healthy, well-educated community-dwelling individuals who came every 2 years for $2\frac{1}{2}$ days of tests (Shock et al., 1985).

PROCEDURE

After respondents signed consent forms, asked them to accompany an experimenter from the starting point day room over a 12-turn course (Figure 5.1) to an ending point test room, where they were asked to remember the route they took and the layout of the floor (see scoring section). Half of the respondents (attention condition) were asked to recall the route.

After presentation, we asked all subjects to draw the actual route presented as well as what he or she perceived to be the shortcut—the most direct route from the start to the goal. The order in which the participants drew these routes was randomly determined by the flip of a coin before their arrival at the testing room. In addition to these two tasks, we asked participants to describe, in their own words, how they remembered what they recalled about the actual route. If respondents needed additional prompting, we instructed them to describe any "memory devices" they used. We then asked respondents to write down the objects they saw in the halls, and the locations of them, all of which we had verified earlier.

Results and Discussion

SCORING

The maze routes drawn by respondents were scored on a variety of measures. We used all measures, with the exception of the sequence index and choice, for scoring both the actual and the short routes. Scoring criteria are described here.

Left index/right index (two measures): The number of left and right turns a respondent produced was subtracted from the expected number of left and right turns.

Turn index: A measure of how many turns a respondent produced divided by the actual number of turns presented, specific to either the actual route (12 turns) or the short route (4 turns).

Length of route index: The maze routes drawn by respondents were measured in centimeters using a ruler in experiments 1 and 2 and using a curvimeter map measurer in the other experiments. This is one "scale of representation" measure.

Drawn to scale index: Scored by placing a transparency with a grid over the respondents' mazes and counting the number of nonshaded squares through which their route passed. Nonshaded squares were intended to outline the expected route through the maze.

Sequence index: For the actual route, the sequence index was scored as a measure of the accuracy of the respondents' series of turns. Respondents scored a point for each correct turn in correct order (expected series of turns = LRRLLLLRRRRR).

Pearson product moment correlations were calculated to determine if age was related to any of the dependent measures. This was not the case. We calculated analyses of variance (ANOVAs) to determine the effect of attention (i.e., intentional use of memory) on performance. To our surprise, *trying* to remember the route did not lead to significantly better performance. All respondents performed with difficulty. Respondents of both ages appeared to attend to spatial layout automatically, supporting the Hasher and Zacks (1979) view. In this naturalistic setting, no reliable age difference appeared, although we had expected that if the task were difficult enough, though naturalistic, age differences would begin to appear. Because many respondents described using visual strategies to learn the layout, another experiment was planned in which visual information was minimal.

Experiment 2

This experiment was conducted in the real building to test the effects of presence or absence of visual cues on memory for the naturalistic route. Our hypothesis was that, without visual information, age differences would appear and that the "nonlooking" version of the tasks would be effortful enough to lead to a significantly poorer response, even in this naturalistic setting. We also expected that encoding was done visually, so that removing the everyday visual information in step-by-step decrements would give us evidence of mechanisms that would compensate as the task was altered to be more laboratory-like.

Data from administrations of the Wechsler Adult Intelligence Scale (Wechsler, 1955)(WAIS) vocabulary scale (number correct), the Benton Visual Retention Test (Benton, 1963) (number of errors), digit span, and from a test of memory for words (immediate free recall, delayed free recall, choice response time, delayed recognition) were also available for these respondents and were used to relate spatial processing to other standard memory processes. These relations were previously reported by Sinnott (1987).

Method

SUBJECTS

Fifty-two members of the Baltimore Longitudinal Study of Aging (Shock et al., 1985) took part in experiment 2. Participating were 29 men and 24 women; their ages ranged from 30 to 85, with a mean age of 60.13; they were community-dwelling individuals in generally good health and well educated (Shock et al., 1985), who came every 2 years for $2\frac{1}{2}$ days of tests.

PROCEDURE

After respondents signed consent forms, we asked them to accompany an experimenter from the starting point day room over the 12-turn course to an ending point test room, where they were asked to remember the route they took and the layout of the floor (see scoring section). Half of the respondents looked only at the floor as they were led by the experimenter; the other half could look around as they wished, obtaining more visual information.

Results and Discussion

Pearson product moment correlations relating age to maze variables were significant and negative for length index of actual path drawing (− .38); actual path drawn to scale variable (− .43); shortcut turns index (− .22); shortcut length index (− .29); and shortcut drawn to scale variable (− .26). Older respondents produced more "compact" or summary maps.

Analyses of covariance, age covaried, demonstrated significant effects for the looking/not looking variable only on the shortcut turns index. Therefore, the manipulation of visual information was not an effective manipulation. Respondents demonstrated equivalent memory for space whether or not they had visual information. This again suggested a somewhat automatic spatial memory function and an encoding process somewhat independent of vision, even in visually unimpaired adults.

We conducted stepwise multiple regression analyses to relate the vocabulary, visual memory, and verbal memory scores to maze variables with age removed first. Significant and reliable predictors were found for several maze variables and for the time taken to walk the path or respond. In the case of time, the better the laboratory cognitive function, the quicker the respondent reacted, irrespective of age. This was as hypothesized. Scores on the drawn to scale index were negatively related to Benton errors (16% of variance accounted for), positively to digit span (16% of variance), and positively to correct hits on choice response time (16% of variance). Length of drawn path was positively predicted by digit span (16%) and choice response time (10%). Digit span was positively related to right turn index (16%) and sequence of turns index (16%). While the laboratory measures were related in expected ways to the spatial memory measures, there were not as many relations as one would expect to find if laboratory measures were robust predictors of everyday performance. The fact that there were so few relations between maze performance and Benton errors was especially confusing. Perhaps very different processes are at work in laboratory versus naturalistic memory.

The next experiment was designed to provide an even more abstract environment in which to learn spatial relations. The lessened naturalism in experiment 2 had been associated with predicted increased age differences (compared with experiment 1), but had not, we speculated, been effortful enough to cause spatial learning to be nonautomatic for most respondents. The next experiment was an even more abstract version of the floor plan, or "maze", which was thought to be more effortful.

Experiment 3

In this experiment, the same floor plan was made into a more abstract styrofoam maze and a paper-and-pencil maze, for use by young and old respondents.

Method

SUBJECTS

The recruitment of respondents for the maze study targeted two groups: "young" respondents, between the ages of 17 and 31, and "old" respondents, ages 59 and older. The total subject pool consisted of 168 participants, 58 in the "young" category, and 110 in the "old" category. Most young participants were undergraduate student volunteers from Towson State University, while older respondents were recruited through an advertisement in a local senior citizens' newspaper. Overall, 114 subjects were women, and 54 were men.

Subjects were randomly assigned to one of two treatment conditions, 70 to the styrofoam maze condition, and 80 to the paper condition. Of the 168 subjects tested, 18 produced data that were not scorable, data ultimately discarded.

MATERIALS

We constructed a human-sized version of the maze in a classroom at Towson State University. It was constructed of 3-ft × 3-ft × 1-in. styrofoam squares, which were pieced together using wooden dowels to form a 30 × 18 × 6-ft rectangular outer boundary. The maze interior comprised five 12 × 3 × 6-ft equidistant rectangular blocks. The maze concluded in an "office," which consisted of a desk placed inside the fourth rectangular block from the entrance. An overview of this layout is depicted in Figure 5.1.

An alternate, "paper" version of the maze consisted of an $8\frac{1}{2}$ × 11 ×-in. scaled diagram proportional to that in Figure 5.1, without the arrowed path pictured.

PROCEDURE

Participants were randomly assigned to either the styrofoam or the paper maze versions. After respondents completed the necessary consent forms, the experimenter read them instructions. In the styrofoam maze condition, respondents stood at the maze entrance and were told that the maze represented an office building that contained five office blocks. They were then asked to follow the experimenter through the maze without talking and to pay close attention because they would be asked to remember the route later. (The experimenter showed each subject the route that is pictured in Figure 5.1.) On reaching the goal, participants were asked to sit at the desk provided.

The paper version of the maze consisted of the subject's visually following the experimenter's forefinger as he or she traced the route across the scaled diagram of the maze.

After presentation, the experimenter asked all subjects to draw the actual route presented as well as what he or she perceived to be the shortest, most direct route from the entrance to the office (goal). We randomly determined the order in which the participants were asked to draw these routes by the flip of a coin before their arrival at the testing site. In addition to these two tasks, participants were asked to describe in their own words how they remembered what they recalled about the actual route. If respondents needed additional prompting, they were instructed to describe any "memory devices" they used.

Results and Discussion

We calculated two-way ANOVAs to test the hypothesis that age and abstractness of maze presentation influenced memory for spatial relations. Older respondents did not perform as well as younger respondents on the right turns index, the sequence of turns index, the drawn to scale measure, or the length of route index for the actual path. For the shortcut path, older respondents drew longer but less accurate paths. Respondents receiving the paper-and-pencil maze performed better than those experiencing the styrofoam maze in that they drew significantly more to scale on the actual and shortcut maps.

These more abstract (and hopefully more effortful) versions of the floor plan were the occasion of more age effects, as predicted. However, although we expected that the greater abstractness of the paper floor plan stimulus (compared with the styrofoam floor plan and the real halls of earlier experiments) would lead to poorer scores on that version, especially by older respondents, the opposite proved to be true. Perhaps responding in the same modality as the stimulus modality made all the difference, because of encoding factors. Experiment 4 was an attempt to explore this further.

Experiment 4

In experiment 4, we gave younger respondents the opportunity to encode the floor plan in three modes: visual, verbal or kinesthetic. The hypothesis was that visual encoding would lead to better performance because the mode of responding was mainly visual.

Method

SUBJECTS

The respondents consisted of 44 younger people, 28 women and 16 men, with ages ranging from 17 to 25 years (mean age = 19.4). The respondents were recruited from Towson State University. They participated in the study to receive extra credits for psychology courses.

MATERIALS

A paper form of the maze (Figure 5.1) was reproduced on an $8\frac{1}{2} \times 11$-in. letter-size paper and was used to present both visual and kinesthetic treatments. At the end of presentation, we gave the subject a blank sheet of letter-size paper and a pencil on which to reproduce the route.

PROCEDURE

After respondents signed consent forms, we assigned them to one of the following three conditions: auditory, visual, and kinesthetic. The instructions for the visual condition are as follows: "The task involves learning your way around a floor plan. Here is the floor plan of a building. Pay close attention because I will ask you to remember the route later." The research assistant went through the route with her finger slowly and only once. At the end of the presentation, the desk was cleared and the respondents were offered a blank sheet paper with the following instructions: "Draw for me the (actual or shortcut) route which we took around the floor plan from the "begin" point to the "end" point. Label where you started and ended." The respondents were instructed not to go through the walls in the shortcut route. Once the maze recall was completed, the respondents were asked to describe how they remembered the actual route on the back of the paper.

The instructions for the kinesthetic condition were the same as previously, except the respondents were blindfolded with a pair of goggles, then the research assistant guided the respondent's dominant index finger through the maze. The respondent then responded, giving actual and shortcut routes as before.

The following verbal instructions were read to the subjects in the auditory condition:

You need to find an office. This rectangular building has five office blocks in it. I am going to give you verbal directions around the building. We will enter the side door and take an indirect route to the office we are looking for. Pay close attention because I will ask you to remember this route later. Ready? Here are the directions. Enter and make a left, go to the end of the block, make a right and go down two blocks and make a right. Go to the end of the block and make a left. Go down three blocks and make a left. Go to the end of this block and make a left. Go to the end of this block and make a right. Go to the end of the block, make a right. Go to the end of this block and make a right, and go into the office you are looking for.

Results and Discussion

One-way ANOVAs were calculated to test the hypothesis that modality of encoding influenced performance so that visual encoding led to the best performance. This proved to be the case in drawn to scale and route length measures on the actual map, and in drawn to scale measures on the shortcut map. No other measures, however, were significantly influenced by encoding mode.

The results were similar to what had occurred in the previous study, that is, that the measures sensitive to encoding modality seemed to be route length and the drawn to scale index. These measures also were the ones most influenced by age earlier, although all measures were difficult for all groups in every experiment. This overall set of results from the first four experiments suggested the possibilities that aging negatively influenced visual encoding more than other modalities, that spatial memory was effortless only if it could rely on visual encoding, and that while aging or impaired visual encoding influenced the scaling of one's spatial representation, it did not significantly influence other indices of spatial memory or even scaling if encoding was in a naturalistic environment. The results of this fourth experiment also suggested explanations for the weak relations among our spatial memory measures and the laboratory measures described in experiment 2. Finally, results suggested that the encoding medium–performance medium match was not the whole reason for good or poor performance, as hypothesized in experiment 4.

Experiment 5

In experiment 4 respondents had received three different types of encoding information, two visual and one verbal, then responded using paper and pencil. In the last experiment reported here, young and old respondents who would respond using paper and pencil received a styrofoam or paper maze version with either visual or visual plus kinesthetic information. In this way we could examine joint effects of age, encoding–performance modality match, and plain visual versus assisted visual stimulus information. We hypothesized that age differences would appear on the styrofoam maze, especially in the visual information-only condition, and that the paper (visual assisted by kinesthetic) version would overall lead to the best scores.

Method

SUBJECTS

One hundred sixty-six urban area respondents voluntarily participated in the study. The subject pool consisted of 83 (22 men and 61 women) students at Towson State University, ages 17 to 30 (mean age = 20.89 years) and 83 (28 men and 55 women) community dwellers, age 60 and over (mean age = 68.29 years).

MATERIALS

We used a human-sized version of the maze identical to that used in experiment 3, with a variation in the height of the walls of the internal rectangular blocks. These walls were 3 ft rather than 6 ft tall such that from the entrance subjects could have an overview of the entire maze. An alternate paper version consisted of an $8\frac{1}{2} \times 11$-in. scaled diagram of the human-sized maze.

A subject information sheet requesting age, sex, and handedness was used along with answer sheets consisting of predrawn rectangles for drawing the maze route.

PROCEDURE

Subjects were randomly assigned to one of four maze conditions. An equal number of young (ages 17 to 30) and old (age 60 and over) participants experienced each condition. The route of the maze was identical to experiment 1; however, the presentation varied for each of the conditions:

1. Actual Maze Involving Both Visual and Kinesthetic Presentations

On being directed to the entrance of the styrofoam maze, participants were told that the maze represented the interior of an office building that was divided into five separate blocks of offices. Their goal was to find a designated office. Respondents were told that they would be asked to recall the route to the office later. At this point, subjects followed an experimenter through the maze corridors until they stopped at the designated office.

2. Actual Maze Involving Only Visual Presentation

The nature of the maze was explained to subjects as in condition 1. While standing at the maze entrance, participants watched as an experimenter walked through the maze corridors until he or she stopped at the designated office.

3. Abstract Paper-and-Pencil Maze Using Both Visual and Kinesthetic Presentations

Respondents were shown a scaled diagram of the maze and were told that it represented a floor plan of a rectangular building with five office blocks in it. Subjects were informed that they needed to find an office. The experimenter maneuvered the subject's finger across the diagram to the designated office. Before the presentation, participants were told that they would be asked to recall the route.

4. Abstract Paper-and-Pencil Maze Using Only a Visual Presentation

The nature of the maze was explained to subjects as in condition 3. This time, the experimenter maneuvered his or her own finger across the diagram to the designated office. Immediately following the maze presentation, participants had to complete three recall tasks identical to experiment 1: draw the route presented to them; draw the shortest, most direct route from the entrance to the designated office; and write down how they remember what they recalled. We scored respondents' maze drawings using the same dependent measures as in experiment 1.

Results and Discussion

We calculated two-way ANOVAs to test effects of age and condition on each of the dependent measures. For the actual route map, age effects favoring the young occurred on the right-turn index, the turns index, the sequence of turn index, and the drawn to scale index. The length of route index was influenced by manipulated maze presentation conditions so that the visual-plus-kinesthetic version led to much shorter maps than the other conditions did. The sequence of turns index also was influenced by conditions so that the styrofoam-visual-plus-kinesthetic version led to the most correct turn sequence and the paper-visual-plus-kinesthetic led to the least correct. For the shortcut map, older respondents made shorter maps. Age interacted with condition for the drawn to scale measure so that the young given either paper stimulus and the old given the paper-visual–only stimulus drew most to scale, whereas the young with styrofoam-visual-plus-kinesthetic and the old with styrofoam visual only drew least to scale. Manipulated experimental condition influenced the right-turns index, too. Conditions leading from worst to best performance, respectively, were styro-foam-visual-plus-kinesthetic; styrofoam-visual; paper-visual-plus-kinesthetic; and paper-visual.

The results did not support the hypotheses for experiment 5. Other interesting and reassuring facts were emerging, however. Age effects seen in earlier experiments were reliable enough to be present again in experiment 5. The most sensitive map measures were still the length, scale, and right-turn measure, as in earlier studies. And the five studies together gave a clearer picture of the processes that are and are not influenced by age and mode of stimulus presentation.

General Discussion

The five studies reported here were conducted to create and explore a new, structured paradigm to test spatial representation and spatial memory aging along the spectrum of stimuli ranging from naturalistic events to laboratory tests. We created this paradigm around variations on a spatial maze design. Many additional variations are possible. This new paradigm proved to be practial, workable, amenable to numerous appropriate manipulations, and linked to laboratory memory studies. This new paradigm for spatial memory measurement permits us to understand not only whether respondents remember but how they do so and why they make the sorts of errors they make at any age. It also permits the use of a naturalistic memory task, which sheds new light on basic memory processes.

Respondent age had more of an impact on performance on certain measures then on others, and the impact was reliable. The most influenced measures were the right-turns index and indices related miniaturization or the drawn-to-scale quality of the remembered spatial layout. Conceptually, the more the maze differed from the totally naturalistic floor plan, the worse the older respondents performed, mainly by forgetting right turns and by miniaturizing their representation. Sequence of turns and left turns were seldom influenced by age. Far from representing a memory loss phenomenon, such a result would seem to indicate that more effective representations of natural spatial environments come with older age. Fewer resources may be needed for miniaturized representation; this would certainly seem to be adaptive for the whole organism in general systems theory terms or in Miller's (1978) terms.

The results of the five studies relate to several of the issues and earlier work described in the introduction to this chapter, but our discussion here must be limited because of space considerations. This new paradigm can speak to both laboratory and naturalistic studies, and can address memory in context. Spatial memory assessed this way seems to be effortless in naturalistic settings and more effortful in the laboratory. Spatial memory encoding may be multimodal with differential emphasis on modalities as a function of age. Clear contextualizing also helps older subjects. Older subjects create more compact "maps" or schematics, treating representations of space as they treat representations of stories, that is, focusing on the gist or the moral. All these and other interpretations suggest further research that can be part of the research program in spatial memory aging.

Acknowledgments. The assistance of Dr. David Arenberg, Diana Bobbi, Dina Cortese, David Dietrich, Patricia Ellison, John Freeman, Dr. Donald Ingram, Judith Plotz, June Saktor, Clifton Santiago, Barbara Skinner, Fran Spencer, Barbara Storyk, Dr. Robin West, and staff of the Baltimore Longitudinal Study of Aging is gratefully acknowledged. Studies 1 and 2 were described at the Cognitive Aging Conference, Atlanta, GA, 1987. This research was supported in part by support to the first author from Towson State University, from the National Institutes of Health, and from the University of Florida.

References

Allen, G.L., & Kirasic, K.C. (1985). Effects of the cognitive organization of route knowledge on judgements of macrospatial distance. *Memory and Cognition, 13,* 218–227.

Baroni, M., Job, R., Peron, E., & Salmoso, P. (1980). Memory for natural settings: Role of diffuse and focused attention. *Perceptual & Motor Skills, 51,* 883–889.

Benton, A.L. (1963). *The Revised Visual Retention Test (3rd ed.).* New York: Psychological Corp.

Bruce, P.R., & Herman, J.F. (1986). Adult age differences in spatial memory: Effects of distinctiveness and repeated experience. *Journal of Gerontology, 41,* 774–776.

Cavanaugh, John C. (1982, November). Memory in everyday life: Theoretical and empirical needs. In J.C. Cavanaugh & D.A. Kramer (Chairs), *On missing links and such: Interfaces between cognitive research and everyday problem solving.* Symposium conducted at the annual meeting of the Gerontological Society, Boston.

Charness, N. (1981). Visual short-term memory and aging in chess players. *Journal of Gerontology, 36,* 615–619.

Evans, G., & Pezdek, K. (1980). Cognitive mapping: Knowledge of real world distance and location information. *Journal of Experimental Psychology: Human Learning and Memory, 6,* 13–24.

Georgemiller, R., & Hassan, F. (1986). Spatial competence assessment of route-finding, route-learning, and topographical memory in normal aging. *Clinical Gerontologist, 5,* 19–37.

Hartley, J., Harker, J., & Walsh, D. (1980). Contemporary issues and new directions in adult development of learning and memory. In L.W. Poon (Ed.), *Aging in the 1980's: Psychological issues* (pp. 239–252). Washington, DC: American Psychological Association.

Hasher, L., & Zacks, R. (1979). Automatic and effortful processes in memory. *Journal of Experimental Psychology, 108,* 356–388.

Hirtle, S.C., & Jonides, J. (1985). Evidence of hierarchies in cognitive maps. *Memory & Cognition, 13,* 208–217.

Hultsch, D.F. (1977). Changing perspectives on basic research in adult learning and memory. *Educational Psychology, 2,* 367–382.

Kausler, D. (1982). *Experimental psychology and human aging.* New York: Wiley.

Kirasic, K. (1983). *Spatial problem solving in elderly adults: Evidence of a home-town advantage.* Paper presented at the annual meeting of the Gerontological Society, San Francisco.

Kozlowski, L.T., & Bryant, K.J. (1977). Sense of direction, spatial orientation, and cognitive maps. *Journal of Experimental Psychology: Human Perception and Performance, 3,* 590–598.

Levine, M., Jankovic, I.N., & Palij, M. (1982). Principles of spatial problem solving. *Journal of Experimental Psychology: General, 111,* 157–175.

Light, L.L., & Zelinski, E.M. (1983). Memory for spatial information in young and old adults. *Developmental Psychology, 19,* 901–906.

Mandler, J.M., & Parker, R.E. (1976). Memory for descriptive and spatial information in complex pictures. *Journal of Experimental Psychology, 2,* 38–48.

McNamara, T.P. (1986). Mental representations of spatial relations. *Cognitive Psychology, 18,* 87–121.

Miller, J. (1978). *Living systems.* New York: McGraw-Hill.

Moore, T.E., Richards, B., & Hood, J. (1984). Aging and the coding of spatial information. *Journal of Gerontology, 39,* 210–212.

Neisser, U. (1982a). *Memory observed.* San Francisco: Freeman.

Neisser, U. (1982b). Memory: What are the important questions? In U. Neisser (Ed.), *Memory observed* (pp. 3–19). San Francisco: Freeman.

Ohta, R.J., Walsh, D.A., & Krauss, I.K. (1981). Spatial perspective-taking ability in young and elderly adults. *Experimental Aging Research, 7,* 45–63.

Perlmutter, M., Metzger, R., Nezworski, T., & Miller, K. (1981). Spatial and temporal memory in 20- and 60-year olds. *Journal of Gerontology, 36,* 59–65.

Pezdek, K. (1983a). *Age differences in memory for items and their spatial locations.* Paper presented at the annual meeting of the American Psychological Association, Los Angeles.

Pezdek, K. (1983b). Memory for items and their spatial locations by young and elderly adults. *Developmental Psychology, 19,* 895–900.

Pezdesk, K., & Evans, G. (1979). Visual and verbal memory for objects and their spatial locations. *Journal of Experimental Psychology: Human Learning & Memory, 5,* 360–373.

Presson, C.C., DeLange, N., & Hazelrigg, M.D. (1987). Orientation-specificity in kinesthetic spatial learning: The role of multiple orientations. *Memory & Cognition, 15,* 225–229.

Salmaso, P., Baroni, M., Job, R., & Peron, E. (1983). Schematic information, attention, and memory for place. *Journal of Experimental Psychology, 9,* 263–268.

Sherman, R., Oliver, C., & Titus, W. (1980). Verifying environmental relationships. *Memory & Cognition, 8,* 555–562.

Shock, N., Andres, R., Arenberg, D., Costa, P., Greulich, R., Lakatta, E., & Tobin, J. (1985). *Normal human aging: The Baltimore Longitudinal Study of Aging.* Washington, DC: National Institute of Aging.

Sinnott, J.D. (1986). Prospective/intentional everyday memory: Effects of age and passage of time. *Psychology and Aging, 1,* 110–116.

Sinnott, J.D. (1987). *Spatial memory and aging: Model linking lab and life, rat and human maze learning.* Paper presented at the Cognitive Aging Conference, Atlanta.

Sinnott, J.D. (1989a). General systems theory: A rationale for the study of everyday memory. In L. Poon, D. Rubin & B. Wilson (Eds.), *Everyday cognition in adulthood and old age* (pp. 358–372). New York: Cambridge University Press.

Sinnott, J.D. (1989b). Prospective memory and aging: Memory as adaptive action. In L. Poon, D. Rubin, & B. Wilson (Eds.), *Everyday cognition in adulthood and old age* (pp. 59–70). New York: Cambridge University Press.

Smyth, M.M., & Kennedy, J.E. (1982). Orientation and spatial representation within multiple frames of reference. *British Journal of Psychology, 73,* 527–535.

Waddell, K., & Rogoff, R. (1981). Effect of contextual organization on spatial memory of middle-aged and older women. *Developmental Psychology, 17,* 878–885.

Wechsler, D.(1955). *WAIS manual. Wechsler Adult Intelligence Scale.* New York: Psychological Corp.

Zacks, R.T. (1982). Encoding strategies used by young elderly adults in a keeping track task. *Journal of Gerontology, 37,* 203–211.

Part 2
Semantic Memory and Speech Processing

6
Adult Age Differences in Script Content and Structure

Thomas M. Hess

It is a well-established fact that our knowledge about the world influences our perceptions and subsequent memory for specific events. Individual differences in relevant background knowledge have been shown to be associated with variations in both the level and type of information remembered about an event. For example, Spilich, Vesonder, Chiesi, and Voss (1979) found that baseball knowledge was positively associated with memory for details from a specific game if the detail were relevant to the goal structure of baseball; no association was observed between memory for irrelevant details and knowledge. Importantly, other more constructive aspects of retention are also related to background knowledge, with the types of inferences and elaborations generated in memory being a function of the individual's interpretation of the event from their particular perspective (e.g., Sulin & Dooling, 1974).

Knowledge effects on performance are of special interest to researchers studying developmental differences in memory (e.g., Chi & Ceci, 1987), which is due to the simple fact that age is correlated with both the level and type of experience possessed by an individual. To the extent that retention is influenced by specific knowledge structures, mechanisms of age-related changes in memory may be discovered by examining the relationship between these structures and performance. Research with children has shown that developmental differences in levels of memory performance are often attentuated and sometimes reversed (e.g., Chi, 1978) when relevant knowledge is manipulated between age groups. The general assumption is that high levels of domain knowledge are associated with more elaborated and integrated cognitive structures, which in turn facilitate the comprehension and retention of domain-related events by providing an interpretive structure for organizing experience (e.g., Chi & Koeske, 1983).

Specific changes in memory processing might also occur in adulthood to the extent that knowledge structures continue to develop and change with age. Age-related experiences might be associated with more elaborative associative networks and variations in categories of knowledge, resulting in changes in the perception and retention of events. Interestingly, this is what appears to happen with increased expertise in various scientific realms, such as physics (e.g., Chi, Feltovich, & Glaser, 1981), and in games of skill, such as chess (e.g., Chase & Simon, 1973). Although limited, some research suggests that knowledge categories do change with age and experience in adulthood. For example, Brewer and Lui (1984) found that older adults have more differentiated knowledge representations of elderly individuals than do young adults, which is apparently due to the increased relevance of specific old-age–related social roles in later adulthood. Similar types of changes may occur in other knowledge domains as well.

Given the importance of knowledge in determining memory performance and the fact that such knowledge may change with age, our understanding of cognitive functioning and aging would benefit from more systematic explorations of developmental changes in knowledge structures. If differences exist in those structures used to interpret specific events, subsequent memory for those events might be affected by aging in a manner that has little to do with negative changes in biologically based processes.

Scripts and Aging

This chapter examines age differences in the nature of one specific type of knowledge structure—scripts. Scripts can be conceptualized as generalized representations of specific activities, such as grocery shopping or going to the doctor, that have been formed with experience over time (Schank & Abelson, 1977). These representations include information about the types of actions associated with the activity, the causal and/or temporal links between these actions, and the objects and actors that can fulfill specific roles within the activity (i.e., slot fillers). It has been demonstrated that these structures have psychological validity in that both the processing of and memory for scripted events have been shown to be influenced by script structure. For example, actions relevant to a scripted activity (e.g., ordering from the menu while dining out) are processed more quickly and recalled better than irrelevant actions (e.g., putting a pen in your pocket during the same activity) (e.g., Hess, Donley, & Vandermaas, 1989). In addition, memories for everyday events appear to be organized in a scripted fashion in that people use script-like structures to guide their retrieval attempts and to constrain these attempts to relevant contexts (e.g., Reiser, 1986). There is even evidence that scripts begin to develop in children as young as 3 years (Nelson & Greundel, 1981) and influence both the development of memory and other cognitive abilities (e.g., Fivush, 1987). Given the general importance of these structures and their influence on memory for everyday events, the examination of age differences in scripts could provide valuable information about potential sources of age-related variation in memory processing.

Unfortunately, few studies have examined scripted knowledge in relation to aging. In one relevant investigation, Light and Anderson (1983) had young and older adults both generate actions associated with specific scripts and then rate each of these actions in terms of their typicality with respect to the script (i.e., how typical or necessary was the action for completion of the scripted activity). They found no age differences in either the number of unique actions or the total number of actions produced, and correlations between age groups for typicality ratings and generation frequencies for specific script actions were in the .7 to .9 range. Based on these findings, they concluded that there are no "systematic differences in the way that scripts are represented in memory" (Light & Anderson, 1983, p. 439). They went on to demonstrate that script structure had similar effects on memory for component actions across age groups.

I have obtained similar findings with respect to age differences in script structure. In one study (Hess, 1985), I found that between–age-group correlations for the mean typicality ratings of individual actions were generally at .84 or above for activities such as getting up in the morning and washing clothes. The least agreement ($r = .72$) was found for the activity of going to the beach, which could conceivably have great potential for age-related variation. The other activities included appeared to be more structured and less likely to change in constituent actions with age, perhaps being more akin to what Abelson (1981) has termed "strong" scripts. In another study (Hess et al., 1989), subjects rated individual actions with respect to their relevance in understanding the scripted sequence. As with typicality, correlations between age groups for these ratings were very high (.86 to .94). Finally, my co-workers and I also found that script structure had similar types of effects on reading times and—with some variation—on memory across age groups (Hess, 1985; Hess et al., 1989). These results appear to reinforce Light and Anderson's (1983) conclusions.

The conclusions that can be made about age differences in scripts, however, are somewhat limited by the methodologies used in these studies. For example, Light and Anderson (1983) constrained subjects to producing about 20 actions per script and also instructed them to include only actions that would be performed by most people. Such instructions appear to have the built-in result of biasing productions toward socially accepted norms. This could result in individuals excluding actions that are specific to their personal script and that might be associated with age-related patterns of script reorganization. Although many scripts are assumed to have a strong socially shared core of information, which in turn serves to facilitate communication, it is still conceivable that interindividual and intergroup differences might exist in specific components, reflecting changes in life contexts with age. For example, bringing a "boom box" and "surfing" might be two highly typical actions in the personal "Going to the beach" scripts of young adults but would probably be less well-represented in those of older adults. (For a more complete discussion of the factors affecting script production, see Chapter 3, this volume.)

Interestingly, even with constraints on production, Light and Anderson

(1983) found significant age differences in typicality ratings on about 10% of the rated actions. Some of my recent work has shown significant age-related variations in ratings associated with specific script actions, the typicality of which I had originally thought to be fairly obvious. These age-related differences, though, tended to be in the degree of rated typicality or atypicality rather than in the assignment to these categories of typicality. Such results, however, suggest that age-related script variations do exist.

With respect to understanding aging and everyday memory, other concerns may be raised about the studies of script memory in which, in the name of experimental control, the stimulus actions were constrained to those exhibiting a high degree of agreement in structural ratings across age groups (Hess, 1985; Hess et al., 1989; Light & Anderson, 1983). While allowing valid inferences to be made about the effects of factors like typicality and relevance on memory processing, this procedure also limits the predictions one can make about age differences in the processing of naturally occurring events.

Finally, in emphasizing actions, other aspects of script-based knowledge have been neglected. Many scripts have different means of goal attainment in different situations. For example, when dining out, one can obtain food by driving up to a window, ordering at a counter, selecting food from a buffet, or ordering from a waiter, depending on the type of restaurant. It is probable that the more experience individuals have with specific scripted activities, the greater will be their knowledge of specific conditions on performance and alternative goal paths, resulting in more elaborate knowledge structures. Thus, it might be hypothesized that relative to young adults, older adults would be more likely to have such information represented in their scripts, owing to their greater experience. Unfortunately, no assessment of these types of knowledge exists in the aging research literature.

An Empirical Investigation of Script Content and Structure

My concern with previous investigations of adult age differences in the nature of scripts led me to conduct a rather simple study in which young and older adults were asked to generate scripts for four common activities. The investigation was carried out with the help of research assistants. The relatively novel aspect of this study was that scripts were generated in narrative fashion with few restrictions placed on their production. This procedure should result in the generation of both more personalized and more elaborate scripts than in earlier studies, thereby allowing assessment of age differences in organizational and content factors not present in lists of actions. Because of age-related variations in experience, it was hypothesized that older adults would be more likely than young adults to include information about conditions on performance and alternative goal paths. I also expected that age differences would be observed in the types of actions produced within a given script.

Method

The original sample consisted of 20 young adults recruited from undergraduate psychology courses at North Carolina State University (NCSU) and 21 older adults recruited from the community. One young adult was dropped from the sample, because her productions were nearly three times as long as those of any of the other subjects. I felt that inclusion of this "outlier" data would distort the differences between age groups. The data of one older adult was also excluded because his productions were recounts of specific events rather than more general descriptions. The remaining young subjects (8 men and 11 women) had a mean age of 20.1 years ($SD = 2.5$), an average of 13.2 years of formal education ($SD = 1.0$), and a mean score of 24.8 ($SD = 7.5$) on the verbal meaning subtest of the Primary Mental Abilities (Thurstone & Thurstone, 1949). The mean age of the remaining older adults (12 men and 8 women) was 70.8 ($SD = 6.0$). These subjects had a higher overall level of education ($M = 15.8$ years; $SD = 2.3$) than the younger adults but were similar in verbal meaning scores ($M = 24.5$; $SD = 7.5$). No age differences existed in self-rated health.

Subjects were tested individually and were told that we were interested in how well they could describe the sequence of events associated with certain common activities. We then presented subjects with the following instructions associated with each of four common activities (in random order):

1. *Getting up in the morning.* In the course of a typical day for a person who has a job or an early class, describe the events that normally occur from the time just before that person wakes up to the time he or she leaves the house.
2. *Going grocery shopping.* Describe the events that normally occur from the time a person decides to go grocery shopping to the time he or she returns home.
3. *Going out to eat at a restaurant with a friend.* Describe the events that normally occur from the time that a person decides to go out to eat with a friend to the time that they leave the restaurant.
4. *Going to the doctor for a minor ailment.* Describe the events that normally occur for someone who is visiting the doctor concerning a minor ailment, such as a cold. Describe the events from the time the decision is made to visit the doctor to the time the person leaves the doctor's office.

Following each set of instructions, subjects gave activity descriptions that were recorded using a tape recorder. In all cases, we asked subjects to describe the activity in detail, using any activity-associated temporal order information as a guide. No time limits were imposed. I selected the four activities based on their general familiarity to individuals in the two age groups. Note that although subjects were not specifically asked to describe what they themselves normally do, the general nature of the instructions allowed great leeway in the information subjects could provide.

Results

Script productions were transcribed, and the information contained in them was classified into the following categories, which are in part based on Katherine Nelson's (1986) work:

1. *An act* was defined as a proposition describing an action (e.g., "The waiter brings the food").
2. *Optional acts* included actions prefaced by probabilistic terms (e.g., sometimes, usually) or alternative actions (e.g., "You either wait to be seated or find your own seat").
3. *Conditional terms* referred to both temporal markers (e.g., before, after) that identify the sequence of actions and enabling conditions (e.g., "If you have a car, then . . . ").
4. *Elaborations* referred to propositions that repeated a previous action with new information (e.g., "You order drinks . . . you order wine").
5. *Optional slot fillers* were defined as specified alternatives for fulfilling particular roles (e.g., "You are seated by the host or hostess").
6. *Descriptions* referred to any statements describing physical setting (e.g., "There is usually a wine list on the table") or affective reactions (e.g., "I dislike waiting").

In the first set of analyses, I examined age differences in the degree to which these six types of information were contained in the script productions. I analyzed the frequency of production of each category of information using a 2 (age group) × 4 (activity) analysis of variance (ANOVA). Mean levels of performance are presented in Table 6.1. In general, few systematic differences were present in the types of information contained in the script productions across both age and activities. The only significant effects obtained were due to activity for optional acts, $F(3,111) = 4.41$, $p < .01$, and for conditional terms, $F(3,111) = 4.57$, $p < .01$. In both cases, significantly more qualifying information was produced in the restaurant script than in either the grocery-shopping or morning scripts and in the doctor script than in the grocery script ($ps < .05$). In addition, significantly more conditional terms were produced in the doctor script than in the morning script. The lack of any age effects provides little support for the hypothesis that older adults would produce more elaborate script information.

A second issue of concern was the extent to which both intergroup varia-

TABLE 6.1. Mean amount of information produced within categories for each script.

			Information category			
Script name	Acts	Optional acts	Conditional terms	Elabora-tions	Descrip-tions	Slot fillers
Going to the doctor						
Young	13.8	1.6	4.5	.7	.6	.5
Old	15.7	2.2	6.8	.5	1.8	.9
Grocery shopping						
Young	13.2	1.1	2.7	.5	1.3	1.1
Old	17.6	1.1	4.8	.7	2.1	2.3
Getting up in the morning						
Young	17.6	1.6	3.9	.5	1.0	.4
Old	15.8	1.3	5.1	.8	1.4	.8
Going to a restaurant						
Young	17.6	3.1	5.3	.7	.6	.7
Old	18.1	1.8	7.0	1.6	1.5	.9

tions and interindividual differences within age groups existed in the types of actions (both acts and optional acts) produced for each activity. To address this concern, the proportions of unique acts produced both between and within age groups was examined. An act was considered age unique if it was produced by one or more subjects in one age group but by none in the other. An act was considered unique within an age group if it was produced by only one individual in that group. We calculated the uniqueness proportions in two different ways, one based on the number of particular actions produced and the other on the total number of actions produced. In the former case, the individual actions produced (excluding repetitions across subjects) within age groups were listed, and then we calculated the proportions of those produced only in that age group or only by one person. This provided a measure of the variability in experience (i.e., the number of different types of actions) associated with specific scripted activities. In the latter case, the same proportions were calculated, but this time based on all the actions produced within groups, including repetitions of specific acts. This provided an estimate of the degree to which individual protocols were composed of shared versus unique actions.

An can be seen in Table 6.2, there is a fair amount of between-age variability in the contents of scripts, and the degree of variability is activity related. In the morning script, where the most intergroup and interindividual variability occurred, approximately 60% of the specific types of ac-

TABLE 6.2. Proportions of unique actions produced between and within age groups.

| | Script and measure[a] | | | | | | | |
| | Doctor | | Shopping | | Morning | | Restaurant | |
Action category	B	W	B	W	B	W	B	W
Specific actions								
Young	.49	.51	.46	.58	.60	.58	.30	.43
Old	.45	.49	.49	.47	.61	.59	.30	.45
Total actions								
Young	.19	.16	.24	.20	.30	.21	.12	.13
Old	.13	.13	.16	.24	.36	.24	.11	.14

[a] B refers to the number of age-unique actions produced (i.e., intergroup variability), and W refers to the number of unique actions produced within age groups (i.e., interindividual variability).

tions produced in each age group were unique to that group, suggesting a great deal of age-related diversity in experience. In addition, an average of 30% of all actions contained in the individual protocols of young adults and 36% in those of the older adults were unique to their age group. In contrast, in the least variable script (i.e., restaurant), only 30% of the specific actions produced were age unique, and only about 12% of the actions contained in an individual's protocol were unique to his or her age group.

What might account for the age differences in script contents? Examination of Table 6.2 reveals that both interindividual and intergroup variability fluctuate similarly across scripts, suggesting that the nature of the activity may be a prime determinant of the degree to which consensus exists on the information making up a script. The activity of eating out at a restaurant may be constrained to a fair degree by external structure, providing little opportunity for individual deviance. In contrast, getting up in the morning may be a fairly idiosyncratic activity with fewer socially prescribed restrictions on performance, thereby accounting for the greater variability in content. Thus, part of the between-age variability may simply be related to factors that influence individual variability.

Interestingly, the data on production of conditional terms are consistent with the preceding characterization of the differences in external constraints on structure across scripts. The script that produced the least variability in productions (i.e., restaurant) also was the one for which the most qualifying information (i.e., conditional terms) was produced, whereas the script with the greatest variability (i.e., getting up) contained the least qualifying information. Conditional terms relating to temporal ordering (e.g., *before, then*) may only be produced in those situations having a relatively well-defined sequence of actions; in less structured situations (e.g., "weak" scripts; see Abelson, 1981), such terms may be unnecessary or inappropriate. For example, many of the acts in the restaurant script (e.g., ordering, paying) are contingent on the occurence of prior events (e.g., reading the menu, getting the check), whereas this contingency is less evident for the morning script (e.g., you can get dressed before or after breakfast).

Further examination of the data, however, suggests that factors that influence script variability in general cannot be the sole explanation for the observed age-related variability. Specifically, 76% of the older adults' age-unique morning actions and 80% of those of the young adults were produced by more than one subject, suggesting that the observed age differences may be based in differential experience between groups. This may result in age-related variations in the emphasis put on different types of script behaviors. For example, some script components may be more relevant to the life circumstances of one age group than to the other, resulting in overrepresentation of those components in the script productions of subjects in the appropriate age group.

One rather superficial way to examine this hypothesis is by calculating the correlations between age groups for production frequencies of individual script actions. To eliminate the positive bias that would result from the inclusion of the relatively large number of items produced by only one subject, we calculated these correlations only for those actions produced by at least two individuals. This procedure also had the result of eliminating some of the non–age-related idiosyncratic aspects of the data. The obtained correlations suggest a fair amount of age-related variation across scripts: .83 for the doctor, .81 for grocery shopping, .67 for getting up, and .76 for dining out. Using Fisher's r-to-Z transformation, comparisons between scripts indicated that the correlation for the morning script was significantly lower than that obtained for either the doctor visit, $Z = 2.24$, $p < .03$, or grocery shopping, $Z = 2.09$, $p < .05$. Thus, consistent with the previous analyses, the getting up in the morning script showed more age-related variation than the others.

It is also interesting to compare between age correlations for generation frequencies in the present study with those of Light and Anderson (1983) for the three scripts common to both studies. The correlations for the doctor's visit and grocery shopping are very similar across studies, whereas that obtained for getting up in the morning is .18 lower in the present study. This suggests that the instructions in the present experiment may have allowed production of more personal scripts, resulting in less agreement between age groups in some situations. The fact that this cross-study variation did not occur in all cases suggests that some scripts may be more socially constrained and therefore less subject to variation across instructional conditions.

To further examine potential age differences in script content, we also broke each script into its component scenes. A scene may be characterized as a group of actions involved in achieving a subgoal within the script. For example, in the restaurant script, specific scenes might relate to the sub-goals of getting to the restaurant, being seated, and ordering food. By identifying both the extent to which different scenes were represented in the production protocols and the amount of information contained in each scene, more specific information about age differences in script content could be obtained.

In identifying possible scenes within scripts, we examined the actions produced by the subjects and the production frequencies for the actions. In doing so, it became obvious that certain general actions referring to sub-goals were produced by a majority of the subjects in both age groups. Using these actions to define scenes, we identified five to seven scenes in each script. For example, the morning script contained the following five scenes: (a) getting up, (b) taking a shower/bath, (c) getting dressed, (d) eating breakfast, and (e) leaving the house/apartment. We then identified the number of actions contained within each scene for each subject as an indication of that scene's importance within the personal script. In general, scene shifts were surprisingly easy to identify, usually beginning with either a shift in physical location (e.g., you then walk to the bathroom) or the actual scene label (e.g., you eat breakfast). Interrater agreement on a subset of 20 scripts in identifying scene shifts was .95.

The proportion of total script actions contained in each scene was then examined using 2 (age) $\times$ 5 $-$ 7 (scene) ANOVAs for the data from each of the four scripts. We observed a fair degree of variability in the specificity with which individual scenes were described, as evidenced by significant scene effects for the doctor, $F(4, 34) = 12.99$, $p < .001$; shopping, $F(4,34) = 4.47$, $p < .01$; morning, $F(4,34) = 5.70$, $p < .01$; and restaurant scripts, $F(5, 33) = 7.23$, $p < .001$. A significant age $\times$ scene interaction, however, was obtained only for the morning script, $F(4,34) = 3.97$, $p < .01$. (Similar results were obtained when number of actions rather than proportions were analyzed.) Further examination of this interaction using between–age-group contrasts for each scene revealed that young adults produced significantly more of their actions than the older adults in the getting up and getting dressed scenes, whereas the opposite was true for the eating breakfast scene ($ps < .05$).

These results are consistent with those previously mentioned in showing that age-related variation in script contents are greatest in the morning script. In addition, however, they have also helped identify more specifically the locus of the age effect by examining relative emphases on the sub-goals associated with the different scenes. Interestingly, the specific pattern of age differences appears to be related to changing life contexts. The young adults produced almost twice as many actions as the older adults when describing the getting dressed scene, suggesting that personal grooming is a relatively important aspect of their morning routine. Such a finding makes sense when viewed in light of the fact that these adults are in, what might be referred to as, the mate-selection stage of life, during which personal appearance concerns might take on increased importance. The older adults, on the other hand, produced almost twice as many actions as the younger adults in the breakfast scene. Much more emphasis was placed on both preparation and the social aspects of mealtime, which often reflected the fact that these individuals lived with a spouse and/or other family.

A final analysis examined the degree to which each scene was represented within each script across age groups. No age differences were observed in the probability of excluding any particular scene across scripts. This suggests that some socially shared script structure is maintained across age groups and that age-related variations in scene content reflected emphasis on, rather than representation of, script components.

Conclusions

The results of this research are relatively straightforward. First, there is a fair amount of age-related and individual variability in the content of script productions, a finding that concurs with that of Ross and Berg (see Chapter 3, this volume). Second, the extent to which this variation occurs is related to event classes. Scripts that are more well specified (i.e., possessing greater external and social constraints on performance) have less between- and within-group variability than less structured scripts. Less structure appears to allow more opportunity for both idiosyncratic and systematic group-related knowledge variation to be observed. Third, when age differences do occur in script knowledge, they appear to be more in content than in structure. Similar amounts of each category of information (e.g., conditional terms, alternative acts) were produced across age groups, whereas the specific actions produced were observed to vary across scripts and ages.

These conclusions should be tempered somewhat by potential limitations of the just-discussed research methodology. First, it should be quite obvious that productions of the sort obtained using the present procedure do not represent the total available script knowledge possessed by an individual. Even with explicit production instructions, subjects may edit out script information that is assumed to be understood across members of the same culture. If asked, most subjects would certainly indicate greater awareness of scripts than that reflected in their productions, thus perhaps limiting the extent to which we can make inferences about age differences in script structure and potential effects on memory. The case can be made, however, that such productions are meaningful in that the information produced must have some lower threshold of activation than other script components in memory that were not generated. This greater accessibility is usually assumed to be related to overall levels or recency of experience with the produced components (see Anderson, 1983). The importance of productions in making inferences about memory effects can also be seen from studies in which generation frequencies for individual actions were found to be the best predictors of later recall for those actions (e.g., Graesser, Woll, Kowalski, & Smith, 1980). Thus, although productions do not contain complete script knowledge, it can be argued that the information contained in them reflects general experience (rather than just social knowledge) and is predictive of the type of information that will be recalled about a scripted event. Indeed, Ross and Berg (1989) have shown that individuals remember more from an activity description when it incorporates components of their personal script (i.e., actions generated by the individual in describing a scripted activity).

A second limitation of the present research is that age-related variation in script knowledge was examined using a cross-sectional rather than longitudinal design. As such, inferences about script development can be made only with caution. More systematic research examining the relationship between changing life circumstances (e.g., social roles) and variations in script knowledge would be extremely useful in further explicating the processes involved in knowledge construction.

If, for present purposes, the results of this study are accepted as valid indications of age effects on scripted knowledge, it seems obvious that potential age differences could occur in memory for common events that are not due to changes in the thinking or processing aspects of cognition but rather to the knowing aspect (see Rybash, Hoyer, & Roodin, 1986). Specifically, age-related variations in the knowledge structures activated during processing could influence the type of information represented in memory, in terms of both veridical information and additions. For example, if young adults possess more differentiated knowledge than older adults relating to a specific script scene, they should retain more specific event information relevant to that scene. In addition, their greater degree of within-scene representation might result in more inferential information being added to the memory trace in the form of, for example, attributions about the actor's behavior. Age differences in knowledge representation might also be used to predict behavior in other circumstances. For example, two different-aged adults might have a more difficult time communicating with each other than two same-aged adults if there is age-related variation in the nature of the background information that each person assumes the other possesses. Thus, our understanding of age-related variations in memory and other functions might be enhanced by more systematic study of developmental changes in common knowledge structures, such as scripts.

Acknowledgments. Preparation of this chapter was supported in part by grant R01 AG05552 from the National Institute on Aging. I would like to thank Jan Donley and Maurean Vandermaas for their assistance in collecting the data reported in this chapter.

References

Abelson, R.F. (1981). Psychological status of the script concept. *American Psychologist, 36,* 715–729.

Anderson, J.R. (1983). A spreading activation theory of memory. *Journal of Verbal Learning and Verbal Behavior, 22,* 261–295.

Brewer, M.B., & Lui, L. (1984). Categorization of the elderly by the elderly: Effects of perceiver's category membership. *Personality and Social Psychology Bulletin, 10,* 585–595.

Chase, W.G., & Simon, H.A. (1973). Perception in chess. *Cognitive Psychology, 4,* 55–81.

Chi, M.T.H. (1978). Knowledge structures and memory development. In R.S. Siegler (Ed.), *Children's thinking: What develops?* (pp. 73–96). Hillsdale, NJ: Erlbaum.

Chi, M.T.H., & Ceci, S.J. (1987). Content knowledge: Its role, representation, and restructuring in memory development. In H.W. Reese (Ed.), *Advances in child development and behavior* (Vol. 20, pp. 91–142). New York: Academic Press

Chi, M.T.H., Feltovich, P.J., & Glaser, R. (1981). Categorization and representation of physics problems by experts and novices. *Cognitive Science, 5,* 121–152.

Chi, M.T.H., & Koeske, R.D. (1983). Network representation of a child's dinosaur knowledge. *Developmental Psychology, 19,* 29–39.

Fivush, R. (1987). Scripts and categories: Interrelationships in development. In U. Neisser (Ed.), *Concepts and conceptual development: Ecological and intellectual factors in categorization* (pp. 234–254). New York: Cambridge University Press.

Graesser, A.C., Woll, S.B., Kowalski, D.J., & Smith, D.A. (1980). Memory for typical and atypical information in scripted activities. *Journal of Experimental psychology: Human Learning and Memory, 6,* 503–515.

Hess, T.M. (1985). Aging and context influences on recognition memory for typical and atypical script actions. *Developmental Psychology, 21,* 1139–1151.

Hess, T.M., Donley, J., & Vandermaas, M.O. (1989). Aging-related changes in the processing and retention of script information. *Experimental Aging Research, 15,* 89–96.

Light, L.L., & Anderson, P.A. (1983). Memory for scripts in young and older adults. *Memory & Cognition, 11,* 435–444.

Nelson, K. (1986) *Event knowledge: Structure and function in development.* Hillsdale, NJ: Lawrence Erlbaum.

Nelson, K., & Greundel, J. (1981). Generalized event representations: Basic building blocks of cognitive development. In M.E. Lamb & A.L. Brown (Eds.), *Advances in developmental psychology* (Vol. 1, pp. 131–158). Hillsdale, NJ: Erlbaum.

Reiser, B.J. (1986). The encoding and retrieval of memories of real-world experiences. In J.A. Galambos, R.P. Abelson, & J.B. Black (Eds.), *Knowledge structures* (pp. 71–99). Hillsdale, NJ: Lawrence Erlbaum.

Ross, B.L., & Berg, C.A. (1989). *The impact of individual differences in scripts on memory for script-related stories in young and older adults.* Unpublished manuscript, University of Utah, Salt Lake City, UT.

Rybash, J.M., Hoyer, W.J., & Roodin, P.A. (1986) *Adult cognition and aging.* New York: Pergamon Press.

Schank, R.C., & Abelson, R. (1977). *Scripts, plans, goals, and understanding.* Hillsdale, NJ: Erlbaum.

Spilich, G.J., Vesonder, G.T., Chiesi, H.L., & Voss, J.F. (1979). Text processing of domain-related information for individuals with high and low domain knowledge. *Journal of Verbal Learning and Verbal Behavior, 18,* 275–290.

Sulin, R.A., & Dooling, D.J. (1974). Intrusion of thematic ideas in retention of prose. *Journal of Experimental Psychology, 103,* 255–262.

Thurstone, L.L., & Thurstone, T.G. (1949). *SRA primary mental abilities test.* Chicago: Science Research Associates.

7
Age Differences in Perceptual Processing and Memory for Spoken Language

ARTHUR WINGFIELD AND ELIZABETH A.L. STINE

Successful memory depends in large measure on the quality of initial stimulus encoding. It is for this reason that the cognitive aging literature has looked to age-related differences in acquisition processes and internal organization as important sources of decreased memory performance in normal aging (Rankin, Karol, & Tuten, 1984; Smith, 1980). These effects have in turn been attributed to presumed differences in working memory or general processing capacity (Craik & McDowd, 1987; Stine & Wingfield, 1987) and to age-sensitive declines in the rate at which new information can be processed (Salthouse, 1985). Less attention has been given to the distinction between cognitive "capacity" versus cognitive "effort" in memory aging, but we predict this to change in future years (cf. Mitchell & Hunt, 1989).

If normal aging is accompanied by diminished input processing capability, one might expect to see elderly adults to have special difficulty with rapid processing of, and memory for, spoken language. As we know from both the experimental literature and from our own experience, however, this is rarely the case. Although serious sensory deficits or neuropathology can produce dramatic impairment, language processing is generally well preserved in normal aging. We are reminded of the engineer who studied the aerodynamic characteristics of insects and concluded that bumblebees (because of their heavy body and small wings) could not fly. Are elderly adults as good at handling rapid spoken language as they appear to be, and if they are, why is this so? Most aging research has focused, not unreasonably, on areas of poor performance in the elderly. In this case we hope to explain, not why the elderly's performance is so poor, but rather, why their performance is in fact excellent. In short, we wish to ask why is it that the bumblebee can fly, and fly so well.

In this presentation we have set three goals. The first is to provide a brief tutorial in the areas under discussion. The second is to introduce several paradigms that we feel can be useful to exploring the questions we raise. Finally, in each area, we introduce recent data to illustrate the use of these paradigms. Whenever, possible, we also suggest promising directions for future research.

Special Characteristics of Spoken Language

Unlike reading, during which one can visually control the rate of word input, speech rate is primarily controlled by the speaker. Miller, Grosjean, and Lomanto (1984) have shown that there is no such thing as a "standard" speaking rate. Their study of 30 speakers in an interview situation showed mean articulation rates ranging from 153 to 336 ms per syllable and considerable variation even within a single speaker. In general, however, ordinary speech rates typically vary between 140 to 180 words per minute (wpm) in normal conversation, to over 200 wpm for a TV newsreader speaking from a prepared script. To comprehend and remember the content of this very rapid spoken discourse, the listener must accomplish a number of complex operations, many of which are performed without conscious control. Although we may describe them sequentially, many of these operations are presumed to be performed concurrently or overlapping in time (Flores D'Arcais & Scheuder, 1983; Marcus, 1984).

Speech processing begins with an initial phase in which the auditory stimulus is encoded, physical features are extracted, and lexical access is achieved. As this occurs, syntactic boundaries are determined and the linguistic content is grouped, or "parsed" into its constituent elements. Some of these processes have been described as "precognitive," in the sense that their performance seems automatic or obligatory. Phonemic processing, lexical access, and surface parsing, for example, may represent encapsulated processes over which one has little voluntary control and cannot refrain from performing (Grodzinsky & Shapiro, 1988; Liberman & Mattingly, 1989). At a still higher stage of analysis, the syntactically identified elements must be grouped into propositions (or "idea units"), in which the meaningful relationships among the words are determined (van Dijk & Kintsch, 1983). Finally, one must establish the relationships between these propositions to construct a coherence structure for the entire utterance. For this to occur, major linguistic elements must be retained and integrated with other elements. In everyday speech, the formation of inferences can be an important part of these processes, as is the ability to distinguish between literal and intended meaning.

Some of the preceding operations are presumed to be conducted on-line, as the speech is being heard. As we have indicated, lexical recognition and parsing of surface syntactic features are probably two examples (Grosjean, 1980; Marslen-Wilson, & Tyler, 1980; Wingfield & Nolan, 1980). If the listening conditions are poor, or the speech is unclear, memory-dependent retroactive analysis based on subsequent context (i.e., off-line processes) may also be required (Groajean, 1985). The integration of propositions and some forms of inference formation may also be conducted off-line, after the speech itself has passed. Therefore, it is undoubtedly true that natural language processing cannot be considered independent of limits on immediate memory capacity (Wingfield & Butterworth, 1984).

One should not assume, however, that the memory systems subserving on-line syntactic parsing and propositional analysis are necessarily the same memory systems as used for storage and recall of what has been heard or for the temporary holding of speech elements for integration across entire discourse-length passages (cf. Caplan, Vanier, & Baker, 1986; Martin, 1987). It is nevertheless the case that age-sensitive limits on working memory capacity, processing rates, or poor organizational strategies would imply decrements in some, if not all, linguistic operations.

Hearing and Age

For most people, age and memory for spoken language raise the immediate question of hearing impairment. We cannot underrate the importance of good hearing to memory for speech or deny that the incidence of hearing impairment does increase with age. Both statements are true. At the same time, the presumption of deafness in older adults is part of a prevailing "ageism" that still maintains at the time of this writing. We see this in the tendency for the young to shout their conversations with all elderly persons, regardless of any evidence of need (cf., Caporael & Culbertson, 1986; Ryan, Giles, Bartolucci, & Henwood, 1986). Even among professional investigators, hearing a report on speech memory and age often raises as the first question whether the elderly subjects could hear the stimuli—often, even when no performance decrements are being reported!

The term for age-related hearing impairment is *presbycusis*, which simply means "old hearing." There are three aspects of note. (a) *High-frequency loss*: the presence of presbycusis is virtually synonymous with a loss of sensitivity across the range of sound frequencies but most noticeably at the higher frequency ranges (e.g., above 3,000 Hz). The frequency range for most speech sounds is between 500 and 2,000 Hz, but losses at 4,000 Hz, which are not uncommon in the elderly, can produce difficulty for the high-frequency (and low-energy) sounds such as *s, th* (unvoiced), *k, f,* and *t.* (b) *Recruitment*: With age, the probability of *recruitment* is increased, an abrupt increase in perceived loudness with an increase in stimulus intensity. (c) *Phonemic regression*: Phonemic regression refers to a loss of intelligibility for speech (and other complex signals) that cannot be accounted for by the loss of sensitivity to tones alone. That is, even when the speech signal is amplified to the level at which pure tones in standard audiometric testing can be heard, when phonemic regression is present, the speech itself sounds garbled. (For a review of physiological and psychophysical factors in elderly hearing, see Olsho, Harkins, & Lenhardt, 1985).

Estimates of the incidence of hearing impairment among the elderly show considerable variability which is due to differences in method and definition of what is considered a significant impairment. Table 7.1 summarizes data on age and impairment taken from health interview surveys conducted by the National Center for Health Statistics (U.S. Congress,

TABLE 7.1. Estimated incidence of hearing impairment across age as taken from health survey interview data (U.S. Congress, Office of Technology Assessment, 1986).

Age group (years)	Reported incidence (%)
under 17	1
45–64	12
65–74	24
75 and over	39

Office of Technology Assessment, 1986, page 14). Data based on audiometric test surveys have given estimates of impaired hearing for speech at 30% for adults between age 65 and 74, and 48% for those between age 75 and 79 (Leske, 1981). Hearing impairment, however, comes in degrees, and estimates suggest that only 2% to 4% of the elderly are truly deaf (U.S. Congress, Office of Technology Assessment, 1986).

Nevertheless, investigators conducting experimental studies of memory for spoken language should be alert to the hearing acuity of their elderly (and young) subjects. Because of the possibility of phonemic regression, this attention should not focus only on pure-tone screening. Speech research with elderly adults should thus include either a pretest or control condition in which accuracy can be demonstrated for speech materials at the intensities of the to-be-remembered stimuli in the various treatment conditions. For example, if we are interested in effects of linguistic structure on speech recall, we should examine a subject's performance under the various experimental conditions or manipulations against that subject's own performance baseline in other conditions.

Aging and Memory for Speech

Under optimal conditions, elderly adults, especially those with good verbal ability and education, traditionally show little memory impairment for meaningful spoken or written prose (Hultsch & Dixon, 1984; Meyer & Rice, 1981). On the other hand, age decrements do appear when listeners are subjected to high speech-input rates (Stine, Wingfield, & Poon, 1986; Wingfield, Poon, Lombardi, & Lowe, 1985; Wingfield & Stine, 1986). There is also a possibility, although still in dispute, that age decrements may also appear when central resources are challenged by competing inputs or the need to do two things at once (Craik & McDowd, 1987; Tun, 1989).

Daneman and Carpenter (1980) have developed a span test of working memory, a measure that implies the manipulation of information being held in store rather than simply a passive buffer storage (Baddeley, 1981).

Interestingly, however, an empirical link between age-related working memory limitations and language-processing deficits have been difficult to establish (e.g., Light & Anderson, 1985). Techniques for estimating working memory (a far more difficult task than measuring simple word or digit spans) may be inadequate. Furthermore, span tests for written materials (the modality used in many experiments) may put a smaller load on working memory capacity than do listening spans (cf. Stine & Wingfield, 1987; Wingfield, Stine, Lahar, & Aberdeen, 1988).

One feature of natural language is the richness of the signal at both the waveform and linguistic levels. It has long been known that, on the waveform level, as much as 50% of the speech signal can be deleted from spoken words without a complete loss of intelligibility. On the lexical level, up to 50% of the words of narrative passages can be randomly removed without the text losing its meaning beyond recovery (see Stine, Wingfield, & Poon, 1989, for a review of evidence). Indeed, human language is so rapidly acquired and so automatic in use, that many theorists have argued that language is special among cognitive functions, that it holds a privileged place in mental processing. There is, for example, a growing consensus that speech processing at the phonemic level is conducted by specialized speech processors distinct from other, nonspeech, auditory processors in the perceptual system (Breedin & Martin, 1989; Liberman, 1982; Liberman & Mattingly, 1989). This is a contentious area, and current trends toward connectionist modeling have attempted to offer alternatives to the more traditional view that, for example, linguistic rules could not possibly develop from simple exposure to exemplars within a complex associationist system (cf. Prince & Pinker, 1988).

Methodological Approaches

In the following sections, we describe four methodologies that can be used to study several different levels of language processing. Each, we believe, can reveal important features underlying language performance in young and elderly subjects. (a) *Propositional density and speech rate:* We look first at effects of speech rate and informational density on recall accuracy. This work demonstrates significant performance declines for elderly subjects hearing sentences at very high input rates but good performance at speech rates closer to those more ordinarily encountered in everyday listening. (b) *Context and gating:* We suggest that an important reason for elderly (and young) subjects' good performance is effective use of linguistic context. We describe a methodological technique new to the aging literature that allows one to examine effects of linguistic context on language processing, even at the level of individual word recognition. (c) *Cross-modal priming and on-line processing:* A third issue we consider is that of inference formation during language processing and the extent to which some types of inference and other semantic connections may be automatically formed on-line as the speech is being heard. (d) *Parsing and recall:* Use of syntactic knowledge offers a final clue to the good performance so often observed for language processing and recall by young and elderly subjects. We describe a method we have used to study the way in which linguistic structure guides subjects' parsing strategies and immediate recall for connected speech.

Propositional Density and Speech Rate

The most explicit formulation of higher level analysis of speech beyond syntax is that of Kintsch (1988; van Dijk & Kintsch, 1983). This model proposes that discourse is processed in cycles on a segment-by-segment basis. As each segment arrives in working memory, the phonological (or orthographic) stream is recoded into a set of propositions (or "idea units"). Propositions are usually defined as having a relational term (a "predicate") and one or more relatable concepts ("arguments"). Connections among propositions are represented by a coherence graph, where the central propositions of the passage are selected ("level 1" propositions), and then other propositions are connected to them on the basis of shared arguments.

Support for this analysis has come from the finding that the number of propositions contained in a passage can increase young subjects' on-line processing loads, as measured by differential reading times across texts (Kintsch & Keenan, 1973). We have shown that propositional density (the number of propositions represented in spoken messages of equivalent word length) also increases processing load for spoken text (Stine et al., 1986).

Figure 7.1 shows data taken from a study in which subjects heard and recalled spoken sentences presented at a several speech rates (Stine et al., 1986). Although all of the sentences contained approximately the same numbers of words (all were between 16 to 18 words in length), they varied in the number of propositions each sentence contained (4, 6, 8, or 10 propositions). (Examples of high- and low-density passages and detail on their construction are given in Stine et al., 1986). Within each density category, subjects heard sentences at 200, 300, or 400 wpm.

Speech rate was varied using the "sampling" method on a Lexicon Varispeech II compressor/expander. In this method, small (20 ms) segments are periodically deleted from the recorded speech, with the remaining segments then abutted in time. The result is speech reproduced in less than normal time but without the distortion in pitch that would, for example, accompany tape-recorder playback at faster than normal speed. The degree of time compression is controlled by the frequency with which the tape segments are deleted (Foulke, 1971).

The subjects' task was simply to listen to each sentence and to recall the sentence as accurately as possible. We asked subjects to attempt verbatim recall but to use their own words if they had to. We scored the proportion

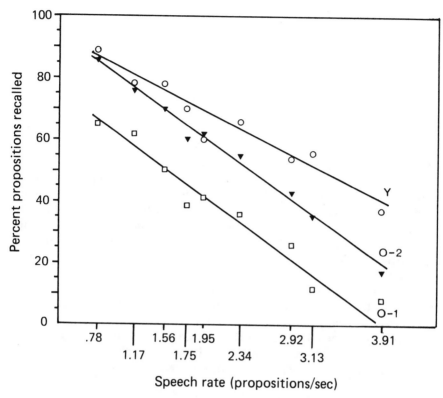

Figure 7.1. Mean percentage of propositions correctly recalled as a function of speech input rate, measured as propositions per second. Performance curves are shown for a group of young adults (Y), a group of elderly adults matched with the young for education level and Wechsler Adult Intelligence Scale (WAIS) vocabulary scores (O–1), and an elderly group with superior education level and WAIS vocabulary (O–2). (*Note.* Data from Stine, Wingfield, Poon, 1986).

of propositions correctly recalled, counting a proposition correct if the gist of it was contained in the recall.

Figure 7.1 shows performance curves for three groups of subjects. These were a young adult group (labeled "Y" on the graph), consisting of 24 university undergraduates and two groups of elderly adults, all tested on the same materials. One of the elderly groups, labeled as "O–1" in Figure 7.1, were 12 elderly adults, ranging in age from 61 to 82, who were closely matched to the young group in terms of years of education and Wechsler Adult Intelligence Scale (WAIS) vocabulary scores. The second elderly group, labeled as "O–2" in the figure, consisted of 24 community-dwelling adults, 61 to 80 years in age, of especially high verbal and educational level. Performance in the figure is plotted as the percentage of propositions recalled for the three groups as a function of speech rate in terms of propositions per second (a composite figure based on the total number of propositions combined with speech rate). As we have shown when we used this metric before (Wingfield & Stine, 1989), recall performance shows an approximately linear decline with increasing speech rate for both young and elderly subjects but with a generally steeper rate of decline with increasing speech rate for the elderly. Note that although the average and high verbal elderly groups differ in their y-intercepts (their overall levels of performance), the rates of decline for the O-1 and O-2 groups are essentially parallel. That is, the elderly group with a higher education and verbal level show overall better performance on recall than the group with lower education and verbal scores. This is consistent with traditional claims that high verbal groups generally show smaller memory deficits with age (Hultsch & Dixon, 1990). On the other hand, regardless of education and verbal ability (at least within these ranges), the two elderly groups responded equivalently to the processing overload represented by increasing speech rates.

Having pointed to this processing deficit, it is equally important to note that the data on the left side of the graph represent input rates closer to those more typically encountered in everyday speech. At these rates, we see virtually no age difference for the O–2 group. It is only under the very high input rates that the age difference begins to appear. Even the performance of the O–1 group is quite good in absolute terms.

Context and Gating

Hearing a word in a sentence context, the listener has two sources of information. One of these is the "bottom–up" information supplied by the build-up of acoustic information over the duration of the word. The second source is derived form the "top–down" information of sentence context. Speech could not be processed at the rate it normally is without this help of prior context. Indeed, the literature shows that words even heard out of context can be recognized long before their full acoustic duration has been completed (Grosjean, 1980; Marslen-Wilson, 1987). This is so because the number of words sharing the same initial sounds (the word-initial *cohort*) is limited, and as more and more of a word onset is heard, the number of potential word candidates decreases at a dramatic rate (Marslen-Wilson, 1984; Tyler, 1984). For example, in a dictionary count we conducted for picturable one- to three-syllable nouns, we found that the amount of phonological information contained in the first 50 ms of a target word was shared, on average, by some 115 other nouns. By the time the first 100 ms of the word onset had been heard, the number dropped to 43 words, then to 11 after 200 ms, and to only 5 by 300 ms. A simple power function relating the number of possible word candidates at each point in word-onset duration, and the percentage of subjects correctly identifying the words, accounted for 94% to 99% of the variance in auditory-recognition data for these words (Wayland, Wingfield, & Goodglass, 1989).

When spoken words are presented in a sentence context, they can be recognized even faster than when they are heard in isolation (Grosjean, 1980; Tyler, 1984). One place to look for an account of elderly adults' excellent abilities with speech processing is to determine whether, like young adults, they also make efficient use of context in on-line speech processing. In this regard, it would be good to seek methodological paradigms that could help identify the mechanisms by which expectations based on context facilitate processing. Studies of spoken word recognition in which word predictability was determined by presenting them within sentence contexts have shown that elderly adults can make use of context to aid word recognition as well as (Hutchinson, 1989), or even better than, the young (Cohen & Faulkner, 1983). Analogous results have also been found for visual recognition of degraded words and for lexical decision latencies (Cohen & Faulkner, 1983; Madden, 1988).

The technique of *gating* was developed by Grosjean (1980) in an attempt to model the ability to recognize words before their full word duration has been heard (see also Tyler, 1984; Tyler & Wessles, 1983). In this methodological paradigm, the duration of word-onset information (i.e., the "gate") is systematically increased across trials until the word can be correctly identified. This technique can be used to illustrate several of the preceding points, and perhaps also can help us understand how elderly subjects may use top-down information to supplement bottom-up processing deficits as may exist.

In a recent experiment using this technique, we recorded a set of 18 words in each of three sentence contexts (Wingfield, Aberdeen, & Stine, 1991; also cited in Wingfield & Stine, 1991). In one case, the sentence context created a high probability environment for the occurrence of one of our target words. An example of a high-context sentence frame was, "She gazed thoughtfully through the window," for which the word *window* was guessed by 89 of 100 people asked to supply the final word to the frame, "She gazed thoughtfully through the. . . ." We also prepared recorded frames with a lower probability of predicting one of our target words. For *window*, for example we used, "She reached up to dust the window," to which only 3 of 100 subjects gave *window* for the last word in the sentence. In the final, no-context case, target words were preceded by a neutral phrase that conveyed no information (e.g., "The word is *window*"). Each of our target words was recorded as the final word in a high-, low-, or no-context sentence frame. (The transitional probability data for our sentence frames and target words were taken from Morton, 1964, who used these stimuli for a study of context effects on visual word recognition.)

To create the "gated" stimuli, recordings of each of the sentence frames and target words were first digitized and then edited using a computer-based speech editing system, to produce a sequence of presentations in which the gate size of the target word from word onset began at 50 ms and then increased by 50-ms increments until the gate included the full word. In the experiment, subjects first heard the first 50 ms of a target word, preceded by its sentence context, and then were asked to say what they thought the word might be. If they were not correct, they would again hear the sentence plus target word, but this time they would hear 100 ms of target-word onset. Trials continued in this manner, with target-word onset duration increased in 50-ms increments, until the word was correctly identified. The gate size at which the word was first correctly identified was defined as the recognition "threshold" for that word. Our interest was to compare thresholds for the same target words when preceded by high-, low-, or no-context frames.

In addition to comparing recognition thresholds across conditions, we were also interested in subjects' errors on presentations that were too short for correct recognition. For example, in the extreme case, an error that matched the word-onset phonology of the gated target word, but did not semantically fit the sentence context, would reflect a solely bottom–up process. Errors that did not match the word-onset phonology but did fit the sentence context, would reflect top–down processes.

Our elderly subjects were 18 community-dwelling volunteers, with ages ranging from 61 to 82 years. As in the previous study, these subjects had good levels of education and WAIS vocabulary. The young subjects were 18 undergraduates ranging in age from 17 to 23 years. Their WAIS vocabulary scores were also good, although somewhat lower than those of the elderly group.

Figure 7.2 shows a series of waveforms printed from the computer screen for the sentence, "The word is *window.*" The target word *window* had a full spoken duration of 750-ms from which we created a series of fifteen 50-ms gates, five of which we show in Figure 7.2. Figure 7.2a shows the carrier phrase, "The word is", followed by the first 50 ms of the spoken target word. The vertical bands represent sound energy over time. The first grouped vertical displacement is the word *the,* which merges into the next vertical displacement which is *word,* spoken with more energy and a longer acoustic duration than *the.* This is followed by a brief flat period of near silence and then a third displacement, which is the word, *is.* This in turn is followed by the onset of the target word *window,* which we have highlighted in white. In this case, the duration of the displacement is very brief, representing only the first 50 ms of the word *onset.* The gate includes only the first part of the first phoneme, a very short /w/. When it was preceded by its high-context sentence frame, "She gazed thoughtfully through the . . .", however, this gate size was sufficient for most of the young and elderly subjects to give the full word correctly. This is a frame, you will recall, that had a probability of .98 of suggesting the word *window* from the context alone.

Figure 7.2b shows the same sentence waveform followed now by the first

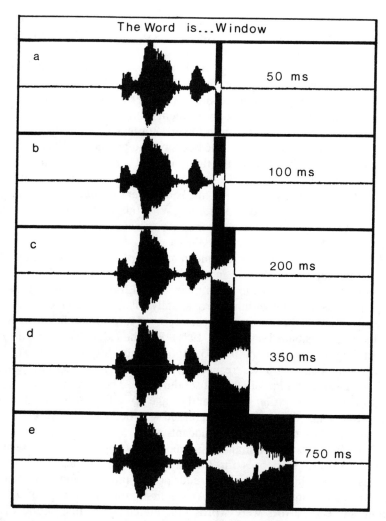

Figure 7.2. Examples of speech waveforms for the spoken sentence, "The word is window," with different word-onset gate sizes for the target word *window*. The time base in milliseconds is shown by the black and white blocked area over the target word.

100 ms of the target-word onset. The gate still includes only the initial phoneme /w/, but now it is heard in a full rich form. When preceded by the context sentence, "She reached up to dust the. . ." (in which "window" had a .30 probablity of being given from context alone), the young subjects were able to correctly identify the target with an average of 58 ms of word onset, and the elderly subjects at an average of 67 ms.

Figure 7.2c skips to a gate size of 200 ms of word onset, at which the gate now includes the first two phonemes, /wɪ/, although the second phoneme /ɪ/ remains short. Figure 7.2d shows 350 ms of word onset. The gate now includes the full word beginning of /wɪ/, plus a hint of the upcoming /n/. That is, although the /n/ cannot be heard, its arrival is signaled by the acoustic coloring of the full /ɪ/ sound in the form it takes when it is going to be followed by an /n/, or similar sound. (The term *coarticulation* is used to refer to variations in articulatory movements and their perceptual consequences, dependent on a particular phoneme context.)

At 500 ms (not shown here), one hears /w ɪ nd/, while at 550 ms, the gate begins to include the onset of the final /o/ but it remains truncated, sounding more like /ə/. At 600 ms the gate gives an unmistakable /o/, but it still sounds unnaturally short. By 750 ms, shown here in Figure 7.2e, the gate includes the full target word, *window*. (With the neutral sentence frame, young subjects gave the correct word with an average gate size of 425 ms, and the elderly at an average of 483 ms.)

Across all stimulus words, the mean gate sizes for word recognition for the young subjects was 108 ms in their high-context frames, 150 ms in their low-context frames, and 296 ms in their neutral frames. These figures correspond to recognition within approximately 20%, 26%, and 52% of word-onset duration and are close to those reported in prior studies with young adults (cf., Grosjean, 1980; Tyler, 1984). For the elderly subjects, the corresponding means were 110, 165, and 328 ms for high-context, low-context, and neutral frames, respectively. These correspond to recognition at 20%, 29%, and 57% of word-onset duration. The data showed a significant effect of context ($p < .001$) and of age ($p < .05$). Although the data suggested an age difference that increased with decreasing context, the age × context interaction was not significant.

There was, however, a major difference in the pattern of errors subjects made. Subjects' responses for the early gates in the neutral sentence frames showed that the elderly were far poorer than the young in identifying the words' initial phonemes. At the first gate, an average of 90% of young subjects' errors were words that matched the first sound of the target, as contrasted with just 65% for the elderly. By a gate size of 200 ms, however, the levels of correct first-phoneme identification for the elderly were very similar to those of the young. From these data for neutral frames, one can see that the elderly subjects were able to make use of within-word context, such as backward-operating coarticulation cues when more of the word onset was heard and perhaps also taking advantage of different sound juxtaposition frequencies as occur in English words (cf. Kinsbourne, 1973).

Of special note was the close similarity of young and elderly subject performance in the high-context condition. Word-onset recognition thresholds were virtually identical (108 ms vs. 110 ms for the young and the elderly). Also, in both context conditions, the majority of both young and elderly subjects' error responses on early gates were words that shared the same initial phoneme as the target word and that represented a reasonable semantic and syntactic fit with the sentence context. We take this as evidence of an effective use of top–down contribution to the recognition process by both subject groups. This was especially interesting in the case of the elderly subjects, who, as we can infer from the lower level of first-phoneme identification in the no-context condition, had less rich bottom–up processing than the young.

The naturalness with which the elderly (and young) subjects supplemented bottom–up processing with contextual, top–down, information, is impressive. We suggest elsewhere that this naturalness comes about because of the inherent context-dependent nature of human speech recognition. That is, the sum of numerous studies in the speech perception literature can be taken to imply a naturally evolved processing system already in place to use multiple sources of information (cf. Liberman & Mattingly, 1989). What gradually changes with age and reduced effectiveness of bottom–up processing is the *ratio* of top–down to bottom–up contributions to the perceptual process. We have suggested, in other words, that the naturalness of top–down compensation reflects only a ratio change, rather than a qualitatively different mode of processing (Wingfield & Stine, 1991).

Cross-Modal Priming and On-Line Processing

On-line methods, such as priming in lexical decisions (e.g., Burke, White, & Diaz, 1987; Howard, Shaw, & Heisey, 1986) and the measurement of on-line reading time (Stine, 1990; Zelinski, 1988) have begun to receive wide use in the cognitive aging literature. In contrast to the findings from retrospective memory measures, these paradigms have produced data showing considerable similarity in the way younger and older adults activate word concepts and process language for meaning. This conclusion may change, however, as more complex forms of language processing are explored.

We said earlier that inference is frequently involved in language comprehension and that it is here that working memory processes might be most taxed. It would be here that effects of any vulnerability at lower level stages might also be expected to accumulate. The picture, however, remains unclear. While some researchers have concluded that the older adult has particular difficulty in processing implied information (Cohen, 1979, 1981), others report a competence in inference making that is maintained over the years (Belmore, 1981; Hess & Arnold, 1986).

It is certainly the case that too much inference formation would not be a good thing in spontaneous language processing. If listeners spontaneously constructed all possible inferences in the ordinary course of comprehension, a virtual "inference explosion" would result (Rieger, 1977). Reading research suggests that readers limit inferences made on-line to those that are absolutely necessary for comprehension, while implied information that is not necessary for immediate comprehension is processed off-line, again when necessary. Some evidence indicates that "plausibility" judgments may also contribute to this process (Reder, 1982).

A primary function of inference in on-line language processing is to enable complete text comprehension (van Dijk & Kintsch, 1983). Language is understood as coherent when its component propositions are rich with referential linkages; that is, when the same concept is repeatedly referenced. This is typically accomplished through anaphoric and bridging inference. The processing of inference is presumed to require not only resources of working memory but also time. For example, reading and verification times show that individuals take longer to process text that contains inferences that must be processed than text that does not (Haviland & Clark, 1974; Kintsch, 1974) and that implied concepts are activated more slowly than explicit ones (Till, Mross, & Kintsch, 1988). In this regard, one may wonder whether some inferences are "expendable" in terms of on-line comprehension. That is, if working memory resources limit the processing of possible inferences, there may be some inferences that would only be partially processed by young adults. Such inferences might not be processed at all by older adults with more limited working memory resources or more limited rates at which they can encode new information into working memory.

An important direction for future research should be to determine the kinds of inferences that are immediately and mandatorily formed during on-line perceptual processing of speech and those that are under voluntary control and may take some time to form. Following Fodor's (1983) views, Swinney and Osterhout (1990) see the former inferences as occurring automatically in language processing as the speech in being heard. In Fodor's terms, such inferences would be an "encapsulated" process occurring so rapidly and automatically that they are independent of, and remain unconstrained by, either real-world or linguistic context. As defined, an automatic encapsulated process would be one in which the processing system performs an immediate and mandatory elaboration of inferences, even if a particular inference is an unlikely one in a particular linguistic context. Swinney and Osterhout suggest that inferences involved in establishing explicit and implicit anaphoric co-reference may be mandatory and automatic.

The question of methodology here is a difficult one, because the demonstration that an inference has been formed by later comprehension testing, direct interrogation, or analysis of recall intrusions, would not tell us when this inference was actually formed. (See McKoon & Ratcliff, 1986, for a review.) Swinney and Osterhout (1990) offer cross-modal lexical priming as a promising method to probe the time course of lexical activation of pronoun references during on-line language comprehension. For example, the subject might hear the sentence, *"The boxer visited the doctor that the swimmer at the competition advised him (*) to see about his injury."* While listening to this sentence, at either the point indicated by the asterisk or at some other point, the subject might see either a random letter string (a nonword), a neutral control word that is semantically unrelated to the sentence, or one of the words, *boxer, doctor,* or *swimmer.* The subjects' task is to press a button to indicate whether the visually presented word is a real word or a nonword. Semantic priming would be reflected by a faster "real-word" response to the pronominal reference than to an unrelated control word. The question, of course, is which word or words are activated by the pronoun *him* (i.e., boxer, doctor, or swimmer) and at which point after the occurrence of *him* this activation occurs. The sooner the activation occurs, the more on-line we can assume the inference formation to be.

As yet unpublished data brought to our attention by Edgar Zurif (personal communication) has used cross-modal lexical priming to explore linguistic "trace" theory, the view that (a) the movement of a linguistic constituent in the course of organizing a sentence for production leaves a "trace" of that original constituent in the surface structure of the sentence and (b) that the detection of this trace is necessary for thematic role assignment in sentence processing (Chomsky, 1981). Using the Swinney and Osterhout (1990) paradigm, he found both young and elderly adults to show a similar temporal pattern in lexical decision responses that implied that both age groups reactivated the semantics of the correct lexical antecedent at the trace position in a similar way. In related work, Zurif and his colleagues have used a priming technique to extend to elderly adults, as well as to young adults, claims for exhaustive access of multiple meanings of polysemous nouns even within a biasing sentence context (Stern, Prather, Swinney and Zurif, 1991).

Parsing and Recall

Processing activity at the level of surface context is important to language processing but only as it subserves organization at the propositional level and, ultimately, higher level organization of these propositions to construct overall coherence. At these levels, working memory may well play a greater role, and subjects' abilities to employ strategic options may become more flexible.

A methodology we have proposed in the past is the technique of *spontaneous segmentation* (Wingfield & Butterworth, 1984; Wingfield & Nolan, 1980), in which subjects hear paragraph-length passages of recorded speech with the freedom to interrupt the spoken input at points of their choosing for immediate recall. It is not dissimilar from the way listeners will often interrupt a rapid speaker to give themselves time to process what has been heard before the arrival of yet more information (Wingfield & Butterworth, 1984; Wingfield & Stine, 1986). It is a method that can help us to explore how young and elderly adults attempt to control the rate of speech input for accurate recall. We can illustrate this technique by demonstrating its use to examine effects of prosody on how subjects spontaneously segment speech input as it is being heard.

The term *prosody* is a general term that includes the intonation pattern (pitch contour) of speech; word stress (a complex subjective variable based on timing, pitch, and loudness); pauses that sometimes occur at the ends of major syntactic elements of sentences; and the lengthening of final vowels in words immediately before clause boundaries (Cooper & Sorensen, 1981; Wingfield, Lahar, & Stine, 1989). Prosody can indicate the mood of a speaker (happy, angry, sarcastic), mark the semantic focus of a sentence, or help disambiguate the meaning of a sentence such as, "I saw a man in the park with a telescope" (Wales & Toner, 1979). Prosodic marking of syntactic boundaries can also aid the listener in perceptually parsing heard speech into its major linguistic constituents as a step to semantic comprehension (Geers, 1978; Wingfield, 1975; Wingfield & Klein, 1971). Some evidence even indicates that prosody can tell us how long a sentence is going to be before all of it has been heard (Grosjean, 1983).

The question of prosody takes on special importance in aging for several reasons. The first comes from suggestions in the literature that elderly adults may make especially good use of prosodic structure in speech processing. We have reported some evidence for this (Stine & Wingfield, 1987), as have Cohen and Faulkner (1986), who have shown elderly adults' recall of spoken utterances to be differentially facilitated by exaggerated stress, as compared with young adults. This latter finding caused these authors to wonder aloud whether the exaggerated intonation young adults and care professionals sometimes use in speaking to elderly adults ("elderspeak") could, in principle, serve to facilitate syntactic parsing and hence sentence comprehension. We say, "in principle," because any such advantage would have to be balanced against the fact that elderspeak can reflect a patronizing attitude toward the elderly that can rob a person of his or her self-esteem (e.g., Caporael & Culbertson, 1986).

In a recent study (Wingfield et al., 1989), we used the spontaneous segmentation paradigm to look more closely at the question of whether the prosody advantage for elderly subjects is due to its help in more effectively parsing (linguistically segmenting) the speech input. This is important because we know that parsing is an essential preliminary step to meaningful organization of the linguistic input.

In one condition, subjects heard 119- to 128-word narrative passages recorded by a speaker in normal prosody at a rate of 114 wpm. In another condition, passages were recorded in "list" prosody, in which the words of the passages were read as if they were a word-list, with each word receiving equal stress, and with no timing, amplitude, or pitch variation across words. The elderly subjects for this experiment were 18 well-educated, community-dwelling volunteers, with ages ranging from 59 to 84 years. The young subjects were 18 university undergraduates ranging in age from 17 to 21 years.

TABLE 7.2. Percentage of interruptions of speech passages occurring at various linguistic boundaries for young and elderly adults hearing prose passages spoken with normal prosody and with "list" prosody.

	Normal prosody		List prosody	
	Young	Elderly	Young	Elderly
Sentence boundaries	60.6	54.5	21.8	14.5
Major clauses	27.1	29.9	38.6	34.1
Constituent components	10.1	11.0	32.9	40.2
Nonconstituents	2.1	4.6	6.7	11.3

Both subject groups selected segments of a variety of sizes, and recall for what had been selected was generally quite good. The mean recall performance across all segment sizes for the normal prose was 98.7% words correct for the young subjects and 93.1% words correct for the elderly subjects. For the passages heard in list prosody, the young averaged 97.6% words correct versus 86.3% words correct for the elderly subjects. Although the recall differences for age and prosody type tended to appear for the longer segments selected (segments more than eight words in length), than for the shorter ones, in absolute terms, recall remained good regardless of segment size selected. That is, within a baseline of generally good recall for all conditions, we observed significant effects of age ($p < .001$) and prosody ($p < .001$) and a significant age × prosody interaction ($p < .001$), indicating that the absence of normal prosody differentially hurt the elderly subjects' recall more than it did the young. Stating this finding in the positive sense, we can say that the elderly subjects made differentially better use of normal prosody when it was there than did the young subjects.

Also of interest was where the subjects chose to interrupt the speech for intermediate recall. Both subject groups interrupted the recorded speech more frequently for passages heard in list prosody than in normal prosody ($p < .001$), and the young and elderly were not markedly different in this regard; the age × prosody interaction was not significant ($p < 1$). More revealing, however, was the pattern of subjects' interruptions in terms of the linguistic structure of the heard speech. Table 7.2 shows the percentage of young and elderly subjects' interruptions that occurred at sentence boundaries and at major clause boundaries that were not also sentence boundaries. It also lists interruptions at points we have called constituent components (e.g., interruptions after nonclausal points such as nouns, verbs, and prepositions that could be used to signal the nature of the following constituents) and, finally, after nonconstituents (those remaining interruptions that did not fall into any of the preceding categories).

As we have found in earlier studies, subjects generally interrupted the speech at structurally determined linguistic points within the passages (e.g., Wingfield & Butterworth, 1984; Wingfield & Nolan, 1980). For the passages heard in normal prosody, just under 88% of all the young subjects' interruptions occurred after sentence or major clause boundaries. For the elderly subjects, this value was just over 84%. When the same passages were heard in list prosody, the numbers were reduced to just over 60% for the young subjects and just under 49% for the elderly. The effects of both age ($p < .01$) and of prosody ($p < .001$) were significant. An age × prosody interaction—which would show that the elderly subjects interrupted the passages differentially less often than the young subjects at sentence and major clause boundaries in list prosody, relative to the normal prosody passages—was only marginally significant ($p < .06$).

The reductions in mean segment sizes when the passages were deprived of normal prosody ("list" prosody) demonstrated that both young and elderly subjects spontaneously adjusted their segmentation strategies according to what we may take to be the processing difficulty of the speech stimuli imposed by the absence of normal prosody. These differences show the elderly to be as sensitive to linguistic structure as the young, the difference being in the relative importance of prosody as a signal to this structure. As we saw, the differences had a subtle effect on place and rate of parsing, but a much larger effect on recall of the segments once they had been selected.

The use of the spontaneous segmentation paradigm brings converging evidence to other data suggesting that elderly adults make especially good use of prosody in sentence processing and recall (Cohen & Faulkner, 1986; Stine & Wingfield, 1987). This returns us to the question of "elderspeak," Cohen and Faulkner's (1986) term for the tendency of young adults to use exaggerated prosodic stress when speaking to the elderly. Our results seem to add support to a growing body of evidence for a communicative benefit from good prosodic marking, and especially so for the elderly subjects. As we have indicated, however, although adjusting one's speech patterns to the individual needs of a particular elderly subject may be of value (e.g., speaking clearly to a person with a known hearing loss), overaccommodation to real or presumed deficits can easily be interpreted as being patronizing (Ryan et al., 1986). This could certainly be counterproductive to effective communication in the broader sense.

Conclusions

In considering how individuals rapidly process and remember spoken language, we have explored a number of methodologies available to examine the effects of age on this important ability. First, the effects of speech characteristics (e.g., informational density, prosody) are useful not only for testing the limits of effective processing but also for teasing apart those aspects of speech to which older adults may be differentially sensitive. Second, we considered the gating technique as a way of exploring the use of linguistic context in the form of top–down and bottom–up interactions. The use of on-line lexical verification was also suggested as a way to understand what elderly listeners comprehend as they listen and, potentially, the point within the text when this may occur. Finally, we examined the technique of spontaneous segmentation as a way of exploring on-line parsing strategies as a precursor to, or reflection of, meaningful organization of linguistic content.

The segmentation paradigm showed how prosody can be added to linguistic context as another source the elderly can use to compensate for processing deficits, so as to end up at a good level of performance. This is so, because the healthy elderly do not lose linguistic skills, and as such, they have an "expertise" in language analogous to expert systems in general (cf. Charness, 1989). The difference here, however, is that expertise in language processing has what appears to be a special place in human cognition. It is not merely that linguistic knowledge is resistant to effects of normal aging. Of special interest is the delicate balance of the speech-processing system in which a fragility of sensory processes that supply bottom–up information is met by corresponding application of top–down sources as derived from this linguistic knowledge. As such, we believe that language processing in normal aging can serve as a useful model for understanding a range of interactive principles as they may operate in complex biological and cognitive systems.

Acknowledgments. This work was supported by PHS Grants AG-04517 and AG-08382 from the National Institute on Aging.

References

Baddeley, A.D. (1981). The concept of working memory: A view of its current state and probably future developments. *Cognition, 10,* 17–27.

Belmore, S. (1981) Age-related changes in processing explicit and implicit language. *Journal of Gerontology, 36,* 316–322.

Breedin, S.D., & Martin, R.C. (1989, October). *Evidence for speech-specific processors*. Paper presented at the 27th annual meeting of the Academy of Aphasia. Santa Fe, NM.

Burke, D.M., White, H., & Diaz, D.L. (1987). Semantic priming in younger and older adults: Evidence for age constancy in automatic and attentional processes. *Journal of Experimental Psychology: Human Perception and Performance, 13,* 79–88.

Caplan, D., Vanier, M., & Baker, C. (1986). A case study of reproduction aphasia: 2. Sentence comprehension. *Cognitive Neuropsychology, 3,* 129–146.

Caporael, L.R., & Culbertson, G.H. (1986). Verbal response modes of baby talk and other speech at institutions for the aged. *Language and Communication, 6,* 99–112.

Charness, N. (1989). Age and expertise: Responding to Talland's challenge. In

L.W. Poon, D.C. Rubin, & B.A. Wilson (Eds.), *Everyday cognition in adulthood and late life* (pp. 437–456). New York: Cambridge University Press.

Chomsky, N. (1981). *Lectures on government and binding*. Dordrecht, The Netherlands: Foris.

Cohen, G. (1979). Language comprehension in old age. *Cognitive Psychology, 11*, 412–429.

Cohen, G. (1981). Inferential reasoning in old age. *Cognition, 9*, 59–72.

Cohen, G., & Faulkner, D. (1983). Word recognition: Age differences in contextual facilitation effects. *British Journal of Psychology, 74*, 239–251.

Cohen, G., & Faulkner, D. (1986). Does 'Elderspeak' work? The effect of intonation and stress on comprehension and recall of spoken discourse in old age. *Language and Communication, 6*, 91–98.

Cooper, W.E., & Sorensen, J. (1981). *Fundamental frequency in sentence production*. Berlin: Springer-Verlag.

Craik, F.I.M., & McDowd, J.M. (1987). Age differences in recall and recognition. *Journal of Experimental Psychology: Learning, Memory and Cognition, 13*, 474–479.

Daneman, M., & Carpenter, P.A. (1980). Individual differences in working memory and reading. *Journal of Verbal Learning and Verbal Behavior, 19*, 450–466.

Flores D'Arcais, G.B., & Scheuder, R. (1983). The process of language understanding: A few issues in contemporary psycholinguistics. In G.B. Flores D'Arcais & K.J. Jarvella (Eds.), *The process of language understanding* (pp. 1–41). New York: Wiley.

Fodor, J.A. (1983). *Modularity of mind*. Cambridge, MA: MIT Press.

Foulke, E. (1971). The perception of time compressed speech. In D.L. Horton & J.J. Jenkins (Eds.), *The perception of language* (pp. 79–107). Columbus, OH: Merrill.

Grodzinsky, Y., & Shapiro, L.P. (1988). Two perspectives on the modularity of language. *Aphasiology, 2*, 295–298.

Geers, A.E. (1978). Intonation contour and syntactic structure as predictors of apparent segmentation. *Journal of Experimental Psychology: Human Perception and Performance, 4*, 273–283.

Grosjean, F. (1980). Spoken word recognition processes and the gating paradigm. *Perception and Psychophysics, 28*, 299–310.

Grosjean, F. (1983). How long is the sentence? Prediction and prosody in the on-line processing of language. *Linguistics, 21*, 501–529.

Grosjean, F. (1985). The recognition of words after their acoustic offset: evidence and implications. *Perception and Psychophysics, 38*, 299–310.

Haviland, S.E., & Clark, H.H. (1974). What's new? Acquiring new information as a comprehension process. *Journal of Verbal Learning and Verbal Behavior, 3*, 512–521.

Hess, T.M., & Arnold, D. (1986). Adult age differences in memory for explicit and implicit sentence information. *Journal of Gerontology, 41*, 191–194.

Howard, D.V., Shaw, R.J., & Heisey, J.G. (1986). Aging and the time course of semantic activation. *Journal of Gerontology, 41*, 195–203.

Hultsch, D., & Dixon, R.A. (1984). Memory for text materials in adulthood. *Life span development and behavior* (Vol. 6). New York: Academic Press.

Hultsch, D., & Dixon, R.A. (1990). Learning and memory and aging. In J.E.

Birren & K.W. Schaie (Eds.), *Handbook of the psychology of aging* (3rd ed., pp. 258–274). New York: Academic Press.

Hutchinson, K.M. (1989). Influence of sentence context on speech perception in young and older adults. *Journal of Gerontology: Psychological Sciences, 44*, P36–44.

Kinsbourne, M. (1973). Age effects on letter span related to rate and sequential dependency. *Journal of Gerontology, 28*, 317–319.

Kintsch, W. (1974). *The representation of meaning in memory.* Hillsdale, NJ: Erlbaum.

Kintsch, W. (1988). The role of knowledge in discourse comprehension: A construction-integration model. *Psychological Review, 95*, 163–182.

Kintsch, W., & Keenan, J. (1973). Reading rate and retention as a function of the number of propositions in the base structure of sentences. *Cognitive Psychology, 5*, 257–274.

Leske, M.C. (1981). Prevalence estimates of communicative disorders in the U.S.: Language, hearing, and vestibular disorders. *Asha, 23*, 229–237.

Liberman, A.M. (1982). On finding that speech is special. *American Psychologist, 37*, 148–167.

Liberman, A.M., & Mattingly, I.G. (1989). A specialization for speech perception. *Science, 243*, 489–494.

Light, L.L., & Anderson, P.A. (1985). Working-memory capacity, age, and memory for discourse. *Journal of Gerontology, 40*, 737–747.

Madden, D.J. (1988). Adult age differences in the effects of sentence context and stimulus degradation during visual word recognition. *Psychology and Aging, 3*, 167–172.

Marcus, S.M. (1984). Recognizing speech: On mapping of sound to word. In H. Bouma & D.G. Bouwhuis (Eds.), *Attention and performance X* (pp. 151–163). Hillsdale, NJ: Erlbaum.

Marslen-Wilson, W.D. (1984). Function and process in spoken word recognition. In H. Bouma & D.G. Bouwhuis (Eds.), *Attention and performance X* (pp. 125–150). Hillsdale, NJ: Erlbaum.

Marslen-Wilson, W.D. (1987). Functional parallelism in spoken word recognition. *Cognition, 25*, 71–102.

Marslen-Wilson, W.D., & Tyler, L.K. (1980). The temporal structure of spoken language understanding. *Cognition, 8*, 1–71.

Martin, R.C. (1987). Articulatory and phonological deficits in short-term memory and their relation to syntactic processing. *Brain and Language, 32*, 159–192.

McKoon, G., & Ratcliff, R. (1986). Inferences about predictable events. *Journal of Experimental Psychology; Learning, Memory and Cognition, 12*, 82–91.

Meyer, B.J.F., & Rice, G.E. (1981). Information recalled from prose by young, middle, and old adult readers. *Experimental Aging Research, 7*, 253–268.

Miller, J.L., Grosjean, F., & Lomanto, C. (1984). Articulation rate and its variability in spontaneous speech: A reanalysis and some implications. *Phonetica, 41*, 215–225.

Mitchell, D.B., & Hunt, R.R. (1989). How much "effort" should be devoted to memory? *Memory and Cognition, 17*, 337–348.

Morton, J. (1964). The effects of context on the visual duration threshold for words. *British Journal of Psychology, 55*, 165–180.

Olsho, L.W., Harkins, S.W., & Lenhardt, M.L. (1985). Aging and the auditory system. In J.E. Birren & K.W. Schaie (Eds.), *Handbook of the psychology of aging* (2nd ed., pp. 332–377). New York: Van Nostrand Reinhold.

Prince, A., & Pinker, S. (1988). Rules and connections in human language. *Trends in Neuroscience, 11,* 195–202.

Rankin, J.L., Karol, R., & Tuten, C. (1984). Strategy use, recall, and recall organization in young, middle-aged, and elderly adults. *Experimental Aging Research, 10,* 193–196.

Reder, L.M. (1982). Plausibility judgments vs. fact retrieval: Alternative strategies for sentence verification. *Psychological Review, 89,* 250–280.

Rieger. C. (1977). Spontaneous computation in cognitive models. *Cognitive Science, 1,* 315–354.

Ryan, E.B., Giles, H., Bartolucci, G., & Henwood, K. (1986). Psycholinguistic and social psychological components of communication by and with the elderly. *Language and Communication, 6,* 1–24.

Salthouse, T.A. (1985). *A theory of cognitive aging.* Amsterdam: North Holland.

Smith, A.D. (1980). Age differences in encoding, storage, and retrieval. In L.W. Poon, J.L. Fozard, L.S. Cermak, D. Arenberg, & L.W. Thompson (Eds.), *New directions in memory and aging: Proceedings of the George A. Talland Memorial Conference* (pp. 23–45). Hillsdale, NJ: Erlbaum.

Stern, C., Prather, P., Swinney, D., & Zurif, E.B. (1991). The time course of automatic lexical access and aging. *Brain and Language, 40,* 359–372.

Stine, E.A.L. (1990). On-line processing of written text by younger and older adults. *Psychology and Aging, 5,* 68–78.

Stine, E.A.L., & Wingfield, A. (1987). Process and strategy in memory for speech among younger and older adults. *Psychology and Aging, 2,* 272–279.

Stine, E.A.L., Wingfield, A., & Poon, L.W. (1986). How much and how fast: rapid processing of spoken language by older adults. *Psychology and Aging, 86,* 303–311.

Stine, E.A.L., Wingfield, A., & Poon, L.W. (1989). Speech comprehension and memory through adulthood: The roles of time and strategy. In L.W. Poon, D.C. Rubin, & B.A. Wilson (Eds.), *Everyday cognition in adulthood and late life* (pp. 195–221). New York: Cambridge University Press.

Swinney, D., & Osterhout, L. (1990). Inference generation during auditory language comprehension. In A. Graesser & G.H. Bower (Eds.), *The psychology of learning and motivation* (Vol. 25, pp. 294–306). Academic Press.

Till, R., Mross, E.F., & Kintsch, W. (1988). Time course of priming for associate and inference words in discourse content. *Memory and Cognition, 16,* 283–298.

Tun, P.A. (1989). Age differences in processing expository and narrative text. *Journal of Gerontology, 44,* 9–15.

Tyler, L. (1984). The structure of the initial cohort: evidence from gating. *Perception and Psychophysics, 36,* 417–427.

Tyler, L., & Wessels, J. (1983). Quantifying contextual contributions to word-recognition processes. *Perception and Psychophysics, 34,* 409–420.

U.S. Congress, Office of Technology Assessment (1986, May). *Hearing impairment and elderly people—A background paper* (OTA-BP-BA-30). Washington, DC: U.S. Government Printing Office.

van Dijk, T.A., & Kintsch, W.A. (1983). *Strategies of discourse comprehension.* New York: Academic Press.

Wales, R., & Toner, H. (1979). Intonation and ambiguity. In W.E. Cooper & E.C.T. Walker (Eds.), *Sentence processing: Psycholinguistics studies presented to Merrill Garrett* (pp. 135–158). Hillsdale, NJ: Erlbaum.

Wayland, S.C., Wingfield, A., & Goodglass, H. (1989). Recognition of isolated words: The dynamics of cohort reduction. *Applied Psycholinguistics, 10,* 475–487.

Wingfield, A. (1975). Acoustic redundancy and the perception of time compressed speech. *Journal of Speech and Hearing Research, 18,* 96–104.

Wingfield, A., Aberdeen, J.S., & Stine, E.A.L. (1991). Word-onset gating and linguistic context in spoken word recognition by young and elderly adults. *Journal of Gerontology: Psychological Sciences, 46,* P127–129.

Wingfield, A., & Butterworth, B. (1984). Running memory for sentences and parts of sentences: Syntactic parsing as a control function in working memory. In H. Bouma & D.G. Bouwhuis (Eds.), *Attention and performance X* (pp. 351–363). Hillsdale NJ: Erlbaum.

Wingfield, A., & Klein, J.F. (1971). Syntactic structure and acoustic pattern in speech perception. *Perception and Psychophysics, 9,* 23–25.

Wingfield, A., Lahar, C.J., & Stine, E.A.L. (1989). Age and decision strategies in running memory for speech: Effects of prosody and linguistic structure. *Journal of Gerontology; Psychological Sciences, 44,* P106–113.

Wingfield, A., & Nolan, K.A. (1980). Spontaneous segmentation in normal and in time-compressed speech. *Perception and Psychophysics, 28,* 97–102.

Wingfield, A., Poon, L.W., Lombardi, L., & Lowe, D. (1985). Speed of processing in normal aging: Effects of speech rate, linguistic structure, and processing time. *Journal of Gerontology, 40,* 579–585.

Wingfield, A., & Stine, E.A.L. (1986). Organizational strategies in immediate recall of rapid speech by young and elderly adults. *Experimental aging research, 12,* 79–83.

Wingfield, A., & Stine, E.A.L. (1989). Modeling memory processes: Research and theory on memory and aging. In G.C. Gilmore, P.J. Whitehouse, & M.L. Wykle (Eds.), *Memory, aging, and dementia: Theory, assessment, and treatment* (pp. 4–40). New York: Springer.

Wingfield, A., & Stine, E.A.L. (1991). Expert systems in nature: Spoken language processing and adult aging. In J.D. Sinnott, & J.C. Cavanaugh (Eds.), *Bridging paradigms: Positive cognitive development in adulthood and aging* (pp. 237–258). New York: Praeger.

Wingfield, A., Stine, E.A.L., Lahar, C.J., & Aberdeen, J.S. (1988). Does the capacity of working memory change with age? *Experimental Aging Research, 14,* 193–107.

Zelinski, E.M. (1988). Integration of information from discourse: Do older adults show deficits? In L.L. Light & D.M. Burke (Eds.), *Language, memory, and aging* (pp. 117–132). New York: Cambridge University Press.

8
Symbolic Processing of Youth and Elders

KATHRYN L. JEPSON AND GISELA LABOUVIE-VIEF

Whereas cognitive aging research often suggests that extensive and irreversible deficits in the information processing system occur as a natural part of aging (Kausler, 1982; Poon, 1985; Salthouse, 1985), several authors recently have asked if, in addition to decremental patterns, aging also may bring adaptive changes. According to that view (for discussion, see Labouvie-Vief & Schell, 1982), some apparent deficits may be the result of an assumption inherent in many information processing approaches— namely, that no major cognitive *qualitative* changes occur after early adulthood. As an inevitable consequence, evidence that mature and older adults process information qualitatively *differently* is interpreted as but another instance of a long list of later-life *deficits*.

Most suggestions that mature adulthood may bring continued qualitative reorganizations are derived in one way or another from critiques of Piaget's theory of social-cognitive maturity, specifically, as these critiques have been formulated by Riegel (1973), and Perry (1968). Contrary to Piaget's notion that adolescence brings the apogee of abstract formal thought, Perry suggested that young college students' ability to handle abstractions still is profoundly limited, because they believe that only one perspective exists on abstract notions such as "truth" or "reality." Hence, they believe that information can be captured in terms of a single, "objective," and outer reality. With continued development, in turn, individuals are able to form a more contextual and integrative understanding, in which the subjective and inner dimensions of information are elaborated, as well. This general finding since has been confirmed with several different methods (Arlin, 1989; Blanchard-Fields, 1986; Commons, Richards, & Armon, 1984; Commons, Richards, & Kuhn, 1982; Kitchener, 1983; Kitchener & King, 1981; Kitchener, King, Wood, & Davison, 1989; Kramer, 1983; Kramer & Woodruff, 1984; Kuhn, Pennington, & Leadbeater, 1983; Labouvie-Vief & Hakim-Larson, 1989; Sinnott, 1989).

This cognitive-developmental perspective, then, suggests that the hypothesized "inward turn" (Neugarten, 1968) with increasing age may be the result of a cognitive and epistemological restructuring. This shift, in turn,

124

may have consequences for how younger and older individuals process information (see Adams, Labouvie-Vief, Hobart, & Dorosz, 1990; Labouvie-Vief & Blanchard-Fields, 1982). For the young, the emphasis is more likely to be on objective, analytical and literal processes, while for the mature and older adults, it is more likely to be on inner, subjective, psychological, and symbolic processes.

Past research (e.g., Labouvie-Vief, DeVoe, & Bulka, 1989) has demonstrated how this restructuring affects such "everyday" cognitions as individuals' efforts at coping and emotion regulation. In this chapter, we focus on another domain—how individuals encode and interpret such "everyday" materials as narratives with symbolic meaning. Using a qualitative method, we provide evidence to show that younger individuals adopt a rather literal approach, whereas older adults focus more on the inner and symbolic.

Evidence to suggest such a literal-to-symbolic restructuring comes from several areas of study. Using free association and a word symbolism task, DeWit (1963) found that categorical style appears to shift with age. Adolescents were prone to use the logical category name (rose-flower), and when their responses were symbolic, they tended to use the association symbol category (rose-spring). Adults made more use of the symbolic categories than did the adolescents, using object–person analogy symbols (rose-mother) and abstract idea analogy symbols (rose-beauty). DeWit proposed that the formal categorical thinking of the adolescent serves as a "developmental bridge" (1963, p. 101) between his or her formerly dominant mode of categorical association to the mode preferred by the adult, which is abstract, analogous, and symbolic. This shift from a reliance on formal systems to more relative systems of thought enables the adult to use broader categories and is the result of the adult's integration of a formal logical approach with more idiosyncratic and personalized ways of thinking.

DeWit's (1963) results also expand other research on categorization in young and old adults. Early studies (see Denney, 1982) suggested that shift in categorical style and problem solving was a regressive phenomenon: Older adults were thought to lose the ability to define categorical boundaries, changing to functional modes of categorization instead. Research such as DeWit's suggests that this trend is integrative, rather than regressive. Indeed, this interpretation is in line with data that suggest category depth increases with age (Birren, 1979; Kogan, 1974; Kramer & Woodruff, 1984).

Another area in which the hypothesized shift from youth to later adulthood appears is metaphor recall and interpretation. Labouvie-Vief, Campbell, Weaverdyck, and Tanenhaus (1980) examined age differences in metaphor recall. Although cue type (literal or symbolic) produced no effect, the *structure* of recall was different. The young (mean age = 23.6) gave predominantly literal responses, while the older adults (mean age =

76.5) primarily responded in terms of meaning-preserving transformations. These response styles could reflect use of different processing styles. When scoring both recall types as correct, age differences disappeared (Labouvie-Vief et al., 1980).

From a somewhat different angle, Boswell (1979) examined age differences in explanations for metaphors. Boswell found that adults (mean age = 70.1) produced significantly more synthesizing (analogous or symbolic, poetic) explanations than the youth (mean age = 18.0), who relied on a primarily analytic (literal or logical) style. Thus, Boswell suggested that later adulthood brings a major shift in organization of thought, from the literal-analytic to the poetic-synthetic (Boswell, 1979). Kramer and Wood-ruff (1984), however, did not replicate this finding.

A third paradigm has been to investigate the recall of narratives by young and older adults. Labouvie-Vief, Schell, and Weaverdyck (1981) had subjects listen to a fable and then recall it under different conditions, "recall" and "summary." The youth (mean age = 22.3) responded the same way under both conditions and provided detailed, faithful reproductions of the text. In contrast, the older adults (mean age = 74.2) responded differentially to the instruction conditions. They performed like younger adults in response to recall, but under summary instructions, they were more likely to give brief protocols focusing on gist. Specifically, they tended to represent the moral, social-normative, and symbolic meaning of the fable. Labouvie-Vief et al. (1981) conclude that knowledge structure differences may account for the age differences seen; that is, that youth and elders process the same information with different modes of processing, thereby yielding different styles of response.

In an extension of the preceding study, Adams et al. (1990) used both a fable and a nonfable text. These authors also found age-related qualitative differences in recall. Protocols of young subjects were heavily text based, while the responses of the older adults were more integrative. In addition, older adults also often offered an interpretive sort of component to their responses, adding moralistic or social-normative information.

These results, however, appeared to depend on text type: They held for the nonfable but not for the fable (Adams et al., 1990). The source of this disagreement with earlier studies is not clear at this time. One possibility is that some themes are more readily interpreted by some age groups. Another possibility is that difficulty level (e.g., whether the text is simple and clear or abstract and filled with detail) may affect interpretation.

In an earlier study, Adams (1986) explored thematic differences in a detailed investigation of two groups of adolescents (13–15, 16–19) and two groups of adults (39–55, 60+). Adams used two different stimulus texts, a narrative story and an expository essay. These texts produced similar yet different patterns of age-related responses to recall and to summarize the texts. In narrative text, adolescents reproduced the story's text fairly literally. A shift in processing style occurred in middle age, however. Middle-aged adults were as good as the young in capturing the literal meaning of the text. But in addition, they added another dimension of the subjective aspects of narrative, imbuing and integrating the propositional content with psychological meanings and becoming more interpretive. The older adults maintained the interpretive style. However, unlike the youth and middle-aged, there was a loss of literal detail.

Thus it appears, from this and other studies, that a shift in mode of processing occurs during adulthood to orient more to symbolic dimensions. At the same time, it is possible that subjects respond differentially to different types of material. The resulting interaction of age and material forms the focus of the present study. Specifically, we hypothesized that age differences would be found in response to symbolic elements of fairy tales, with adolescents relying more on verbatim representations of the text and mid-life and older adults more likely to interpret the tales symbolically. We also expected, however, that this effect would be moderated by story type. Thus, we used two tales, one representative of youth and one of aging.

Method

Subjects

A total of 60 subjects from three age groups (early adolescence, 13–15 years; midadulthood, 40–55 years; later adulthood, 65–88 years) participated in this study. An equal number of males and females were in each group. The sample was drawn from middle- to upper-middle-class communities and neighborhoods in a large Midwestern metropolitan area, and it was homogeneous with regard to occupational status (for adolescents, parent's status was used), education, and self-rated health.

Procedure

All subjects read two fairy tales and were subsequently interviewed about the symbolic content of these tales. In addition, we administered a background interview and a measure of verbal ability (Jastak & Jastak, 1964).

The fairy tales used are representative of the thematically distinct youth and elder tales that Chinen (1987, 1989) described. Tales that feature young protagonists reflect the ego in formation. They focus on "personal" development, paralleling the psychology of youth who are attempting to become individuals in the real world. In contrast, Chinen argues that tales that feature old adults as protagonists are centered on themes of poverty, self-reformation, transcendence, wisdom, emancipated innocence, and mediation with the supernatural.

On the basis of these considerations, we chose two tales. These tales were abbreviated versions of tales which had been edited into narrative form. The youth tale, "The Tale of the Faraway Islands" (from "The Tale of the Oki Islands" in Cole, 1982), focused on a young girl's quest to be reunited with her father, a lord who was unjustly banished. The girl encounters many obstacles to her goal, which she overcomes one by one. The final obstacle, a monster that has terrorized the islands, is slain by the girl, who has found a totem of the king in the monster's possession. The king, who recovered from a long illness as these events took place, links them, and finally, father and daughter are reunited. As an example of the style and readability of the text, the first paragraph follows:

Many, many years ago there lived a tyrannical and dictatorial king. One of his lords had displeased him, and the king, to punish him, banished the lord to a wild rocky group of islands off the coast which were known as the Faraway Islands. He was lonely there, for he'd been forced to leave his beautiful young daughter behind.

In contrast, "How an Old Man Lost His Wen," the elder tale, is an account of one man's fortunate encounter with the supernatural world (the full text can be found in Chinen, 1985, 1987, 1989). The man, who has resigned himself to a disfiguring growth, happens on some demons in the woods. The demons are in need of entertainment, and the old man's love of dance is stronger than his fear of the demons, so he dances for them—they remove his growth to ensure his return. This old man's greedy neighbor, afflicted with a similar growth, takes the old man's place the next day and suffers an unfortunate fate. The first paragraph of the text follows:

Many years ago there lived a good old man who had a wen like a tennis-ball growing out of his right cheek. The lump disfigured the old man and he tried in vain to get rid of it. Finally, he resigned himself to the wen and even joked about it.

These tales were moderately abbreviated versions of Chinese fairy tales (about 600 words each). The stories were at the same level of readability—high seventh grade—according to the Fry (1968) readability formula. Subjects were simultaneously presented with both typewritten and audiotaped versions of the stories. The typewritten version was presented in Orator font, and the audiotaped stories were presented over headphones.

Subjects were tested individually in a quiet room in their own homes or at a neutral location, by one of four female interviewers. Story condition was counterbalanced across age and sex, so that each story appeared as story 1 an equal number of times. Following presentation of the first story, the interviewer removed the stimulus materials and administered a background questionnaire. Next, the written version of the story was returned, and subjects responded to an interview about the symbolic meaning of specific events and characters of the tales. To construct the interview, 10 graduate students familiar with text processing were asked to nominate the most salient symbolic events of each story. From this list, five interview questions per story were generated. This study focuses on one question per story; a majority of subjects rated these questions as the "most important" aspect of the story.

After subjects completed the first symbolic interview, they were presented with the second story. Story 2 was followed by the verbal abilities test. Next, the second symbolic interview was administered. Total testing time was $1\frac{1}{2}$ to $2\frac{1}{2}$ hours.

Scoring

Responses to the symbolic interview were audiotaped and transcribed. Unitization used the "idea unit" (e.g., Adams, 1986; Brown & Smiley, 1977; Johnson, 1970) as the basic unit of analysis. Idea units expressed a single action, event, or state as an explicit or implicit subject-verb-object clause. In the case of protocol unitization, we assigned each protocol an arbitrary number to blind the coder as to age and sex of the subject. Notwithstanding the flow of speech reflected in the interview protocols, every attempt was made to segment distinct ideas within that flow.

Next, we classified protocol units into one of five categories that were mutually exclusive. The first category included comments not relevant to how individuals interpret, while the remaining four categories represented levels of symbolic understanding, from literal to complex symbolic.

CATEGORY 0: COMMENTS

The category 0 statements did not directly answer or respond to the interviewer's questions or comments; therefore, they could not be coded with a particular "level" of response or abstraction from the text. Comments consisted mainly of inquiries for clarification and "I don't know" statements. The general rule was to try to code in any other category before this.

CATEGORY 1: TEXT-BASED STATEMENTS

The category 1 statements were literal responses, that is, repetitions or paraphrases of the text units themselves. To qualify as a text-based statement, the unit could be tied to only one of the units in the text (e.g., Island story: "it just says she found a wooden statue of the king"; Wen story: "it says they decided the old man would return if they took his wen").

CATEGORY 2: TEXT-BASED INFERENCES

The category 2 responses went beyond simple literal text repetitions but involved some inference. These inferences remained very concrete and were directly tied to the text. Unlike category 1 responses, however, they were not mere paraphrases but synthesized two or more text units. Nevertheless, these inferences were not abstract or symbolic because individuals were concerned only with inferences directly called for by the text. Specifically, three types of category 2 statements were coded: Statements about actions and events (e.g., Wen story: "They [the demons] were looking for anything that would bring the man back"); statements referring to psychological attributes (e.g., Island story: "she had a strong will"); and simple speculations, attempting to put a story event into perspective (e.g., Wen story: "maybe they were judged before").

CATEGORY 3: SIMPLE SYMBOLIC INFERENCES

The main difference between category 2 and 3 inferences was that the latter were not concerned merely with literal extensions of the text. Rather, the objects, events, and people referred to in the text were taken to stand for something outside the text per se, that is, as a symbol of real-life events or objects. Nevertheless, the symbols in this category remained fairly concrete and/or undifferentiated. Specifically, one or both of the following conditions must have been present for inclusion into this category: (a) The symbol referred to a general but concrete and physical character event, as when interpreting the "wen" as referring to any physical disfigurement, (e.g., Wen story: "Well, I think of it as like The Elephant Man. A facial ugliness"); or (b) the symbol referred to absolute opposing forces, such as good versus evil (e.g., Islands story: "We have to be taught to think of others. It has to be instilled in us somehow. So there has to be good and bad. We are basically not good people").

CATEGORY 4: COMPLEX SYMBOLIC INFERENCES

Like category 3, the inferences in category 4 were symbolic, but they were less concrete and more abstract because they referred to more general psychological aspects of human functioning. For example, many interpretations of "wen" no longer referred to it as a general physical disfigurement but rather highlighted its psychological dimensions. These dimensions were generalized to refer not only to the story characters but to humanity in general. (E.g., Wen story: "We have other aspects of our lives. We have a mental aspect of our lives that we can concentrate on. And we have a spiritual aspect of our lives that we can concentrate on. If we happen to have shortcomings in a physical aspect, why let our whole life go down the drain because of that? We can develop other areas.") More generally, statements at this level referred to an inner, psychological reality rather than one that is outer and physical (e.g., Islands story: "But, alot of times things that appear to be situations outside ourselves are really things that we need to be conquering inside. But we have to have that outside confrontation to find out who we are and what we're made of"). Overall, statements integrated dualistic themes, asserted that opposing forces can coexist, and/or integrated concrete and symbolic dimensions of reality.

Coding

The preceding scheme was applied to each unit of each protocol. The 60 protocols for each story were randomly divided into six batches of 20 (10 Wen and 10 Islands protocols). The coding system was refined on the first batch, with the first author and two advanced undergraduate students acting as coders. After the coding system was trained, it was applied to the remaining five batches. We derived two reliability measures. Both were based on intraclass correlations, computed on a randomly selected subsample of 20% of the protocols. Using the method suggested by Shrout and Fleiss (1979), the first measure was one of intrarater reliability, and yielded $r = .86$ for the Wen, and $r = .86$ for the Islands stories. Second, we calculated a measure of interrater reliability across the three coders. Reliability coefficients were .89 for the Wen story, and .87 for the Island story.

Verbal Ability Measure

Because verbal ability is correlated with overall intellectual ability, an index of this was obtained. The Jastak and Jastak (1964) is an objectively scored, 20-item version of the Wechsler Adult Intelligence Scale-Revised (WAIS-R) vocabulary scale, which can be administered in written form. Items were scored 0, 1, or 2, depending on whether the response was incorrect, partially correct, or completely correct, respectively.

Results

Several preliminary analyses were performed on variables that may have been related to outcome variables of interest. We conducted these analyses to examine possible confounds that may have been due to interviewer location, story order, and the effect of other background variables. None of these variables was significantly related to the interview levels.

Because the interview protocols varied in length, data analyses were based on the interview protocol's percentage of responses in each category. To examine the effects of age and story type for each category, we calculated separate 3 (age-group) $\times$ 2 (sex) $\times$ 2 (story) analyses of variance (ANOVAs), resulting in five ANOVAs. (The dependent variables of percentage of responses at category levels were treated in simple ANOVAs, rather than as a multivariate ANOVA, because of the linear dependence of the levels.)

Main effects of age-group occurred for category 2, text-based inferences, $F(2,51) = 4.35, p < .02$; category 3, simple symbolic inferences, $F(2,51) = 11.20, p < .00$; and marginally at category 4, complex symbolic inferences

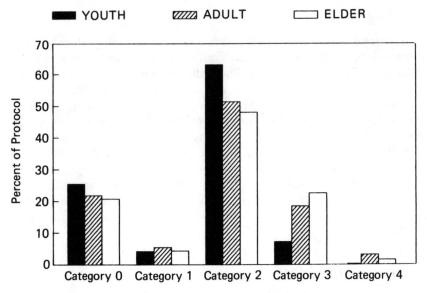

FIGURE 8.1. Percentage of protocol at each category by age.

$F(2,51) = 3.09$, $p < .054$ (see Figure 8.1). Although age groups did not differ in the number of comments or text-based statements (categories 0 and 1), with increasing age, individuals made fewer text-based inferences (category 2), while increasing in simple symbolic inferences (category 3).

Overall, the percentage of use of categories 2 (text-based inference) and 3 (simple symbolic inference) suggests that across age, there was an almost perfect trade-off of the type of inferential category used. As use of category 2 declined, this decrease was almost exactly compensated by the increase in category 3; and overall, all age levels used categories 2 and 3 about 70% of the time. Youth used category 2 on the average 63.2%, and category 3 an average of 7.2% of the time. Adults used category 3 more than twice as often as the youth, using category 2 an average of 51.3% and category 3 an average of 18.4%. Finally, elders used category 2 an average of 48.0% and category 3 an average of 22.5%.

We found a main effect for story at category 2 $F(1,51) = 7.22$, $p < .01$, and category 4, $F(1,51) = 7.21$, $p < .01$. The story effect indicates that more text-based inferences and fewer complex symbolic inferences were made for the Islands story.

A significant three-way interaction of age-group × sex × story occurred at category 1, text-based statements, $F(2,51) = 4.0$, $p < .02$. The pattern of this relationship was inverse for each story. For the Wen story, males appeared to have an age-related increase, while females had an age-related decrease in the use of this category. For the Islands story, the middle-aged men were lower, while the middle-aged women were higher in the use of this category than other age groups. However, because this finding bears no impact on the outcomes of interest here (i.e., categories 2, 3, and 4), it will not be discussed further.

A final analysis concerned the relationship between verbal ability and symbolic inferencing. One-way ANOVA results showed that verbal ability distinguished the youth from the adult groups. The adult groups scored on the average twice as high as the youth; the mean score for midlife adults = 30.9, for elders = 33.75, and for adolescents = 16.6, $F(2,57) = 31.86$, $p < .001$. In addition, verbal ability correlated negatively with category 0 for the Wen story ($-.31, p < .05$), and positively for both stories with categories $3 + 4$ (Wen story, .51, $p < .01$, Islands story, .34, $p < .05$). When verbal ability was used as a covariate, the age-group effect at category 4 was eliminated, but the effect remained at the other levels. That is, significant age-group differences still exist for categories 2 and 3 when verbal ability was held constant.

Discussion

The main hypothesis of this research was that a processing shift would occur with increasing age. Specifically, in the processing of a fairy tale, older adults would have more symbolic responses, while relying less on literal interpretations of the text. The results provide clear support for the main hypothesis that there are age-group differences in symbolic processing. With age, subjects were less likely to respond with text-based inferences (category 2) and were more likely to use simple symbolic inferences (category 3). Adults also tended to use complex symbolic inferences (category 4) more often than adolescents.

These results support the notion that symbolic processing is different at varying points in the life span. Overall the data suggest that although there is the same overall *amount* of inferencing (at categories 2, 3, and 4), the *type* of inferencing shifts. In fact, there is an almost perfect trade-off: As category 2 use declined with age, that of categories 3 and 4 increased. Thus, qualitative change, not deficit, appears to be responsible for the difference in response between these age groups.

While the age-group effect was significant across the stories, there were, however, story differences. The Wen story appeared to be a simpler tale, easier for subjects of all ages to understand. Furthermore, some evidence indicated that hearing and reading the Islands story first had an interfering effect. While our assumption was that each story spoke to different age groups, overall, the Islands story seemed to be more difficult for *all* age groups. The Wen story appeared to be clearer and more involving, while the Islands story was confusing and difficult to follow. Results may have been different if stories were more precisely matched in terms of variables such as number of adjectives and the like.

One possible limitation of the results of this study relates to the type of text used. Our results contradict those of other researchers who have explored age-related changes in semantic integration (see Hultsch & Dixon, 1984). A basic difference between these two lines of research, however, is that we used a different genre, narrative, which may call for symbolic responses (see Adams, 1986). In addition, the coding system is unlike most that are used in research on semantic integration, which focus on the amount of direct correspondence between the text materials and subject responses. In contrast, we have found such systems to be biased in favor of the responses of youth, while our system specifically includes the symbolic, generalizing responses found in mature and older age groups. Thus, the meaning of "semantic integration" clearly differs for the two lines of research.

Another potential limitation of the results of this study is that for our "young" group we chose adolescents rather than the age group most often used in research on inference and aging, namely college-aged youth. Available research, however, suggests that our selection has not invalidated the results. For instance, Adams (1986) included both early and late adolescent groups in her study yet found no differences in interpretive responses between these two groups. Rather, the tendency to make interpretations appears to develop in adulthood.

One interesting aspect of this study was the inclusion of a middle-aged group. Our results indicated a gradual transfer or shift in processing style from youth to midlife and beyond. This finding raises an interesting issue of interpretation. Sometimes it is claimed that later life brings a more global style of processing as a compensation for accumulating processing deficits (see Denney, 1982). Another possibility, and one in line with our data, is that the symbolic style develops continuously throughout adulthood and is then maintained as major late-life deficits occur.

This second possibility is also congruent with Adams's finding that only later-life adults have a significant loss of text *detail*, yet these older adults still show evidence of an understanding of the text base (1986). In addition, this interpretation is supported by the work of Kemper, Kynette, and Norman (see Chapter 9, this volume), who suggest that personal interpretations interfere with working memory as the mechanisms that control access to working memory fade. The fact that the use of symbolic processing is related to verbal ability seems to further contradict a simple deficit interpretation. Higher verbal ability was related to higher incidence of use of a higher level of inferencing—simple symbolic inferences (category 3). Adolescents, whose verbal ability was lower, did not use this level to the extent that midlife and older adults did.

Interestingly, no age-related changes were apparent in the use of the literal base (category 1). Subjects made about the same amount of mediating comments and literal repetitions of the text. This result further lends support to the conclusion that the difference between the groups appears to relate to processes of inferencing and semantic integration rather than an inability to process the text base, per se—a result similar to the findings of Adams (1986).

Finally, it should be noted that the differences between age groups are *between,* not within-subjects differences (see Schaie, 1990). Although the current interpretation suggests that qualitative changes occur in the information processing system, this hypothesized change has yet to be demonstrated over time, within subjects.

A further question raised by the data is whether they can be generalized beyond specific aspects of the coding scheme. Unlike many schemes that code text, our scheme does not give subjects an "overall score" of the highest category they used but rather examines the proportions of use of each category. Therefore, the low rate of frequency of response using category 4, (complex symbolic inferences) is not surprising. This relatively low frequency is in line with other research on qualitative changes in adulthood. Generally, use of the highest levels is very rare, as evidenced by studies of ego level (Loevinger, 1976), cognitive development (Kitchener & King, 1981), moral development (Colby, Kohlberg, Gibbs, & Lieberman, 1983), and emotional maturity (Labouvie-Vief et al., 1989).

In conclusion, processing appears to change in quality throughout adulthood. In youth, interpretations rely heavily on concrete, external, verifiable propositions. With age, these interpretations are transformed to aspects of human functioning and motivation and to general regularities of human life. These responses become increasingly symbolic. This suggests that changes in the more general information processing system are not necessarily all a matter of quantitative deficit. Rather, it appears that the nature of processing—at least in the symbolic realm—may change in a positive way. These data, therefore, lend additional support to recent views that suggest that aging brings not only deterioration but important adaptive changes as well.

References

Adams, C. (1986). *Qualitative changes in text memory from adolescence to adulthood.* Unpublished doctoral dissertation, Wayne State University, Detroit, MI.

Adams, C., Labouvie-Vief, G., Hobart, C., & Dorosz, M. (1990). Adult age group differences in story recall style. *Journal of Gerontology, 45,* pp. 17–27.

Arlin, P. (1989). Problem solving and problem finding in young artists and young scientists. In M.L Commons, J.D. Sinnott, F.A Richards, & C. Armon (Eds.), *Adult development: Vol. 1. Comparisons and applications of developmental models* (pp. 197–216). New York: Praeger.

Birren, J.E. (1979). Age and decision strategies. In A.T. Welford & J.E. Birren (Eds.), *Decision making and age: Interdisciplinary topics in gerontology* (Vol. 4, pp. 23–36). Basel Switzerland: S. Karger.

Blanchard-Fields, F. (1986). Reasoning on social dilemmas varying in emotional saliency: An adult developmental perspective. *Psychology and Aging, 1,* 325–333.

Boswell, D.A. (1979). Metaphoric processing in the mature years. *Human Development, 22,* 373–384.

Brown, A.L., & Smiley, S.S. (1977). Rating the importance of structural units of prose passages: A problem of metacognitive development. *Child Development, 48,* 1–8.

Chinen, A.B. (1985). *Fairy tales and transpersonal development in later life.* Unpublished manuscript, University of California, San Francisco.

Chinen, A.B. (1987). Fairy tales and psychological development in late life: A cross-cultural hermeneutic study. *The Gerontologist, 27,* 340–346.

Chinen, A.B. (1989). *In the ever after: Fairy tales and the second half of life.* Willmette, IL: Chiron Publications.

Colby, A., Kohlberg, L., Gibbs, J., & Lieberman, M. (1983). A longitudinal study of moral development. *Monographs of the Society of Research in Child Development, 49,* (2, Serial No. 206).

Cole, J. (1982). *Best-loved folktales of the world,* New York: Doubleday.

Commons, M.L., Richards, F.A., & Armon, C. (1984). *Beyond formal operations.* New York: Praeger.

Commons, M.L., Richards, F.A., & Kuhn, D. (1982). Systematic, metasystematic, and cross-paradigmatic reasoning: A case for stages of reasoning beyond Piaget's stage of formal operations. *Child Development, 53,* 1058–1068.

Denney, N.W. (1982). Aging and cognitive changes. In B.B. Wohlman (Ed.), *Handbook of developmental psychology* (pp. 807–827). Englewood Cliffs, NJ: Prentice-Hall.

DeWit, G.A. (1963). *Symbolism of masculinity and femininity: An empirical phenomenological approach to developmental aspects of symbolic thought in word associations and symbolic meanings of words.* New York: Springer Publishing.

Fry, E. (1968). A readability formula that saves time. *Journal of Reading, 11,* 513–516, 575–578.

Hultsch, D.F., & Dixon, R.A. (1984). Memory for text materials in adulthood. In P.B. Baltes & O.G. Brim, Jr. (Eds.), *Life-span development and behavior* (Vol. 6, pp. 77–108). New York: Academic Press.

Jastak, J., & Jastak, S. (1964). Short forms of the WAIS and WISC vocabulary subtests. *Journal of Clinical Psychology, 20,* 167–199.

Johnson, R.E. (1970). Recall of prose as a function of the structural importance of the linguistic unit. *Journal of Verbal Learning and Verbal Behavior, 9,* 12–20.

Kausler, D.H. (1982). *Experimental psychology and human aging.* New York: John Wiley & Sons.

Kitchener, K.S. (1983). Cognition, metacognition, and epistemic cognition. *Human Development, 26,* 222–232.

Kitchener, K.S., & King, P.M. (1981). Reflective judgment: Concepts of justification and their relation to age and education. *Journal of Applied Developmental Psychology, 2,* 89–116.

Kitchener, K.S., King, P.M., Wood, P.K, & Davison, M.L. (1989). Consistency and sequentiality in the development of reflective judgment: A six year longitudinal study. *Journal of Applied Developmental Psychology, 10,* 73–95.

Kogan, N. (1974). Categorizing and conceptualizing styles in young and older adults. *Human Development, 17,* 218–230.

Kramer, D.A. (1983). Post-formal operations? A need for further conceptualization. *Human Development, 26,* 91–105.

Kramer, D.A., & Woodruff, D.S. (1984). Breadth of categorization and metaphoric processing: A study of young and older adults. *Research on Aging, 6,* 271– 286.

Kuhn, D., Pennington, N., & Leadbeater, B. (1983). Adult thinking in developmental perspective. In P.B. Baltes & O.G. Brim, Jr. (Eds.), *Life-span development and behavior* (Vol. 5, pp. 158–195). New York: Academic Press.

Labouvie-Vief, G., & Blanchard-Fields, F. (1982). Cognitive aging and psychological growth. *Ageing and Society, 2,* 183–209.

Labouvie-Vief, G., Campbell, S.O., Weaverdyck, S.E., & Tanenhaus, M.K. (1980). *Metaphoric processing in young and old adults.* Unpublished manuscript, Wayne State University.

Labouvie-Vief, G., DeVoe, M., & Bulka, D. (1989). Speaking about feelings: Conceptions of emotion across the life span. *Psychology and Aging, 4,* 425–437.

Labouvie-Vief, G., & Hakim-Larson, J. (1989). Developmental shifts in adult thought. In S. Hunter & M. Sundel (Eds.), *Midlife myths: Issues, findings, and practical implications* (pp. 69–96). Newbury Park, CA: Sage.

Labouvie-Vief, G., & Schell D.A. (1982). Learning and memory in later life. In B.B. Wohlman (Ed.), *Handbook of developmental psychology* (pp. 828–846). Englewood Cliffs, NJ: Prentic-Hall.

Labouvie-Vief, G., Schell, D.A., & Weaverdyck, S.E. (1981). *Recall deficit in the aged: A fable recalled.* Unpublished manuscript, Wayne State University.

Loevinger, J. (1976). *Ego development.* San Francisco: Jossey-Bass.

Neugarten, B.L. (1968). The awareness of middle age. In B.L. Neugarten (Ed.), *Middle age and aging* (pp. 93–98). Chicago: University of Chicago Press.

Perry, W.G. (1968). *Forms of intellectual and ethical development in the college years.* New York: Holt, Rinehart, & Winston.

Poon, L.W. (1985). Differences in human memory with aging: Nature, causes and clinical implications. In J.E. Birren & K.W. Schaie (Eds.), *Handbook of the psychology of aging* (2nd ed., pp. 427–462). New York: Van Nostrand Reinhold.

Riegel, K.F. (1973). Dialectical operations: The final period of cognitive development. *Human Development, 16,* 346–370.

Salthouse, T. (1985). *A theory of cognitive aging.* Amsterdam: North Holland.

Schaie, K.W. (1990). Intellectual development in adulthood. In J. E. Birren & K.W. Schaie (Eds.), *Handbook of the psychology of aging* (3rd ed., pp. 291– 309). New York: Academic Press.

Shrout, P.E., & Fleiss, J.L. (1979). Intraclass correlations: Uses in assessing rater reliability. *Psychological Bulletin, 86,* 420–428.

Sinnott, J.D. (1989). Life-span relativistic postformal thought: Methodology and data from everyday problem solving studies. In M.L. Commons, J.D. Sinnott, F.A. Richards, & C. Armon (Eds.), *Adult development: Vol. 1. Comparisons and applications of developmental models* (pp. 239–278). New York: Praeger.

9
Age Differences in Spoken Language

Susan Kemper, Donna Kynette, and Suzanne Norman

Despite the prevalence of the view that language abilities show little decline across the adult years (Bayles, Boone, Tomoeda, Slauson, & Kaszniak, 1989; Kempler, Curtiss, & Jackson, 1987), ample evidence indicates that older adults speak differently than young adults. Significant differences in the basic characteristics of the oral language of young and elderly adults have been reported in studies using a wide range of research methodologies. A variety of hypotheses have been advanced to account for these age differences in spoken language including cohort differences in the amount or nature of the adults' formal education, functional differences in adults' choice of topic or conversational style, sensory impairments (presbycusis), and age-group differences in memory, attention, and motivation (see Obler, 1985; Obler & Albert, 1985, for reviews).

This chapter surveys age differences in spoken language and focuses on the use of complex syntactic constructions. The review documents an age-related decline in syntactic complexity and discusses whether a loss of linguistic *competence* must be evoked to account for this decline in syntactic complexity but concludes that *performance* factors arising from limitations of working memory are responsible for the loss of syntactic complexity in elderly adults' speech. To support this conclusion, we analyze language samples and working memory measures, collected over a 3-year period from a panel of adults 60 to 92 years of age, to reveal the relationship between working memory and speech complexity. Finally, the chapter examines the implications of this research for elderly adults' everyday conversation by considering alternative accounts of the source of working memory limitations and the nature of speech production limitations.

Loss of Complexity

In a series of studies, Kemper and her colleagues (Kynette & Kemper, 1986; Kemper, Kynette, Rash, O'Brien, & Sprott, 1989) have carried out extensive analyses of the spontaneous speech of elderly adults. Kynette

138

and Kemper (1986) compared adults 50 to 90 years of age on six different aspects of speech: their use of simple and complex syntactic structures, their use of different auxiliary verb constructions, their production of grammatical forms (parts of speech), their lexical diversity, and their speech disfluencies including sentence fragments and lexical fillers. Across the age range, Kemper et al. noted a reduction in the variability and accuracy of the adults' production of syntactic structures, auxiliary verb, and grammatical forms. In contrast there was no age-related change in the incidence of speech disfluencies or in the measures of lexical diversity. Kynette and Kemper (1986) suggested that adults' use of complex linguistic forms, such as embedded sentences and sentences with multiple auxiliary verbs marking modality and aspect, were susceptible to age-related impairments while adults' use of simple forms, such as single-clause sentences, were buffered from age-related loss.

This hypothesis, that aging affects adults' use of complex linguistic structures, was pursued in a related study by Kemper et al. (1989). They compared measures of the sentence length, syntactic complexity, and fluency for speech samples collected from college students 18 to 28 years of age and elderly adults 60 to 92 years of age. They obtained three different language samples: (a) oral samples from an interview about the participants' employment history and current activities, (b) oral samples describing the person the participants most admired, and (c) written samples describing the most significant event in the participants' lives. In all three samples, Kemper et al. noted overall decrements in syntactic complexity attributable to an age-related loss of sentence embeddings yet observed no age-group differences in vocabulary or measures of speech disfluency. This analysis also revealed that the age-related decline in syntactic complexity was greatest for the language samples obtained from the written statements, perhaps because the overall complexity of written language exceeds that of oral language. A "floor" effect may have reduced the age-group differences in syntactic complexity for the oral interviews, because even the young adults used few complex sentences in answering the questions. Thus, some aspects of language, such as vocabulary, show little change with advancing age, while other aspects of language, particularly the use of complex, multiclause sentences in written language, decline with advancing age.

This loss of complexity cannot be attributed to cohort differences in language or education, because it is also apparent in longitudinal language samples. Kemper (1987, 1990) has analyzed the written diary entries made by adults across a seven-decade period; an age-related loss of sentence embeddings was also characteristic of these diary entries. Thus, it appears that elderly adults use a simplified style characterized by simple sentences with few embeddings and few auxiliary verbs. However, Kemper found no evidence for a pervasive deterioration of adults' language; these studies have not revealed a consistent age-related increase in sentence fragments or ungrammatical constructions or any loss of lexical diversity or vocabulary.

Other age-related changes have also been observed in the oral language of elderly adults. Gold, Andres, Arbuckle, and Schwartzman (1988) have observed that verbosity or prolonged, unfocused, off-target speech is characteristic of older adults, especially those who are extraverted, under stress, and experiencing cognitive decline. Increased errors in the use of pronominal anaphors (Ulatowska, Hayashi, Cannito, & Fleming, 1986), a loss of discourse cohesion (Kemper, 1990; Kemper, Rash, Kynette, & Norman, 1990), and increased hesitation phenomena such as false starts, repetitions, and word-finding problems (Burke, MacKay, Worthley, & Wade, in press; Walker, Roberts, & Hedrick, 1988) have also been reported as characteristic of the speech of elderly adults. Of interest would be research investigating whether elderly adults have similar production problems during writing.

These findings must be interpreted cautiously: (a) Hoyt (1989) suggested that age-group differences in language may not be observed when exceptionally well-educated and healthy elderly adults are compared to younger adults; conversely, age-group differences may be exacerbated in studies of adults in poor health, those socially isolated in health-care facilities, or those with severe depression (Emery, 1986, 1988). (b) Intergenerational differences in conversational style (Coupland, Coupland, Giles, & Henwood, 1988; 1991) also may contribute to age-group differences in spoken language. Older adults may follow conversational conventions during face-to-face conversations that differ from those of young adults. Age-group differences in the rate or pacing of conversations and in the use of gestures, gaze, or other forms of nonverbal communication may contribute to the observed differences in spoken language. Further, elderly adults may weigh competing communication needs differently than young adults (Ryan, Giles, Bartolucci, & Henwood, 1986) and prefer to maximize, for example, message clarity rather than efficiency. (c) Some aspects of spoken language may be less vulnerable to age-related change than others. The dissociation of syntax and semantics, as suggested by modularity theories of language (Fodor, 1987; Garfield, 1987), is consistent with the findings of Kynette and Kemper (1986) and Kemper et al. (1989) that the complexity of adults' syntax declines with advancing age, yet adults' semantic knowledge of word meanings is preserved. The reverse asymmetry of syntax preservation and semantic loss is observed in the linguistic deterioration that accompanies Alzheimer's disease. Kempler et al. (1987) compared the speech of healthy elderly adults with adults, matched for age and gender, with a diagnosis of Alzheimer's disease. Kempler et al. (1987) did not find that the syntax of the Alzheimer's patients was any less complex than that of the healthy elderly adults. A similar conclusion was reached by Blanken, Dittman, Hass, and Wallesch (1987). Yet Alzheimer's disease is characterized by the progressive deterioration of semantic abilities (Bayles

& Kaszniak, 1987), leading to a loss of lexical diversity and increased word-finding problems, verbal paraphasias, circumlocutions, and naming deficits.

Why might the syntactic complexity of adults' speech decline with advancing age? First, it is tempting to conclude that adults' basic syntactic competence gradually deteriorates with advancing age. A loss of syntactic competence might follow a "last learned, first lost" principle such that the most complex aspects of syntax, such as sentence embeddings, are most vulnerable to age-related loss. Other aspects of syntactic competence, such as phrase structure, selectional restrictions, and morphology, may be more resistant to loss but not immune. Such a loss of syntactic competence itself might arise indirectly from a reorganization or restructuring of the syntactic rule system (Hyams, 1986).

In contrast, syntactic competence may be preserved over the life span. If so, performance factors, such as age group differences in memory, attention, and motivation, may account for the observed loss of syntactic complexity. One way in which linguistic competence can be distinguished from linguistic performance is to examine metalinguistic judgments (Linebarger, Schwartz & Saffran, 1983). Pye, Cheung, and Kemper (in press) collected grammaticality ratings from college students and adults 60 to 92 years of age. They found that adults of all ages are able to detect violations of grammatical rules with equal accuracy, although older adults rate long and complex sentences as ungrammatical. All of the adults were able to recognize that sentences such as "Whom did you see the woman from the apartment house next door and?" and "John is expected the woman from the city treasurer's office to help" violated grammatical rules, but the older adults, particularly those in their 80s, also rated some grammatical sentences as ungrammatical. For example, "You saw the woman from the apartment house next door and whom?" and "The woman from the city treasurer's office is expected to help John" are grammatical although the older adults typically rated these sentences as ungrammatical. These results suggest that linguistic competence is preserved across the life span and that performance limitations on adults' syntactic processing contribute to their rejection of the long, multiple-embedded sentences and, by extension, the loss of syntactic complexity in adults' spoken language.

Kemper (1988) and Kemper and Rash (1988) suggested that age-related limitations on working memory are responsible for the loss of complexity in adults' speech. Kemper and Rash (1988) and Kemper et al. (1989), working with different groups of adults, reported that adults' backward digit span, a measure of working memory, is positively correlated with their use of complex syntactic constructions. In both studies, adults with larger backward digit spans used more sentence embedding, particularly left-branching embeddings. Further, Kemper and Rash (1988) and Cheung and Kemper (in press) applied a variety of formal measures of syntactic complexity to adults' language samples; these complexity metrics were based on theoretical models of language processing. In a series of regression analyses, the adults' backward digit spans, not their age, emerged as the better predictor of syntactic complexity regardless of which metric was employed. Thus, working memory limitations, as measured by the backward digit span, appear to constrain adults' production of complex syntactic constructions and contribute to the observed age-group differences in syntactic complexity.

Measuring Working Memory and Syntactic Complexity

The relationship between adults' syntactic complexity and working memory was examined in an extension of the study by Kemper et al. (1989). The hypothesis that limitations of adults' working memory constrain their production of complex syntactic constructions comprises three assumptions (a) adults should evidence age-group as well as individual differences in measures of working memory and (b) there should be age-group as well as individual differences in measures of syntactic complexity, (c) working memory should be correlated with linguistic complexity such that a loss of working memory leads to a loss of linguistic complexity. To examine this hypothesis, we have extended the study by Kemper et al. (1989) over a 3-year period. Multiple language samples have been collected from the same group of adults, initially 60 to 92 years of age. In addition, we have administered annual span tests of working memory to these adults. This study will be extended over additional years; the results reported here are, hence, preliminary and await further analysis pending the completion of the project.

Initially, 78 elderly adults were recruited for the project. During the first year, participants consisted of 37 adults 60 to 69 years ($M = 65$ years), 26 adults 70 to 79 years ($M = 74$ years), and 15 adults 80 to 92 years ($M = 84$ years). By year 3, subject attrition was 21%, leaving 23 adults ($M = 67$ years), 27 ($M = 74$ years), and 12 ($M = 84$ years), respectively, in each of the three age groups.

Year 1

Initially, the participants were interviewed to collect basic background information including educational and employment histories and self-report assessments of health including ratings of overall health, vision, hearing, and mobility. At this time the vocabulary test from the Wechsler Adult Intelligence Scale (WAIS, Wechsler, 1958) and the digits forward and digits backward subtests were administered. Three different language samples were also collected: oral answers to a series of questions about occupations and hobbies, an oral statement about "the person you most admire," and a written statement about "the most significant event in your life." The complete analysis of this data was published by Kemper et al. (1989).

Year 2

As part of an on-going series of experimental studies of geriatric psycholinguistics, additional language samples were obtained from many of the same adults. Two language samples were obtained in the second year: an oral story that was either a personal narrative, an original fantasy, or a retelling of a familiar story and an oral statement about "changes you have observed in your life-time [sic]." The complete analysis of the narratives is reported in Kemper et al. (1990). In addition, WAIS digit spans were again collected from these adults during year 2.

Year 3

Two additional language samples were also collected in year 3. The adults provided an oral account of "a trip or vacation you have taken" and an oral description of their family. WAIS digit spans were also collected during year 3.

Attrition

To determine whether attrition had differential effects affecting the composition of the participants, a series of analyses of variance (ANOVAs) were performed, contrasting those who remained in the project with those who had dropped out. These ANOVAs compared these two groups on two sets of measures: the initial WAIS vocabulary and digit span (forward and backward) scores and the initial self-reported measures of health (overall health, hearing, vision, and mobility). Most of these comparisons were not significant, except that those adults who remained in the project reported that their overall health, $F(1,75) = 2.05$, $p < .05$, and mobility, $F(1,75) = 3.11$, $p < .05$, were somewhat greater than those who dropped out of the project. These differences may account for the loss from year 1 to year 3 of some of the participants.

Working Memory

Figure 9.1 summarizes the results of the annual digit span tests. These data were examined using a 3 age group × 3 years × 2 spans repeated measures ANOVA. No overall effect of year was observed; however, the main effect for age group, $F(2,75) = 8.75$, $p < .01$; and the main effect for span, $F(1,75) = 7.51$, $p < .01$; and their interaction, $F(2,75) = 4.65$, $p < .01$, were significant. Performance on the digit span tests declined across the

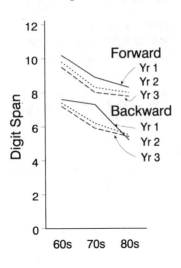

FIGURE 9.1. Wechsler Adult Intelligence Scale forward and backward digit spans for the 60-, 70-, and 80-year-olds collected in years 1 to 3.

age groups, forward digit span exceeded backward digit span, and the age decline was somewhat greater by year 3 for backward digit span than for forward digit span.

Table 9.1 provides the matrix of correlations among these digit spans, partialling out the linear effect of age. Most of the correlations are significant, indicating that these tests measure a common component of working memory. All of the correlations are of moderate strength, however, accounting for no more than 36% of the variance.

A regression analysis using the residual-gain score procedure advocated by Cronbach and Furby (1970) was used to identify three groups of participants. Residualization removed from the year 3 scores that portion linearly

TABLE 9.1. Correlations among the forward and backward digit spans obtained in years 1 to 3.

Digit span and year	Forward			Backward		
	Year 1	Year 2	Year 3	Year 1	Year 2	Year 3
Forward digit span						
Year 1	—					
Year 2	.53**	—				
Year 3	.45**	.55**	—			
Backward digit span						
Year 1	.56**	.36*	.58**	—		
Year 2	.25	.55**	.40**	.60**	—	
Year 3	.41**	.46**	.66**	.47**	.59**	—

*$p < .05$. **$p < .01$.

FIGURE 9.2. Mean clauses per utterance (MCUs) and the incidence of left-branching (LEFTS) clauses in the speech samples collected in years 1 to 3.

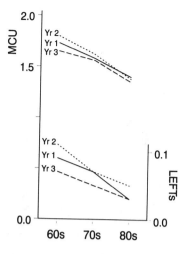

predicted from the year 1 scores. Thus, it identified individuals who improved or declined more than would have been expected on the basis of their initial performance. In this analysis, a residual gain (or loss) of 3 or more points was significant at $p < .05$. Therefore, three groups of participants were identified: (1) Those whose composite digit spans were relatively unchanged from year 1 to year 3; 46 participants were in this group. (2) Those whose composite digit span showed an unexpectedly large increase from year 1 to year 3; 3 participants' digit spans improved significantly. (3) Those whose composite digit span showed an unexpectedly large decrease from year 1 to year 3; 12 participants' digit spans decreased significantly.

Language Samples

A variety of measures can be obtained from language samples (Kemper et al., 1989, 1990). For this analysis, only two will be used: the mean number of clauses per utterance (MCU) and the proportion of clauses that were left branching (LB). These two measures appear to be sensitive measures of the complexity of adults' language, they can be readily computed from the language samples following transcription, and the measures appear to be compatible with formal measures of linguistic complexity derived from theoretical models of language production and processing (Cheung & Kemper, in press).

Figure 9.2 presents the MCUs and LBs for the participants averaged over the three language samples from year 1 and the two samples collected in each of years 2 and 3. A 3 age groups × 3 years repeated measures multivariate analysis of variance (MANOVA) was performed on these data. A significant main effect of age and a marginally significant main effect for

TABLE 9.2. Correlations among measures of linguistic complexity with the effect of age removed.

Complexity measures	Mean clauses per utterance			Left-branching clauses		
	Year 1	Year 2	Year 3	Year 1	Year 2	Year 3
Mean clauses per utterance						
Year 1	—					
Year 2	.63**	—				
Year 3	.79**	.39*	—			
Left-branching clauses						
Year 1	.29*	.19	.19	—		
Year 2	.36*	.59**	.14	.74**	—	
Year 3	.20	.39*	.32*	.64**	.63**	—

$*p < .05.$ $**p < .01.$

year were observed, but no interaction was noted in the multivariate analysis. In the univariate analyses, the main effect for age was significant for both MCU, $F(3,75) = 5.42$, $p < .01$, and LB, $F(3,75) = 4.87$, $p < .01$. The main effect for year was not significant for MCU, $F(2,75) < 1.0$, $p > .05$, nor was the interaction. MCUs declined with age, yet equivalent averaged MCUs were obtained from the various language samples. The main effect for year was marginally significant for LB, $F(2,75) = 2.97$, $p < .06$, as was the interaction, $F(2,75) = 3.04$, $p < .06$. Left-branching clauses declined with age; however, the narratives collected in year 2 from the 60- and 70-year-olds contained a greater incidence of LB sentences than did the other language samples. The incidence of LB sentences did not vary with language sample for the 80-year-olds.

Table 9.2 presents the matrix of correlations among these complexity measures, partialling out the effect of age. In general, the MCUs are positively correlated across years, as are the LB clauses. Because LB clauses as well as sentences with right-branching clauses and those with conjoined main clauses all contribute to MCU, MCUs and LB clauses are not, in general, significantly correlated. The use of multiclause sentences, especially those with LB clauses, appears to be a stable characteristic of some speakers although there is an age-related decrease in MCUs and LB clauses.

As in the analysis of the working memory measures, three groups of participants were identified on the basis of their residual gain (or loss) scores when the year-3 data were regressed on the year-1 data. For this analysis, a residualized gain (or loss) of 30% was significant at $p < .05$; this procedure produced three groups: (1) 40 participants whose LB scores were unchanged from year 1 to year 3. (2) 4 participants whose LB scores

TABLE 9.3. Correlations among working memory measures and linguistic complexity measures with the effect of age removed.

Linguistic complexity measures	Digit span		
	Year 1	Year 2	Year 3
Mean clauses per utterance			
Year 1	.41*	.43*	.41*
Year 2	.43*	.48**	.40*
Year 3	.49*	.61**	.61**
Left-branching clauses			
Year 1	.57**	.58**	.37*
Year 2	.57**	.68**	.46**
Year 3	.71**	.72**	.65**

*$p < .05$.   **$p < .01$.

improved from year 1 to year 3. (3) 17 participants whose LB scores declined from year 1 to year 3.

Working Memory and Linguistic Complexity

We performed a preliminary test of the hypothesis that a decline in working memory leads to a loss of linguistic complexity in adults' speech by computing correlations between the digit span scores and the linguistic complexity measures. Table 9.3 provides the first-order correlations, removing the linear effect of age. In general, digit span is positively correlated with linguistic complexity, especially with the incidence of LB clauses in adults' speech. Because the effects of age are partialled out, the pattern of correlations suggests that chronological age per se is not the mediating factor in these correlations. Of particular interest is the finding that year 1 digit spans correlate somewhat more strongly with year 3 MCUs and LB clauses than with year 1 MCUs and LB clauses. This suggests that adults with working memory limitations will gradually lose MCUs and LB clauses over time, resulting in higher correlations between the working memory measures and the linguistic complexity measures.

The relationship between working memory and linguistic complexity was also examined by comparing those participants who had no change, a gain, or a loss of digit span over the 3-year interval with those who showed no change, a gain, or a loss of LB clauses over this interval. Table 9.4 summaries these results.

Most of the adults did not have a significant change in working memory over the 3-year interval or a change in linguistic complexity. More interestingly, of those 12 adults whose digit spans were significantly lower after 3

TABLE 9.4. Relationship between change in working memory and change in linguistic complexity.

	Working memory measure		
Left-branching clauses	Loss	No change	Gain
Loss	11	5	1
No change	1	38	1
Gain	0	3	1

years, 11 (91%) also had LB scores that were significantly lower in year 3 than in year 1. These 11 adults were between 76 and 83 years of age ($M = 76$ years) in year 1, suggesting that the late 70s and early 80s are a critical period for language development. During this period, a decline in working memory appears to foretell a loss of linguistic complexity. These results must be viewed cautiously, but they suggest a cause–effect relationship between the loss of working memory and the loss of linguistic complexity.

The converse relation between working memory decline and syntactic complexity does not appear to be true; an increase in adults' working memory does not appear to lead to an increase in linguistic complexity. The three adults whose digit spans increased were 64, 67, and 68 years of age. These "young-old" adults may have benefitted from the repeated digit span testing but this benefit does not appear to carry over to the production of LB clauses.

Conclusion

The research summarized here suggests that limitations of working memory may constrain elderly adults' speech production. Two aspects of this hypothesis are unresolved: First, what is the source of the working memory limitations? Second, what is the extent of the linguistic limitations?

Working Memory Limitations

Working memory limitations on processing and storage are commonly evoked to account for a variety of age-related linguistic phenomena (see Light & Burke, 1988, for a review). Most accounts of working memory limitations assume that there is an age-related decline in the *capacity* of working memory. Working memory is required to process complex syntactic constructions involving multiple clauses, thematic roles, and syntactic relations while processing complex discourse structures with many anaphoric references, pragmatic inferences, and semantic implications. Given such simultaneous processing demands, working memory capacity limitations will result in processing inefficiencies, hence, production or comprehension deficits such as the loss of LB sentences.

Alternatively, Hasher and Zacks (1988) have suggested that the capacity of working memory remains constant across the life span but that there is a revision or reevaluation of inhibitory mechanisms that control access to working memory. As inhibition wanes, performance becomes less task centered, as personal interpretations, individual experiences, and emotional reactions intrude into working memory. Such intrusions interfere with discourse production or comprehension, including the production of LB sentences.

One implication of this account is that elderly adults ought to be more likely to produce LB sentences under some circumstances but not others. For example, Kemper et al. (1989) observed marked genre differences in the complexity of adults' speech. It may be that linguistic interactions, such as face-to-face conversation and question answering, increase the likelihood that personal reminiscences and emotional associations may intrude into working memory and, hence, block the production of LB sentences. Other sorts of linguistic interactions, such as formal statements or impersonal writings, may be characterized by a greater incidence of LB and multiclause sentences because such subjective intrusions are less likely.

Linguistic Limitations

There is a widespread ageist myth that development is u-shaped, such that elderly adults resemble children. Under this assumption, the incremental nature of language development in children might be used to predict a systematic decrement in the language of elderly adults. Hence, the loss of LB structures and multiple clauses might foretell other syntactic impairments, leading inevitably, albeit gradually, to adults' use of telegraphic speech. However, although care givers have been observed to use "baby talk" in addressing elderly adults, particular the ill or infirm (Caporael, 1981), no evidence suggests that elderly adults come to use baby talk themselves. That is, the loss of syntactic complexity appears to be restricted to a loss of sentence embeddings rather than a pervasive simplification or disruption of syntax. Although some researchers (e.g., Walker et al., 1988) have reported that elderly adults' speech is characterized by increased disfluencies, including sentence fragments, others (e.g., Kynette & Kemper, 1986) have not observed a systematic decrease in elderly adults' fluency.

This issue is complicated by the existence of genre differences in linguistic complexity. Whereas written language is characterized by the use of complex grammatical constructions, oral question answering is characterized by the use of simple, elliptical forms. Hence, an age-related loss of syntactic complexity or an age-related increase in disfluencies may not be apparent in all language samples.

The life-span development of other semantic or pragmatic aspects of speech may run counter to a u-shaped developmental curve. Wingfield and Stine (Chapter 7, this volume) have suggested that older adults develop compensatory mechanisms for speech processing to overcome sensory limitations. Jepson and Labouvie-Vief (Chapter 8) suggest that older adults may develop a symbolic approach to information processing at the expense of objective or analytical processing styles. In the domain of spoken language, adult development may also be characterized by adaptive change. For example, elderly adults' may employ a greater diversity of lexical items in their speech than young adults. Although type-token ratios do not appear to vary with age (Kemper et al., 1989; Kynette & Kemper, 1986), increased lexical diversity may be manifested in elderly adults' use of familiar figurative expressions such as metaphors, proverbs, idioms, or other formulatic expressions. Elderly adults may also be more adept at using inversions, such as "Was he mad!", subtle markers of status, role, and politeness, context, or other linguistic devices (Green, 1988) than young adults.

For example, Kemper (1990) and Kemper et al. (1990) have observed that elderly adults produce structurally complex narratives with multiple embedded episodes and evaluative codas; they suggest that elderly adults sacrifice syntactic complexity to preserve narrative complexity, given working memory limitations. Alternatively, elderly adults may use complex narrative forms to indicate the causal and temporal connections among events that young adults convey through the use of sentence embeddings. Hence, complex pragmatic structures may compensate for syntactic limitations.

Indeed, one implication of the modularity thesis (Fodor, 1987) is that other linguistic modules may compensate for limitations of the syntactic module. Hence, elderly adults may compensate for their inability to process complex syntactic constructions by relying on semantic and pragmatic devices to serve the same functional goals. Thus, the speech of elderly adults might by characterized simultaneously as syntactically simple but semantically or pragmatically complex.

Acknowledgments. We thank Shannon Rash and Hintat Cheung for their assistance with this project. This research was supported by grants R01AG06319 and K04AG0043 from the National Institute on Aging to S. Kemper.

References

Bayles, K.A., Boone, D.R., Tomoeda, C., Slauson, T., & Kaszniak, A.W. (1989). Differentiating Alzheimer's patients from the normal elderly and stroke patients with aphasia. *Journal of Speech and Hearing Disorders, 54*, 74–87.

Bayles, K.A., & Kaszniak, A.W. (1987). *Communication and cognition in normal aging and dementia.* Boston: Little, Brown.

Blanken, G., Dittman, J., Hass, J-C., & Wallesch, C-W. (1987). Spontaneous speech in senile dementia and aphasia: Implications for a neurolinguistic model of language production. *Cognition, 27,* 247–275.

Burke, D.M., MacKay, D.G. Worthley, J.S., & Wade, E. (in press). On the tip of the tongue: What causes word finding impairments in young and older adults? *Journal of Memory and Language.*

Caporael, L. (1981). The paralanguage of caregiving: Baby talk to the institutionalized aged. *Journal of Personality and Social Psychology, 40,* 876–884.

Cheung, H., & Kemper, S. (in press). Competing complexity metrics and adults' production of complex sentences. *Applied Psycholinguistics.*

Coupland, N., Coupland, J., Giles, H., Henwood, K. (1988). Accommodating the elderly: Invoking and extending a theory. *Language in Society, 17,* 1–14.

Coupland, J., Coupland, N., Giles, H., & Henwood, K. (1991). Formulating age: Dimensions of age identity in elderly talk. *Discourse Processes, 14,* 87–106.

Cronbach, L.J., & Furby, L. (1970). How should we measure "change"—or should we? *Psychological Bulletin, 74,* 68–80.

Emery, O. (1986). Linguistic decrement in normal aging. *Language and Communication, 6,* 47–64.

Emery, O. (1988). *Pseudodementia: A theoretical and empirical discussion.* Cleveland, OH: The Western Reserve Geriatric Education Center.

Fodor, J.A. (1987). Modules, frames, fridgeons, sleeping dogs, and the music of the spheres. In J.L. Garfield (Ed.), *Modularity in knowledge representation and natural-language understanding* (pp. 25–36). Cambridge, MA: MIT Press.

Garfield, J.L. (1987). Introduction: Carving the mind at its joints. In J.L. Garfield (Ed.), *Modularity in knowledge representation and natural-language understanding* (pp. 17–24). Cambridge, MA: MIT Press.

Gold, D., Andres, D., Arbuckle, T., & Schwartzman, A. (1988). Measurement and correlates of verbosity in elderly people. *Journal of Gerontology: Psychological Sciences, 43,* 27–33.

Green, G.M. (1988). *Linguistic pragmatics for cognitive science.* Hillsdale, NJ: Erlbaum.

Hasher, L., & Zacks, R.T. (1988). Working memory, comprehension, and aging: A review and a new view. In G.H. Bower (Ed.), *The psychology of learning and motivation,* (Vol. 22, pp. 193–226). New York: Academic.

Hoyt, M.J. (1989). *Language production skills of high functioning elderly women.* Unpublished doctoral dissertation, Boston.

Hyams, N.M. (1986). *Language acquisition and the theory of parameters.* Dordrecht, The Netherlands: D. Reidel.

Kemper, S. (1987). Life-span changes in syntactic complexity. *Journal of Gerontology, 42,* 323–328.

Kemper, S. (1988). Geriatric psycholinguistics: Syntactic limitations of oral and written language. In L. Light & D. Burke (Eds.), *Language, memory and aging* (pp. 58–76). Cambridge, England: Cambridge University Press.

Kemper, S. (1990). Adults' diaries: Changes to written narratives across the life-span. *Discourse Processes, 13,* 207–223.

Kemper, S., Kynette, D., Rash, S., O'Brien, K., & Sprott, R. (1989). Life-span changes to adults' language: Effects of memory and genre. *Applied Psycholinguistics, 10,* 49–66.

Kemper, S., & Rash, S. (1988). Speech and writing across the life-span. In M.M.

Gruneberg, P.E. Morris, & R.N. Sykes (Eds.), *Practical aspects of memory: Vol. 1. Current research and issues* (pp. 107–112). Chichester, England: Wiley.

Kemper, S., Rash, S.R., Kynette, D., & Norman, S. (1990). Telling stories: The structure of adults' narratives. *European Journal of Cognitive Psychology, 2,* 205–228.

Kempler, D., Curtiss, S., & Jackson, C. (1987). Syntactic preservation in Alzheimer's disease. *Journal of Speech and Hearing Research, 30,* 343–350.

Kynette, D., & Kemper, S. (1986). Aging and the loss of grammatical forms: A cross-sectional study of language performance. *Language and Communication, 6,*43–49.

Light, L.L., & Burke, D.M. (1988). Patterns of language and memory in old age. In L.L. Light & D.M. Burke (Eds.), *Language, memory and aging* (pp. 244–272). Cambridge, England: Cambridge University Press.

Lingbarger, M.C., Schwartz, M.F., & Saffran, E.R. (1983). Sensitivity to grammatical structure in so-called agrammatic aphasics. *Cognition, 13,* 361–392.

Obler, L.K. (1985). Language through the life-span. In J. Berko Gleason (Ed.), *The development of language* (pp. 227–306). Columbus, OH: Charies E. Merrill.

Obler, L.K., & Albert, M.O. (1985). Language skills across adulthood. In J.E. Birren & K.W. Schaie (Eds.), *Handbook of the psychology of aging* (pp. 463–473). New York: Van Nostrand Reinhold.

Pye, C., Cheung, H., & Kemper, S. (in press). Islands at eighty. In H. Goodluck (Ed.), *Psycholinguistic studies of island constraints.*

Ryan, E.B., Giles, H., Bartolucci, G., & Henwood, K. (1986). Psycholinguistic and social psychological components of communication by and with the elderly. *Language and Communication, 6,* 1–24.

Ulatowska, H.K., Hayashi, M.M., Cannito, M.P., & Fleming, S. (1986). Disruption of reference in aging. *Brain and Language, 28,* 24–41.

Walker, V.G., Roberts, P.M., & Hedrick, D.L. (1988). Linguistic analyses of the discourse narratives of young and aged women. *Folia Phoniatica, 40,* 58–64.

Wechsler, D. (1958). *The measurement and appraisal of adult intelligence.* Baltimore, MD: Williams & Wilkins.

Part 3
Intervention and Instruction

10
Memory Interventions in Alzheimer's-Type Dementia Populations: Methodological and Theoretical Issues

CAMERON J. CAMP AND LESLIE A. McKITRICK

In this chapter, we will consider methodological and theoretical issues encountered while implementing memory interventions in individuals with Alzheimer's-type Dementia (AD). The severe memory impairments associated with AD have profound impact on the ability of afflicted individuals to carry out daily activities, and any new learning (or relearning) tends to be limited and specific. Interventions in this population must address the practical needs of individuals as they cope with a reality configured by impairments in everyday memory (i.e., memory tasks encountered in the real world). Previous attempts to modify the memorial abilities of individuals with AD have met with little success, when they have been tried at all, and we will discuss the problems associated with using traditional mnemonic training with this population. We will then describe a relatively new intervention—spaced retrieval—which seems to overcome many of these difficulties. Results from recent studies using this technique with individuals having AD will be reported.

Memory Loss in Alzheimer's-Type Dementia

Memory loss is one of the earliest and most characteristic signs of AD. Individuals suffering from AD often show such loss in a variety of ways. Some common memory problems associated with AD include dysphasia, consolidation failures for new information, difficulty retrieving information after delays, and high rates of proactive interference (old learning interfering with new learning) for different types of memory (Butters, Salmon, Heindel, & Granholm, 1988; Butters, Salmon, Cullum, et al., 1988; Morris & Kopelman, 1986).

These memory deficits associated with AD have important implications for the ability of individuals to function effectively in ordinary living situations. Afflicted individuals forget locations of objects; routes to follow; to keep appointments; to pay bills; the names of friends or relatives; how often they have asked the same question; whether or not they have eaten;

and so on. It is very common to see these people write notes to themselves (including statements such as "My name is Joe") and forget where they placed the notes. Such problems are the everyday behavioral manifestations of the memory deficits seen in both research settings and neuropsychological examinations.

Morris and Kopelman (1986) review memory loss associated with AD and document evidence of both severe deficits and preserved abilities across different memory systems. Peripheral components of iconic memory (which are relatively unprocessed sensory images) seem to be generally spared in AD, while central processing of iconic memory is compromised. Individuals in the early stages of AD also show deficits on a variety of tasks involving primary memory, such as a reduction in memory span (Morris & Kopelman, 1986). (Primary refers to a substage of the memory process in which small amounts of information are retained for a brief period of time and then are retrieved without substantial transformation.)

Memory models often include a stage of memory that follows primary memory and that involves relatively active processing of new information. This stage appears under many names, depending on the model of memory used. Most researchers agree that individuals with AD show substantial decrements in the active processing of new information. Such decrements severely limit the transfer of new information into a permanent store, or "long-term memory." In research with individuals suffering from AD, deficits have been documented in a variety of tasks, including free recall, pictorial and facial recognition memory, story recall, and paired associate learning (Butters, Salmon, Cullum et al., 1988; Morris & Kopelman, 1986).

Morris & Kopelman (1986) note that while persons with AD show decrements in memory, the end product of information processing, some of the processing mechanisms (such as articulatory rehearsal) function normally. This may suggest impairment in central executive functioning (Morris & Kopelman, 1986) or reduced processing resources (see Craik & Rabinowitz, 1983). Morris and Kopelman (1986) discuss these decrements of memory in terms of a theoretical distinction between explicit and implicit memory systems (see Graf & Schacter, 1985).

Explicit Memory

Explicit memory involves the conscious recollection of personally experienced events. There are several possible theoretical explanations for the widespread deficits apparent in this system. Individuals with AD may be impaired in the ability to transfer information from short-term to long-term storage. A classic finding for AD participants is little or no retention of information in delayed recall tests. This could be due to problems in memory consolidation (cf. Butters, Salmon, Heindel et al., 1988, p. 85) and/or rates of forgetting (Hart, Kwentus, Taylor, & Harkins, 1987; see Squire,

1986, for a discussion of the relationship between consolidation and forgetting in memory).

Kopelman (1985) studied rates of forgetting in demented (AD and alcoholic Korsakoff's) individuals. Recognition memory for pictures was measured 10 min, 24 hr, and 7 days after initial learning. Demented and control participants showed generally equivalent recognition memory at the 10-min recall interval. This was accomplished by giving demented individuals longer initial exposure to experimental stimuli. Memory was then assessed at the latter two retention intervals. Rates of forgetting were parallel across these time spans for demented and control participants. A similar finding was reported by Corkin, Growdon, Nissen, Huff, Freed, and Sagar (1984; cited in Morris & Kopelman, 1986) for retention intervals between 10 min and 72 hr.

Morris and Kopelman (1986) summarized results from these studies and stated that rates of forgetting are normal in AD when adjustments are made for the amount of learning. This suggests that the recall deficits in AD are caused by deficient mechanisms of acquisition rather than storage.

Hart et al. (1987) compared the forgetting rates in normal controls, individuals with AD, and those with depression after all groups learned a set of line drawings to criterion. Their procedures were similar to those described here except that they compared recognition performance at 90 s, 10 min, 2 hr, and 48 hr. To equate initial levels of learning, individuals whose performance was less than near ceiling at 90 s were given additional training until their performance reached criterion at that retention interval. Even though initial levels of learning had been equated in all groups, Hart et al. found that their AD participants showed significantly faster rates of forgetting in the first 10 min than either depressed individuals or normal controls. Rates of forgetting after the first 10 min, however, were comparable for all groups, a result similar to that found by Kopelman (1985). Hart et al. speculate that individuals with mild AD may retain some newly learned information at the expense of very rapid forgetting of the remainder of the material.

This focus on a consolidation deficit seems compatible with the acquisition deficit suggested by Morris and Kopelman (1986). Thus, individuals with AD may experience more rapid initial forgetting (and therefore acquire a smaller amount of consolidated material) after exposure to new information. However, consolidated material (e.g., whatever is retained for 10 min after initial exposure) demonstrates similar forgetting rates in both AD and normal aging.

It is important to note at this point that research findings on rates of forgetting in AD are important to the gerontologist interested in designing interventions in this population. This line of research has three important implications: (a) Forgetting is not an all-or-none phenomenon in AD. Though levels of memory performance are markedly lower than in normal aging, individuals with AD do show the capacity to learn and retain some new information. (b) Learning and retention of new information in AD can be influenced by experimental manipulation. Researchers have equated delayed memory performance by manipulating exposure to experimental stimuli (e.g., Hart et al., 1987). Manipulations carried out in real-world environments might also influence learning and forgetting of new information in AD populations. (c) The critical period for consolidation of new information appears to occur within 10 min of initial exposure. Information that can be retained after that period should show similar forgetting rates in AD and normal aging. The key is to find an intervention that can increase the chances that information will not be forgotten within 10 min of initial exposure. A learning method that does not rely on the extensive use of explicit memory may be a likely candidate.

Implicit Memory

Implicit memory refers to information that is encoded without conscious awareness, and it is expressed without conscious recollection (Schacter, 1987). The functioning of this memory system is commonly measured as the facilitation of test performance by previous exposure to material.

Several researchers have found that persons with AD demonstrate impaired verbal priming abilities, relative to both normal controls and to amnesics (Butters, Salmon, Heindel et al., 1988; Salmon, Shimamura, Butters, & Smith, 1988; Squire, 1986). Verbal priming involves increased accessibility to previously presented material without explicit awareness of prior exposure. For example, amnesics can be shown a list of words such as "MOTEL". Though unable to consciously recall or recognize words from the list, participants complete word stems such as "MOT--" using words from the list in preference to more common words with the same initial letters.

In contrast to the researchers cited previously (Butters, Salmon, Heindel et al., 1988; Salmon et al., 1988), Morris and Kopelman (1986) cited evidence that persons with AD show normal priming effects in lexical decision tasks, word-stem completion and semantically related word generation. They concluded that implicit memory functioning is relatively preserved in the early stages of AD (Morris & Kopelman, 1986). Similarly, Mitchell (1988) reported that individuals with AD showed savings in the time it took to name pictures a second time that were equivalent to those of both younger and older normal adults. Increased naming speed as a function of prior exposure to materials is another method used to measure priming.

There are several possible reasons for the discrepant conclusions regarding verbal priming effects in AD. Differences in participants' stage of disease or level of impairment across experiments could create discrepancies in outcomes. Another reason involves the way in which implicit memory is conceptualized and measured. If the purpose of an implicit memory task is to help differentiate AD from other memory disorders, interest will be focused on level of performance. For example, in Mitchell's (1988) study, individuals with AD were slower in their overall name-generation speeds than other groups.

However, if a researcher's interest is in designing an intervention, the focus of research will be very different. An attempt will be made to find tasks or manipulations to eliminate performance differences or to find out if the relative amount of performance facilitation by preserved abilities is similar across groups (as was the case in Mitchell's, 1988, study).

Subtle variations in experimental procedures, even when using the same task, can create very different outcomes. Evidence in the general area of amnesia research indicates that the amount of verbal priming displayed by amnesics can vary greatly according to task. For example, Squire (1986) stated that verbal priming in amnesia generally vanishes within a short period of time. However, he also noted that "priming might well last longer under more natural conditions, such as when subjects have frequent encounters with the same stimuli" (Squire, 1986, p. 1615).

Experimental research has already demonstrated that long-term verbal priming can be induced in amnesics. A "natural conditions" analogue task was used in a study demonstrating long-term priming effects in severely amnestic individuals. McAndrews, Glisky, and Schacter (1987) demonstrated strong verbal priming effects lasting up to 1 week in two individuals who demonstrated no preservation of explicit memory across that span.

The task used by McAndrews et al. (1987) involved sentences associated with the "aha" effect—a shift from lack of comprehension to sudden understanding of sentence meaning. A flash of sudden insight is a relatively common phenomenon in natural settings. This may have made such sentences especially amenable to retention, at least in implicit memory (e.g., as seen in priming). The saliency of information to be remembered in priming tasks may critically influence whether evidence of priming is obtained. This is probably true for both general amnestic and AD populations. If verbal implicit memory can be demonstrated in AD populations, it may serve those attempting to design memory interventions for them.

The implicit memory system is also involved in nonverbal abilities (Heindel, Salmon, Shults, Walicke, & Butters, 1989; see also Squire's discussion of procedural knowledge, 1986). Individuals with AD show learning of motor skills (Heindel et al., 1989; Martone, Butters, Payne, Becker, & Sax, 1984), demonstrating preservation of at least some aspects of implicit memory functioning. For example, the ability to become quicker and more accurate with repeated practice in a pursuit rotor task has been used as an index of motor priming (in the absence of explicit memory for previous task performance).

Heindel et al. (1989) used this preservation of motor priming to distinguish AD from Huntington's disease (HD). They found that motor priming was not preserved in HD for the task they presented but was preserved in their AD participants. In addition to the traditional use of the preservation of motor priming as a diagnostic marker, evidence of such a preserved ability in AD implies that the use of motor cues (perhaps in combination with other interventions) may be a useful tool in designing memory interventions for this population. Motor cues have been shown to be effective in improving the memory of amnesics (Moffat, 1984; Wilson, 1987).

In the absence of a cure for the disease, memory loss in AD is inevitable. It may, however, be possible to design interventions that enhance the remaining capabilities of persons with AD and prolong their independent functioning. To date, a wide range of techniques has been used to facilitate memory functioning in normal and impaired aging populations. We will now review some of these interventions and discuss their usefulness for AD populations.

Memory Interventions

Internal Mnemonics

Mnemonic strategies are traditional internal memory aids. These strategies include visual imagery techniques, semantic elaboration, and a variety of methods of verbal organization. Visual imagery is the most established and frequently used technique of memory enhancement (Glisky & Schacter, 1986; Schacter, Rich, & Stampp, 1985). This technique involves the formation of distinctive mental images of the item to be remembered. Visual imagery and organizational strategies have been used by some individuals with memory impairments, with varying degrees of success. Not all have been able to benefit from them; the ability to use mnemonic strategies seems closely related to degree of impairment (Glisky & Schacter, 1986).

Hill, Evankovich, Sheikh, and Yesavage (1987) attempted to train a man with primary degenerative dementia to use a visual imagery mnemonic to learn face–name associations. They found that the client was unable to retain more than two face–name pairs at one time. Before training, face–name associations for new faces could be retained for no more than 4 min. After training, the retention intervals rose to 7 min. However, the client generally had great difficulty remembering all three steps of the mnemonic strategy, with the interactive component of the strategy being the most difficult step to retain.

As just described (Hill et al., 1987), individuals with degenerative dementia may be unlikely to learn to use a complicated strategy, even during a clinical training session. Learning the spontaneous use of an internal strategy in the real world requires even greater cognitive effort (c.f., Schacter et al., 1985). The need for the strategy must be recognized in those situations where it would be useful, and the strategy itself remembered. The procedures involved in using the strategy must be understood and held in memory while they are applied. These great demands on cognitive resources are required by most traditional mnemonics and may severely limit the usefulness of such strategies as interventions in AD populations (Glisky & Schachter, 1986).

Research in this area has made it clear that there is an immediate need for an intervention that can be used to teach limited and specific pieces of information important to individuals with AD. For an internal mnemonic to be effective in AD populations, it must involve little or no conscious allocation of effort on the part of the individual.

External Aids

Because the use of internal memory strategies appears to be difficult for individuals with AD to maintain, the potential of external memory aids becomes more important. In informal interviews, some individuals in the early stages of AD report an increase in the spontaneous use of simple external memory aids (a behavior that seems to parallel that of normal older adults). For instance, many write more notes to themselves than they used to. Most increase their reliance on family members or other care givers. However, many problematic memory failures involve intentions that are perceived by the individual as either too trivial or too salient to warrant the use of an external aid. Many of those who see the value of external aids may be unable to judge when their use is appropriate or may be unable to remember to use them.

Repetition

A common intervention to improve memory in impaired and normal individuals is the simple practicing or repetition of information (Glisky & Schacter, 1986). There is no real evidence, however, that practice improves memory itself (Glisky & Schacter, 1986) or that the specific information learned generalizes well to items not directly practiced (Woods, 1983).

Little, Volans, Hemsley, and Levy (1986) presented patients with senile dementia a series of paired associate lists and assessed learning performance repeatedly over 6 months (at baseline, and then later after 1, 2, 4, and 6 months). Some lists were repeated at each testing, and some were new. Performance on changing items progressively declined. Performance on repeated items showed no improvement (no practice effect), but likewise did not show decline. The authors concluded that "same" information could be retained over 1- and 2-month intervals. Memory practice alone, however, is an ineffective way to increase the general memory ability of individuals with AD (Camp, 1989; Little et al., 1986).

Training in Domain-Specific Knowledge

The goal of many memory-training interventions is to improve general memory functioning, by enhancing internal strategy use or perhaps increasing memory capacity itself (Glisky & Schacter, 1986). Glisky and

Schacter (1986) propose an alternative emphasis on the acquisition of specific information that is useful in a person's everyday life. It was noted earlier that individuals with degenerating memory ability, such as those with AD, may lose the ability to use external aids effectively. Specific training in the use of an external aid may benefit these individuals.

Glisky, Schacter, and Tulving (1986) describe an intervention designed to train memory-impaired individuals to remember the vocabulary required for the use of a microcomputer. A second study (reported by Glisky and Schacter, 1986) extended this training to interactive use of the computer. The ability to successfully use a microcomputer as an external storage device could be of great potential benefit to a person with an impaired memory. Their intervention made use of a fading technique—the method of vanishing cues. The definition of a targeted vocabulary word was presented, followed by a fragmented prompt for the correct response (i.e., "SOF-----" as a cue for the word "SOFTWARE"). The cue was extended as needed (i.e., "SOFT----") until the participant successfully recalled the response, and then was withdrawn gradually. The participants in these studies were able to learn a small vocabulary of computer commands and to perform a variety of computer operations.

The fading technique just described was designed to tap the implicit memory abilities that are preserved in amnesic individuals (Glisky & Schacter, 1986). The presentation of a fragmented cue for the correct response is similar to a word-stem completion priming task, a task in which amnesics perform well without explicit memory for previous exposure to the target. The authors (Glisky & Schacter, 1986) noted that this new learning remained very specific to the training situation and that many repetitions were required before error-free performance was achieved. However, this research does point to the ability to make use of preserved implicit memory channels in designing useful memory interventions. Another line of research has explored the role of active retrieval processes in enhancing the memorability of information (e.g., Landauer & Bjork, 1978; Rabinowitz & Craik, 1986).

Retrieval Practice

Retention has been shown to be improved more by repeated attempts to retrieve items from memory than by repeated exposure alone (Moffat, 1984; Modigliani, 1976; Rabinowitz & Craik, 1986). The act of attempting to retrieve information maintains access to that information in memory and facilitates subsequent retrieval attempts (Bjork, 1988). Bjork (1988) states that memory is altered by the act of retrieval; the items retrieved become increasingly more retrievable, while other related items may become less accessible. This capacity for improved memory performance associated with retrieval practice has been used in the design of a new type of memory intervention—spaced retrieval.

The Spaced Retrieval Intervention

Development of the Technique

The spaced retrieval technique of memory intervention, first described by Landauer and Bjork (1978), is a method in which to-be-remembered information is repeatedly retrieved at increasingly longer intervals of time. Landauer and Bjork developed the technique while investigating optimal methods with which normal individuals could learn new information. Their subjects (college students) were asked to learn name–name or face–name paired associates in one of several conditions. Their studies compared the effects of uniform intertrial intervals separating retrieval attempts, expanding intervals separating retrieval attempts, and expanding intervals separating study trials. The expanding schedule of active retrieval attempts produced the best performance and was related to good long-term retention of new associations (Landauer & Bjork, 1978).

In addition to its development with normal subjects, the spaced retrieval technique has been used successfully with subjects having memory impairments of varying underlying causes (Schacter et al., 1985). Schacter et al. noted that the technique involved little cognitive effort and might be more useful in work with memory-impaired individuals than traditional interventions.

Bjork (1988) noted that in the first study using spaced retrieval (Landauer & Bjork, 1978), the fast pace of stimulus presentation precluded the use of traditional mnemonic techniques. Bjork concluded that "expanding retrieval practice is a nonsemantic mnemonic technique that questions our typical characterization of storage in long term memory" (1988, p. 400). Spaced retrieval, a form of expanding retrieval practice, might be a useful technique in aiding the acquisition of domain-specific information in AD populations. Research that corroborates this position will be discussed next.

Technique Revisions for AD

Moffat (1989) described a case study in which a woman in her late 50s with AD was given expanded rehearsal (spaced retrieval) training to improve picture naming. Moffat incorporated some new procedures in his intervention, compared to the original implementations of spaced retrieval. Moffat trained only one item at a time. In addition, he established the intervals between recall trials by interjecting actual time segments rather than by using varying numbers of intervening stimuli.

In previous studies, intervals between tests were manipulated by showing a target and then showing the target again after a varying number of other stimuli had intervened. For example, after showing a target picture, Landauer and Bjork (1978) presented either 1, 4, or 10 other pictures before retesting memory for the target.

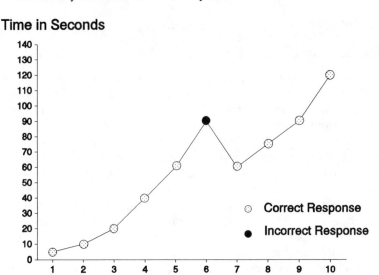

FIGURE 10.1. Hypothetical performance in a spaced retrieval training session.

Moffat's (1989) interval expansions were created by doubling successive recall test intervals (e.g., 2 min, 4 min). After an unsuccessful recall attempt, the time of that trial was halved to determine the length of the next recall test interval. Moffat reported success in his intervention, with some evidence of generalization of training.

Following the example of Moffat (1989), Camp (1989) used time intervals to separate recall trials. These intervals were filled with conversation to prevent rehearsal. As described, Moffat's expansion schedule began with an initial 2-min retention interval that doubled after each successful retrieval. This rate of expansion was too rapid for the AD participants in Camp's early pilot work; and was modified as illustrated in Figure 10.1.

Camp (1989) made another procedural change while using the spaced retrieval technique to train individuals with AD to retain face–name associations. Following the procedures of Moffat (1989), single-target stimuli were used. Landauer and Bjork as well as Schacter et al. (1985) used multiple stimuli. Schacter et al. concluded that this may have hampered retention in their client populations. Camp used single photographs as target stimuli to train single face–name associations.

Spaced Retrieval as Shaping of Memory

The use of an expansion schedule in this paradigm is a form of shaping (Bjork, 1988; Landauer & Bjork, 1978). The desired response is long-term retention (e.g., over weeks or years) of information. Retention intervals are increased at a rate determined by the participant's performance, thus producing closer and closer approximations to the ultimately desired goal. If an expansion interval leads to a failure, the next testing interval is reduced to a previous level of successful recall, and following intervals are increased at a slower rate.

An Example of Spaced Retrieval Training

As described previously, the spaced retrieval training procedure is a shaping paradigm (see Figure 10.1). Memory for target behaviors is tested after successively longer intervals. When a retrieval failure occurs, the learner is told the correct response and asked to immediately repeat it. The next intertest interval is shortened to that of the last interval at which retrieval was successful. The expansion rate is then decreased until the individual successfully retains information over the interval during which failure previously occurred. Recall intervals are then expanded at usual rates until the next recall failure.

In Figure 10.1, data indicate that a hypothetical participant remembered the target behavior after 60- and 90-s intervals (30-s expansion increments). Recall failure occurred after 120 s, and the next retrieval interval returned to 90 s (the last previously successful retrieval interval). Recall was again successful, and the expansion of the testing intervals continued. However, the expansion was increased in shorter (15 s) increments (105 s followed by 120 s) until the participant was able to retain the target information over the interval at which failure had previously occurred (120 s). The testing interval then returned to a 30-s increment schedule (150 s for the next retrieval test).

Expansion schedules are now controlled by laptop computers, which record responses and adjust schedules accordingly. Training sessions generally last for 30 min (cf. Camp, 1989; McKitrick & Camp, 1989). In our experience, longer sessions can lead to fatigue and reduced levels of performance at the end of the session. We usually give training once a week, though frequency of sessions may vary (McKitrick & Camp, 1989).

The optimal number of sessions per week has yet to be established. One might argue that multiple sessions per week would facilitate faster initial learning and/or overlearning. However, Bjork (1988) suggests that an optimal spacing for recall attempts should present the recall trial just before the point when the individual is unable to recall the information. The days between sessions may quickly become part of an effective expansion schedule if Bjork is correct.

From the second training session on, we test the participant at the beginning of each session for retention of the trained response from the previous training session. (If the participant cannot exhibit intersession retention, the first training interval used is the longest successful retention interval from the previous session). If this intersession recall attempt is successful, no further training is given in that session, because the interval of retention already obtained is longer than the highest possible interval (30 min) that could be obtained within a session. Again, this is a shaping paradigm with the purpose of generating closer and closer approximations to an extended (permanent?) retention interval.

INITIAL STUDY

Camp (1989) conducted a pilot study that used the spaced retrieval technique with a woman diagnosed as having AD. In the initial testing session, she was unable to retain new face–name associations for more than 20 to 30 s. After four weekly training sessions using spaced retrieval, she was able to retain a new face–name association for 7-min intervals. At the 7th week of training, she demonstrated the ability to remember the association from the previous training session (i.e., she demonstrated a 1-week retention interval). Control procedures indicated that the effect was not due solely to repetition of the stimuli.

SECOND STUDY

Camp (1989) undertook a second study to replicate these initial results with two additional male subjects (ages 67 and 68). Both regularly attended an adult daycare facility in New Orleans and were diagnosed as having AD. The associations to be learned by the subjects were the names and faces of staff members at the daycare center.

For the first subject, the retention interval for naming the photograph of the targeted staff member reached $3\frac{1}{2}$ min by the end of the first session. On the 4th day after the session, he was shown the actual staff member at the center and asked to name her, which he did. On the 6th day after the initial session, he failed to name the staff member. The next day, at the beginning of the second session, he correctly named the target photograph. Thus, the participant was able to retain the name–face association for the photograph for 1 week. The ability to generalize the training to the naming of the actual staff member was of a more limited duration.

At the second training session, Camp (1989) presented a new target photograph. In a slightly extended session, the longest testing interval reached was 5 min. At no time did the participant mistakenly use the name of the first staff member when naming the second target photograph. In other words, the second piece of new information did not elicit intrusion errors from the original learning. Generalization of training for the second target staffer was displayed when tested on the floor during the following week.

At the start of the third and last training session, the first participant correctly recognized and named the second target photograph but not the first. Training was then reinstated for the original target. The same procedure was used except that the first interval lasted $3\frac{1}{2}$ min rather than 5 s, because $3\frac{1}{2}$ min represented the longest retention interval during the first training session. Again, no recall failures were found within the training session.

For the second subject, the initial training session elicited a 4-min maximum interval of retention. Generalization the following week was not obtained, nor was the subject able to name the target at the start of the second session. The first interval used in the second session was 4 min (the highest retention interval during the first training session). From this point, the subject eventually attained a 6-min retention interval. The following week, generalization was found after 4 days, but not after 6 days. At the third training session, the subject accurately named the target at the beginning of the session and proceeded to learn a new target, reaching a maximum retention interval of 5 min. Again, Camp found no intrusion errors from initial learning.

To summarize, Camp (1989) was able to teach individuals with AD to remember new associations and retain them over extended time periods. This was found in people who normally have difficulty retaining new learning for minutes or even seconds. Some generalization of training also was found. These results were obtained by using relatively brief training sessions (30 min per weekly session).

THIRD STUDY

McKitrick & Camp (1989) conducted a study to assess the utility of spaced retrieval techniques with an AD population to improve memory for the locations of objects, as well as the names of faces. Six individuals with AD participated over an 8-week training period, with a 5-week follow-up.

The experiment produced several interesting results. As might be expected, participants found it easier to remember a verbal association (e.g., "I left my glasses on the bed") than a face–name association. Face–name associations seem to be one of the most difficult types of associations to remember for any population (West, 1985). In addition, participants seemed to be able to translate the verbal association of location into action (e.g., when the experimenter actually had difficulty locating her glasses, a participant joked "Don't look in your purse, look on the bed").

Initially, all six participants failed to retain the memory for a new association for 60 s on three consecutive trials embedded within a 30-min interview. All participants significantly increased their recall performance after training. Half (three) of the participants demonstrated the ability to retain new associations over a 1-week interval during the 8 weeks of training, and three demonstrated maintenance of new associations at the final follow-up session 5 weeks later.

Advantages of Spaced Retrieval

Social Context

An important point to remember is that training sessions have been embedded within the context of a social visit (conversing, playing cards or checkers, etc. in the intervals between testing), and thus participants have looked forward to the sessions. This context greatly diminishes the test anxiety normally associated with interventions in individuals having AD (Camp & Stevens, 1990).

Shaping and Success Rates

As a result of using a shaping technology, participants experience high frequencies of success with this training procedure. One individual remarked that she looked forward to the training sessions because they made her feel "smarter" (Camp & Stevens, 1990).

Effortless Learning

Finally, the learning occurred "effortlessly." In fact, participants commented that it was easy to remember what we were teaching. During one training session, after a successful recall following a 3 1/2-min testing interval, a participant remarked "Don't worry, I'm not going to forget" (Camp & Stevens, 1990).

Given the success of initial research efforts, the positive experiences and lack of anxiety associated with the procedure, and the fact that large amounts of cognitive effort do not have to be expended by individuals with this training, the spaced retrieval intervention seems an ideal form of memory intervention for AD populations. As we noted, new information that can be remembered over an initial 10-min interval does not show differential rate of forgetting in AD individuals compared to normals. If spaced retrieval can allow such initial learning to occur, its effects may be truly long-term.

Why Does Spaced Retrieval Work?

We have documented that long-term retention of new information can be achieved by individuals with AD through spaced retrieval training (Camp, 1989; McKitrick & Camp, 1989). But why should this procedure work? Our current speculation is that spaced retrieval accesses implicit memory systems. We have several pieces of anecdotal evidence that support this assumption. The clearest is the source amnesia for the newly learned information displayed by participants. Correct recalls are often followed by

the question "Did you tell me that before?" More commonly, correct recalls are spoken with a questioning voice, as if participants were unsure
why they were giving that response.

In a similar vein, after incorrect responses are given, we supply participants with the correct response. A typical reaction to this is "That was
what I thought of at first, but I wasn't sure so I guessed something else."
Our impression is that such a response is not an attempt to cover up a
memory loss to save face. Instead, it reflects the deeper trust that individuals have in explicit memories retrieved from tertiary memory as
opposed to newly learned information coupled with source amnesia. This
represents an interesting situation in that success in our recall tasks may
necessitate the repression of explicit memories.

If implicit memory is the underlying basis for success using spaced retrieval, which implicit process is involved? We are currently investigating
two candidates—priming and classical conditioning. These were both
categorized by Squire (1986) as components of a memory system not involving conscious (i.e., "declarative" or explicit) mechanisms. To address
this issue, we are about to engage in a series of studies in which multiple
priming tasks and/or classical conditioning tasks are used together with
spaced retrieval in the same AD individuals.

Directions for Future Research

The immediate goal of spaced retrieval training is to allow individuals with
AD to remember a specific verbal association. Evidence from past research
(Camp, 1989; McKitrick & Camp, 1989; Moffat, 1989) using this technique
indicates that such associations may be learned successfully. We are now
engaged in pilot studies that involve attempts to train individuals to remember a strategy rather than a specific association. If a general strategy
can be learned, it would maximize the clinical importance of the training
procedure, and the strategy could be used with a variety of specific memory
tasks. Older adults seem to use external memory aids in preference to internal mnemonics (Camp, 1988; Camp & McKitrick, 1989a; 1989b), but
individuals with AD forget how to use them effectively, as we stated.
Spaced retrieval training might be used to train a strategy that would allow
external aids to be used effectively. Our current research is designed to
explore this possibility.

Finally, we would like to encourage researchers to investigate the general area of implicit memory from the perspective of memory intervention
and remediation. We need to determine which components of implicit
memory are preserved in AD and to track the deterioration or maintenance of these components across the course of the disease. We need to
determine what types of stimuli and/or task manipulations maximize reten-

tion of new information. We need to determine the relationship between spared implicit and explicit memory systems, and how they interact.

It is becoming increasingly clear that some memory systems remain functional in AD, such as motor priming and possibly some forms of verbal priming. We need to devise ways to use such spared memory abilities to enhance interventions for AD populations in real-world settings.

Acknowledgment. The writing of this chapter was partially supported by a grant from the Alzheimer's Disease and Related Disorders Association to the first author.

Note: The order of authorship was decided by a coin flip. Requests for additional information should be addressed to: Cameron J. Camp, Ph.D., Department of Psychology, University of New Orleans, New Orleans, LA 70148.

References

Bjork, R.A. (1988). Retrieval practice and the maintenance of knowledge. In M.M. Gruneberg, P. Morris, & R. Sykes (Eds.), *Practical aspects of memory* (Vol. 2, pp. 396–401). London: Academic Press.

Butters, N., Salmon, D.P., Cullum, C.M., Cairns, P., Troster, A., Jacobs, D., Moss, M., & Cermak, L.S. (1988). Differentiation of amnesic and demented patients with the Wechsler Memory Scale—Revised. *The Clinical Neuropsychologist, 2,* 133–148.

Butters, N., Salmon, D.P., Heindel, W., & Granholm, E. (1988). Episodic, semantic, and procedural memory: Some comparisons of Alzheimer's and Huntington's disease patients. In R.D. Terry (Ed.), *Aging and the brain* (pp. 63–85). New York: Raven Press.

Camp, C.J. (1988). In pursuit of trivia: Remembering, forgetting, and aging. *Gerontology Review, 1,* 37–42.

Camp, C.J. (1989). Facilitation of new learning in Alzheimer's disease. In G.C. Gilmore, P.J. Whitehouse, & M.L. Wykle (Eds.), *Memory, aging, and dementia* (pp. 212–225). New York: Springer.

Camp, C.J., & McKitrick, L.A. (1989a). The dialectics of remembering and forgetting across the adult lifespan. In D.A. Kramer & M.J. Bopp (Eds.), *Transformation in clinical and developmental psychology* (pp. 169–187). New York: Springer-Verlag.

Camp, C.J., & McKitrick, L.A. (1989b). Memory interventions in old age. *The Southwestern, 5,* 62–73.

Camp, C.J., & Stevens, A.B. (1990). Spaced-retrieval: A memory intervention for dementia of the Alzheimer's type (DAT). *Clinical Gerontologist, 10,* 58–61.

Craik, F.I.M., & Rabinowitz, J.C. (1983, August). *Processing resources in relation to memory encoding and retrieval.* Paper presented at the annual convention of the American Psychological Association, Anaheim, CA.

Glisky, E.L., & Schacter, D.L. (1986). Remediation of organic memory disorders: Current status and future prospects. *Journal of Head Trauma Rehabilitation, 1,* 54–63.

Glisky, E.L., Schacter, D.L., & Tulving, E. (1986). Learning and retention of computer-related vocabulary in memory-impaired patients: Method of vanishing cues. *Journal of Clinical and Experimental Neuropsychology, 8,* 292–312.

Graf, P., & Schacter, D. (1985). Implicit and explicit memory for new associations in normal and amnesic subjects. *Journal of Experimental Psychology: Learning, Memory, and Cognition, 11,* 501–518.

Hart, R.P., Kwentus, J.A., Taylor, J.R., & Harkins, S.W. (1987). Rate of forgetting in dementia and depression. *Journal of Consulting and Clinical Psychology, 55,* 101–105.

Heindel, W.C., Salmon, D.P., Shults, C.W., Walicke, P.A., & Butters, N. (1989). Neuropsychological evidence for multiple implicit memory systems: A comparison of Alzheimer's, Huntington's, and Parkinson's disease patients. *The Journal of Neuroscience, 9,* 582–587.

Hill, R.D., Evankovich, K.D., Sheikh, J.I., & Yesavage, J.A. (1987). Imagery mnemonic training in a patient with primary degenerative dementia. *Psychology and Aging, 2,* 204–205.

Kopelman, M.D. (1985). Rates of forgetting in Alzheimer-type dementia and Korsakoff's syndrome. *Neuropsychologia, 23,* 623–638.

Landauer, T.K., & Bjork, R.A. (1978). Optimal rehearsal patterns and name learning. In M.M. Gruneberg, P. Morris, & R. Sykes (Eds.), *Practical aspects of memory* (pp. 625–632). London: Academic Press.

Little, A.G., Volans, P.J., Hemsley, D.R., & Levy, R. (1986). The retention of new information in senile dementia. *British Journal of Clinical Psychology, 25,* 71–72.

Martone, M., Butters, N., Payne, M., Becker, J., & Sax, D.S. (1984). Dissociations between skill learning and verbal recognition in amnesia and dementia. *Archives of Neurology, 41,* 965–970.

McAndrews, M.P., Glisky, E.L., & Schacter, D.L. (1987). When priming persists: Long-lasting implicit memory for a single episode in amnesic patients. *Neuropsychologia, 25,* 497–506.

McKitrick, L.A., & Camp, C.J. (1989, August). *Name and location learning in SDAT with spaced-retrieval.* Paper presented at the annual convention of the American Psychological Association, New Orleans.

Mitchell, D.B. (1988). Memory and language deficits in Alzheimer's disease. In R.L. Dippel & J.T. Hutton (Eds.), *Caring for the Alzheimer patient* (pp. 81–93). Buffalo, NY: Prometheus Books.

Modigliani, V. (1976). Effects on a later recall by delaying initial recall. *Journal of Experimental Psychology: Human Learning and Memory, 2,* 609–622.

Moffat, N.J. (1984). Strategies of memory therapy. In B.A. Wilson & N. Moffat (Eds.), *Clinical Management of memory problems* (pp. 63–88). Rockville, MD: Aspen.

Moffat, N.J. (1989). Home-based cognitive rehabilitation with the elderly. In L.W. Poon, D.C. Rubin, & B.A. Wilson (Eds.), *Everyday cognition in adulthood and late life* (pp. 659–680). New York: Cambridge University Press.

Morris, R.G., & Kopelman, M.D. (1986). The memory deficits in Alzheimer's-type dementia: A review. *The Quarterly Journal of Experimental Psychology, 38A,* 575–602.

Rabinowitz, J.C., & Craik, F.I.M. (1986). Prior retrieval effects in young and old adults. *Journal of Gerontology, 41,* 368–375.

Salmon, D.P., Shimamura, A.P., Butters, N., & Smith, S. (1988). Lexical and semantic priming deficits in patients with Alzheimer's disease. *Journal of Clinical and Experimental Neuropsychology, 10,* 477–494.

Schacter, D.L. (1987). Implicit memory: History and current status. *Journal of Experimental Psychology: Learning, Memory and Cognition, 13,* 501–518.

Schacter, D.L., Rich, S.A., & Stampp, M.S. (1985). Remediation of memory disorders: Experimental evaluation of the spaced-retrieval technique. *Journal of Clinical and Experimental Neuropsychology, 7,* 79–96.

Squire, L.R. (1986). Mechanisms of memory. *Science, 232,* 1612–1619.

West, R.L. (1985). *Memory fitness over 40.* Gainesville, FL.: Triad.

Wilson, B.A. (1987). *Rehabilitation of memory.* New York: Guilford.

Woods, R.T. (1983). Specificity of learning in reality-orientation session: A single-case study. *Behavioral Research and Therapy, 21,* 173–175.

11
Applications of Psychological Research for the Instruction of Elderly Adults

Dennis N. Thompson

For most of its history, American education has focused on the instruction of children and adolescents. In spite of this, historically, there was some education directed toward adult populations (Charles, 1976, 1980). Instruction in English for immigrants, agricultural classes for rural people, and night schools in business, all existed at the turn of the century, but were small and local enterprises. Educational psychologists, however, concentrating on the problems of public schools, paid little attention to these efforts. Thorndike (1928), for example, in his review of the existing literature cited fewer than 30 studies on learning during adulthood and old age.

In more recent years, the involvement of middle-aged and older adults in adult education programs has been expanding. Surveys conducted by the National Center for Education Statistics (1978) found that in 1969 approximately 10% of the adult population was involved in organized instruction. In the same report, the figure rose to 11.3% in 1972, and 11.6% by 1975. More recently, Withnall (1989) estimates that 20% of the 2.5 million adult students in the United Kingdom are over 60.

As the proportion of active elderly individuals in the population has changed, so has our concept of their functional ability. The once popular belief that age is correlated with decreased learning capacity is being replaced by a new belief that older adults are both interested in and capable of continued education. Discovering the conditions under which older learners are at their best is an increasingly important goal for educational gerontologists.

This chapter is organized into three sections. The first section examines the educational setting in which older adults learn. In this section, variables will be discussed that adult educators may wish to consider in creating a match between the needs and interests of the older adult learner and the programs that are offered. In addition, instructors may wish to use particular approaches with older adults to maximize the effectiveness of classroom instruction. These are presented in the second section. The discussion focuses on findings that are of greatest relevance to program planners, instructors, and administrators. More detailed presentations on the cognitive capabilities of the elderly can be found in the *Handbook of the Psychology of Aging*, edited by James Birren and Warner Schaie (1990), or recent volumes of the *Annual Review of Gerontology*. Third, research in a relatively new area will be presented, the applications of computer technology to the instruction of older adults.

The Educational Setting

Andragogy is the term coined by Knowles (1980) to describe the instructional process appropriate for adults, as opposed to *pedagogy*, which describes instructional processes for children. Instead of the traditional view that education is the dissemination of knowledge from the teacher, andragogy emphasizes the development of skills rather than facts and encourages a cooperative planning, instructional, and evaluative climate between student and teacher.

Bolton (1976) concurs that such concepts are of particular importance to the older learner. He maintains that some older people have internalized negative stereotypes of the capabilities of older people, and bring a low self-concept to the learning situation. They enter with the expectation that they are too old to learn and unlikely to keep up (also see Rebok & Offermann, 1983; West, 1985). Okun and Siegler (1977) argue that by choosing a passive role, and not committing themselves, older learners are protected from the responsibility of failure. Bolton found, however, that the elderly can perceive themselves as successfully investing in the learning experience if the means for involvement are provided and a supportive group atmosphere develops. Belbin and Belbin (1972) emphasize the role of the instructor in this regard. They argue that adults perceive the instructor as a colleague. An effective instructor supports the efforts of the learner rather than sets an example that has to be followed.

In spite of the evidence that involvement in adult education is increasing rapidly (National Center for Educational Statistics, 1978: Percy, 1989, Withnall, 1989), the majority of older people continue to remain uninvolved with adult education programs. While a number of reasons have been suggested for this lack of involvement, there is a growing consensus that current approaches to the instruction of the elderly do not fully address the diversity of needs and backgrounds of this population. Some researchers (e.g., Cross, 1979: Percy, 1989) have argued that socioeconomic status and educational attainment are directly related to participation. In addition, goals differ along class lines, with lower income participants wanting vocational help from classes, while more advantaged adults are interested in the intrinsic rewards of education. Others (Cranton, 1989; Peterson, 1983) have focused on cognitive style variables. Peterson (1983), for example, argues that,to date,most programs directed to the elderly have assumed that they are almost universally field dependent, preferring discussion and discovery methods, and methods that involve social inter-action (Witken, 1976). However, at least some elderly appear to be field independent, preferring traditional classroom settings.

One major framework has addressed the educational interests of older people. The framework has grown out of the work of Talcott Parsons (cited in Londoner, 1978). Parsons looked at the gratification people received from participation in social settings and concluded that this can be either immediate or delayed. In applying Parson's work to education, Londoner (1978) has termed these needs as *expressive* versus *instrumental*. Courses that are immediately enjoyable without specific future value are termed *expressive*. Courses that are designed for a practical end such as a future job or promotion, are referred to as *instrumental*. Contradictory results have been reported in the literature regarding the instrumental and expressive interests of older learners. Basically, however, the research indicates that adult learners from lower income levels, and with limited educational backgrounds, prefer instrumental courses with a more practical orientation (Marcus, 1978). Adults from white-collar occupations with higher levels of formal education indicate expressive interests (Burkey, 1975; Percy, 1989). They see education as a means toward intellectual stimulation rather than as a way of solving practical problems (also see Peterson, 1983). While the instrumental–expressive distinction provides a fairly broad means for tying together value judgments and available data, continued research should provide greater specificity and insight into this area.

Designing Effective Instruction

Once the content of a course has been determined in terms of the needs of the participants, the next step in planning instruction is the selection of the methods to be used. A great deal of research is available addressing the cognitive capabilities of older people and the conditions under which they are at their best. Although this research is detailed and sometimes contradictory, some general principles for instruction can be derived from the results obtained to date. This review will focus on five major areas of concern in designing instructional programs for the elderly: (a) presentation time, (b) climate, (c) meaningfulness of material, (d) introduction of new material, and (e) organization of information.

PRESENTATION TIME

Older adult learners often take longer than young people to learn new material (Botwinick, 1984). In the classroom, new information may have to be presented at a fairly slow rate, and because there is wide variability among older adults, self-paced instruction is often recommended (Brookfield, 1986). Presenting material over several sessions rather than one session may prevent "swamping" effects.

Peterson (1983) argued that instruction should be paced in such a way as to provide ample time for both intake and retrieval. Because lecture is a form of timed instruction, it should be organized so that material is presented, examined, and then reviewed. And because older adults do not organize new information as well as younger adults, the initial presentation of an outline of the topics to be covered is extremely helpful. Ample time needs to be devoted to answering questions as well. In a classroom setting, this will typically require the instructor to reduce the breadth of content presented and to offer greater specificity and depth, to enhance understanding.

CLIMATE

A light atmosphere and a supportive climate should be maintained to reduce tension. This may be especially helpful with older people who have been out of school for many years and who may need to overcome a fear of not being able to compete (Bolton, 1976). Engaging the older learner in information-oriented, collaborative evaluations may also prove to have clear benefits (Hayslip & Kennelly, 1985).

MEANINGFULNESS OF MATERIAL

The conditions for learning should use the background of the older adult, so that new material can be assimilated with what has already been learned. The use of concrete examples and illustrations will also be useful. In this regard, Cranton (1989) presents a step- by-step approach to task analysis that can enable the planner to arrange instruction from the simple and otherwise familiar to the complex.

INTRODUCTION OF NEW MATERIAL

Instruction should be designed so that material is relevant and provides positive feedback. Brookfield (1986) recommends that instructional units be organized so that potentially interfering materials are spaced far apart from each other. The careful use of objectives can help provide a clear understanding beforehand of what class participants are expected to learn or be able to do after instruction (Cranton, 1989).

ORGANIZATION OF INFORMATION

New information should be presented in a carefully organized fashion. Section headings, handouts, and summaries may be used to help delineate the main concepts and ideas presented. Conditions should be arranged so that attention is held on clearly defined sections of instruction, because the introduction of irrelevant information and digressions may be difficult for older learners (Botwinick, 1984).

Advance organizers and embedded questions are two instructional strategies that may help older people organize the information they receive in the classroom. Advance organizers are designed to be highly abstract introductions that provide an anchor around which main ideas can be organized. Ausubel, Novak, and Hanesian (1978) and Glover, Ronning, and Bruning (1990) review general applications of this method. In working with older learners, Thompson (1988) and Thompson and Diefenderfer (1986) found support for the use of advance organizers with the elderly, especially with adults of limited verbal ability.

Embedded questions placed in text are designed to direct learners to the most salient parts of the material (Rothkopf, 1976). They also have the potential advantage of actively involving the learner in the process of reading text-based material. According to Rothkopf, embedded questions inserted in text may encourage deeper verbal processing and have been shown to be effective with young subjects (e.g., Boker, 1974). While comparatively little work in this area has been directed toward older learners, several recent studies have investigated their use with the elderly (Doll & Thompson, 1987; Woods & Bernard, 1987)

Computer Applications with the Elderly

As Charness and Bosman (1990) have pointed out, desktop computers, virtually unknown 10 years ago, have become commonplace in our lives. Still, relatively little is known regarding applications with the elderly. For several years, researchers interested in this area have focused their attention on two basic questions. The first question concerns the extent to which the elderly are willing to incorporate computer-based technology into their lives. The second asks whether barriers exist that would prevent use by large numbers of this age group. The answers to both of these questions are encouraging.

The elderly, especially the better educated, appear to be increasingly open to computer technology. Kerschner and Hart (1984) found computer use among older adults to be greater among those with higher education, higher income, and those living in large communities. In this investigation, an important factor determining favorable attitudes was the level of experience that elderly individuals had with the computer. Addressing the area of computer-assisted instruction (CAI) Doll (1986) found that the attitudes of the elderly were favorable toward CAI and that the attitudes of the sample improved further with practice. Evidence in support of Doll's conclusion can be found in a recent investigation by Ansley and Erber (1988). They found that in general, the attitudes of the elderly toward computer technology were highly similar to the young. Of several areas surveyed, however, the elderly were most highly receptive to the use of computers in education.

Several authors have addressed the issue of potential physical barriers to the use of computers with the elderly (Hoot & Hayslip, 1983; Office of Technology Assessment, 1984). Individuals with visual or motor impairments may find currently available hardware (keyboards, monitors, etc.) difficult to use. Others may find inadequate typing skills a hindrance. Weisman (1983), for example, found that elderly individuals with Parkinson's disease, multiple sclerosis, moderate senile dementia, and moderate visual impairments were able to play computer games with the Apple II. To facilitate use by this population, the games (i.e., the software) were modified by slowing down the action on the screens, increasing the length of the "bats" used in the games, and increasing the probability of mastery early in the session.

More recent research addresses the issue of design variables in developing CAI for the elderly. Doll and Thompson (1987) investigated the instructional effectiveness of pictorial highlighting of key material versus verbal highlighting in CAI lessons. Verbal highlighting involved placing key ideas from the text on a separate screen. Pictorial highlighting included animation to illustrate the same points as in the verbal highlighting condition. The results indicated that both forms of highlighting showed significant improvement over a nonhighlighted condition, but there was a particular advantage for verbal highlighting with the elderly. The authors cautioned, however, that more work needs to be done to determine circumstances for which each form of highlighting is best suited.

Studies addressing video display terminal characteristics and computer input devices have yielded results relevant to the design of CAI lessons. Charness, Graham, Bosman, and Zandri (1988) found that reading from a monitor was easiest for older adults if the monitor was set up with a black-on-white display. Also, Doll (1986) suggested that CAI lessons should be written in the 40-character mode provided with many authoring systems rather than the standard 80-character mode. She found it best to leave screens relatively uncluttered by presenting a maximum of eight or nine lines of text per screen. In her study, placing the monitor on an adjustable platform allowed the elderly to choose the most comfortable viewing angle. This was found to be especially helpful to the elderly with bifocals.

In addressing the use of input devices, Charness et al., (1988) found that the elderly adjusted readily to a mouse, while Doll (1986) reported that the numeric pad made selecting choices to multiple-choice questions much easier for the elderly than letter alternatives, because letter alternatives forced subjects to search the keyboard.

Only one study to date has addressed the design of audio feedback. Charness et al. (1988, study 4) found that the default audio frequencies incorporated with many computers may not be heard by elderly users. He recommended that lower frequencies be used whenever this option is available.

Some studies have investigated approaches to teaching new software packages to the elderly. Nearly all of this research indicates that it takes the elderly longer to learn software than the young, with the general conclusion that instructors should budget about twice as much time (see Charness & Bosman, 1990, for a review).

Jaycock and Hicks (1976) provide one of the more persuasive arguments for introducing computer technology, instructional or otherwise, to the elderly. That is, computers can increase the number of options open to the elderly. For example, networking with peers through the computer may be particularly valuable for the home-bound individual. Older adults with physical problems can use the computer for home employment. Instruction presented visually via the computer can be particularly effective for deaf individuals. Each of these applications represents one or more means by which individuals can cope with the aging process.

Conclusion

Adult educators interested in the instruction of older adults will not lack consumers in the future. For those adults choosing to remain in the workplace, updating and retraining are necessary to keep up with rapid technological change. Many other elderly individuals, outside the requirements of employment, are actively involved in learning new things and meeting new people in an educational environment. Given the heterogeneity of the elderly population, the programmatic and instructional decisions of the educational gerontologist will depend on the goals and outcomes of the educational setting, careful consideration of the needs and characteristics of the learner, and an appreciation of the ever-expanding technology available to the field.

References

Ansley, J., & Erber, J.T. (1988). Computer interaction: Effects on attitudes and performance in older adults. *Educational Gerontology, 14,* 107–119.

Ausubel, D., Novak, J., & Hanesian, H. (1978). *Educational psychology: A cognitive view.* New York: Holt, Rinehart & Winston.

Belbin, E., & Belbin, R.M. (1972). *Problems in adult retraining.* London: Heinemann Educational Books.

Birren, J.E., & Schaie, K.W. (Eds.). (1990). *Handbook of the psychology of aging* (3rd ed.). New York: Academic Press.

Boker, J.R. (1974). Immediate delayed retention effects of interspacing questions in written instructional passages. *Journal of Educational Psychology, 66,* 96–98.

Bolton, C.R. (1976). Humanistic instructional strategies and retirement education programming. *Gerontologist, 16,* 550–555.

Botwinick, J. (1984). *Aging and behavior* (3rd ed.). New York: Springer.

Brookfield, S. (1986). *Understanding and facilitating adult learning.* San Francisco: Jossey-Bass.

Burkey, F.T. (1975). *Educational interests of older adult members of the Brethren Church in Ohio.* Unpublished doctoral dissertation, Ohio State University.

Charles, D.C. (1976). An historical overview of educational psychology. *Contemporary Educational Psychology, 1,* 76–88.

Charles, D.C. (1980). Educational psychology and the adult learner. *Contemporary Educational Psychology, 5,* 289–297.

Charness, N., & Bosman, E.A. (1990). Human factors and design for older adults. In J.E. Birren & K.W. Schaie (Eds.), *Handbook of the psychology of aging* (3rd ed., pp. 446–463). New York: Academic Press.

Charness, N., Graham, G., Bosman, E., & Zandri, E. (1988, April). *Computer technology and age.* Poster presented at the second Cognitive Aging Conference, Atlanta.

Cranton, P.A. (1989). *Planning instruction for older adult learners.* Toronto: Wall and Thompson.

Cross, K.P. (1979). Adult learners: Characteristics, needs and interests. In R.E. Peterson and Associates (Eds.), *Lifelong learning in America: An overview of current practices, available resources, and future prospects* (pp. 75–141). San Francisco: Jossey-Bass.

Doll, L.S. (1986). *The instructional effectiveness of the microcomputer with an elderly population.* Unpublished doctoral dissertation, Georgia State University, Atlanta.

Doll, L.S., & Thompson, D. (1987, April). *The instructional effectiveness of the microcomputer with an elderly population.* Paper presented at the American Educational Research Association Convention, Washington, DC.

Glover, J., Ronning, R., & Bruning, R. (1990). *Cognitive psychology for teachers.* New York: Macmillan.

Hayslip, B., Jr., & Kennely, K. (1985). Cognitive and noncognitive factors affecting learning among older adults. In B. Lumsden (Ed.), *The older adult as learner* (pp. 73–98). Washington, DC: Hemisphere.

Hoot, J.L., & Hayslip, B. (1983). Microcomputers and the elderly: New directions for self-sufficiency and life-long learning. *Educational Gerontology, 9,* 493–499.

Jaycox, K., & Hicks B. (1976). *Elders, students. and computers—background information* (No. 8). Illinois Series on Educational Applications of Computers. (ERIC Document Reproduction Service No. ED 138285 IR004714).

Kerschner, P.A., & Hart, K.C. (1984). The aged user and technology. In R.E. Dunkle, M.R. Haug, & M. Rosenberg (Eds.), *Communications technology and the elderly* (pp. 135–144). New York: Springer.

Knowles, M.S. (1980). *The modern practice of adult education.* Chicago: Associate Press.

Londoner, C.A. (1978). Instrumental and expressive education: A basis for needs assessment and planning. In R.W. Sherron & D.B. Lumsden (Eds.), *Introduction to educational gerontology* (pp. 75–92). Washington, DC: Hemisphere.

Marcus, E.E. (1978). Effects of age, sex and status on perception of the utility of educational participation. *Educational Gerontology, 3,* 295–319.

National Center for Education Statistics. (1978). *Participation in adult education: Final report.* Washington, DC: U.S. Government Printing Office.

Office of Technology Assessment (1984). *Technology and aging in America.* Washington, DC: Congress of the United States.

Okun, M.A., & Siegler, I.C. (1977). The perception of outcome–effort covariation in younger and older men. *Educational Gerontology, 2,* 27–32.

Percy, K. (1989). Participation of older people in learning activities in the United Kingdom. *Educational Gerontology, 15,* 133–150.

Peterson, D.A. (1983). *Facilitating education for older learners.* San Francisco, CA: Jossey-Bass.

Rebok, G.W., & Offermann, L.R. (1983). Behavioral competencies of older college students: A self-efficacy approach. *The Gerontologist, 23,* 428–432.

Rothkopf, E.Z. (1976). Writing to teach and reading to learn: A perspective on the psychology of written instruction. In W.L. Gage (Ed.), *The psychology of teaching methods* (pp. 91–129). Chicago: University of Chicago Press.

Thompson, D.N. (1988, April). *Use of advance organizers to improve reading comprehension of older adults.* Paper presented at the second Cognitive Aging Conference, Atlanta.

Thompson, D.N., & Diefenderfer, K. (1986, April). *The use of advance organizers with adults of limited verbal ability.* Paper presented at the American Educational Research: Association Convention, San Francisco.

Thorndike, E.L. (1928). *Adult learning.* New York: Macmillan.

Weisman, S. (1983). Computer games for the frail elderly. *The Gerontologist, 23,* 361–363.

West, R.L. (1985). *Memory fitness over 40.* Gainesville, FL: Triad Publishing.

Withnall, A. (1989). Education for older adults: Some recent British research. *Educational Gerontology, 15,* 187–198.

Witken, H.A. (1976). Cognitive style in academic peer performance and in teacher–student relations. In S. Messick (Ed.), *Individuality in learning: Implications of cognitive styles and creativity for human development* (pp. 35–89). San Francisco: Jossey-Bass.

Woods, J.H., & Bernard, R.M. (1987). Improving older adult's retention of text: A test of an instructional strategy. *Educational Gerontology, 13,* 107–120.

12
Bridging the Gap Between Researchers and Clinicians: Methodological Perspectives and Choices

KATHRYN PEREZ RILEY

The emergence of everyday memory and aging as a major field of study has resulted from the combined efforts of investigators from a variety of backgrounds, interests, and disciplines, including experimental researchers as well as practicing clinicians. While the findings of everyday memory research are clearly relevant to the development of intervention programs, efforts to implement laboratory-based research methods and designs in clinical settings are still in the relatively early stages of development. This chapter will discuss the contributions that can be made by practicing clinicians to the field of everyday memory and aging, focusing on two themes. First, the methodological choices made by experimental researchers will be considered in terms of their utility and relevance to the practitioner who wishes to apply these methods in training programs with clinical populations. A second issue to be discussed is the role of the clinician in initiating interventions that may then be examined on a larger scale by experimental researchers in the field of everyday memory and aging. A small number of recent studies on memory skills training programs will be used to illustrate these themes, emphasizing my work and the work of others with persons who have been diagnosed as memory impaired. The interested reader is referred to recent reviews of the literature on memory-training programs for a more detailed discussion of findings in this area (West, 1990; West & Tomer, 1989; see also Chapter 10, this volume).

Methodological Issues: Application of Research Designs

The very nature of everyday or practical memory research signifies a shift from the study of some aspects of memory functioning that may be limited in generalizability beyond the lab to a consideration of older adults' abilities in more naturalistic settings (West, 1986). An examination of the research in this area reveals that some changes in method and design are often made in the move away from strictly laboratory-based studies, particularly when research is conducted on memory skills training programs (Hill, Storandt, & Simeone, 1990; Poon et al., 1986; Riley, 1990; Scogin,

Storandt & Lott, 1985; Yesavage, Sheikh, Friedman & Tanke, 1990). Nevertheless, the practitioner who wishes to apply experimental training procedures in controlled clinical trials may have difficulty in replicating some of the methods described in the research studies. Some of these difficulties arise from the limited time and resources the clinician may have to devote to this kind of project, while other problems are likely to be related to the type of patients who will be involved in the training program. In developing a memory skills training program for older adults diagnosed as having either Age-Associated Memory Impairment (AAMI) (Crook et al., 1986; Crook & Larrabee, 1988) or early Alzheimer's type dementia (AD), I found that the time frames of most published studies posed the greatest single barrier to the clinical application of empirical designs (Riley, 1990). Many of these research procedures involve 2- to 3-hour sessions occurring two or more times per week, held for as many as 10 weeks (cf. Hill, Evankovich, Sheikh, & Yesavage, 1987). Although it would be desirable to replicate the procedures of a successful program when possible, the clinician may have to modify the design by using shorter training sessions and reducing the number of sessions to make a training program feasible. This streamlining of procedures may be particularly essential when one is working with cognitively impaired or frail elderly patients who, along with their care givers, may be unable to withstand lengthy training sessions or to commit to an 8- or 10-week training program.

One way in which memory training programs can be modified and yet remain comprehensive is to employ homework or self-directed training materials (West, 1990). Recent research has shown that older adults (Baltes, Sowarka, & Kliegl, 1989; Hill et al., 1990; Scogin et al., 1985) can benefit from training programs that rely heavily on homework materials. Using these procedures may make the intervention more cost-effective for the practitioner, while also reducing wear and tear on the older clients. It is helpful that many of the studies that have employed self-training or homework assignments have described their procedures in some detail, making the application of these methods in clinical settings more feasible (cf. Hill et al., 1990).

A final methodological issue of relevance here is the failure of most memory skills training programs to document either the generalizability or long-term maintenance of the training (West, 1990). Although there are some exceptions (Camp, 1989; Sheikh, Hill, & Yesavage, 1986), this general lack of evidence for the enduring, practical utility of training in daily life may make it difficult for the practitioner and his or her patients to invest in an intervention program.

This issue is especially critical in light of the practitioners' obligation to avoid raising false hopes in elderly clients who are mildly cognitively impaired. It seems reasonable, then, to suggest that this is an area in which practitioners can make a meaningful contribution to the everyday memory literature by conducting field trials of intervention programs that include long-term follow-up and methods designed to enhance the generalizability of the mnemonic techniques (Poon, Fozard, & Treat, 1978; West & Tomer, 1989).

Clinical Intervention Programs and Everyday Memory

It has been suggested that the gerontological practitioner may be in a unique position to design and carry out both quantitative and qualitative work in a manner that will be of use and interest to fellow clinicians and to experimental researchers (Kahana, Kahana, & Riley, 1988; Rowles & Reinhartz, 1988; Poon et al., 1986). As the field of everyday memory and aging matures, it seems likely that more attention will be paid by investigators to the clinical utility of their research paradigms (West, 1990). As more researchers include comments on how modifications in their designs might affect the outcome of a training program (see Willis, 1987), discuss the clinical applications of the designs (Scogin et al., 1985; Yesavage et al., 1990), or conduct studies with clinical populations (Hill et al., 1987; Zarit, Cole, & Guider, 1981; see also Chapter 10, this volume), the "gap" between experimental and clinical investigators will begin to close. Yet much remains to be done, and the practitioner may have a special role and responsibility in helping to expand on current knowledge and stimulate further research. Clinical intervention programs that are based on experimental methods can meet some of the recommendations made by cognitive aging researchers for accomplishing these goals (Baltes et al., 1989; Erickson & Howeison, 1986; Riley, 1990; West & Tomer, 1989).

The Development of a Training Program for the Memory Impaired

In attempting to develop and evaluate a memory skills training program for use with persons diagnosed as having AAMI or early AD, Riley (1990) reviewed the relevant literature to find an approach that had some documented success, was relatively simple to teach and use, and would be relevant to the everyday memory demands of the mildly memory-impaired client. Some of the more complicated methods such as the method of loci (see Yesavage & Rose, 1984) and others (West, 1990) did not seem appropriate for this population, although they had documented success. I chose the spaced retrieval method of memory enhancement (Camp, 1989; Landauer & Bjork, 1978) as the strategy to be trained because it had been used with cognitively impaired subjects and because this technique seemed particularly amenable to the kinds of modifications that would be helpful in working with AD or AAMI patients. A case study design was used with two subjects, both of whom were diagnosed as having very mild AD. Extensive baseline data were gathered for each participant, including neuropsychological test data, detailed histories, performance on the Rivermead Behavioral Memory Test and the Geriatric Depression Scale, and reports of individual memory problems and use of internal or external memory aids in daily life. I held four weekly, 1-hour training sessions, with the care giver of each Alzheimer's patient participating as an active member of the research intervention team. A major goal of the study was to see if the spaced retrieval technique would be useful to the patient and care giver in the home environment once the training sessions were completed. Each session focused on using the technique to learn a face–name pair; both patients had reported this as a particularly difficult area of everyday memory. During the third training session, the care givers were instructed to use the technique at home in the coming week, and both care givers and patients were asked to use it in the month before a 1-month follow-up session. Homework assignments and daily or weekly diaries were used throughout the study. The results of the study, including a 6-month follow-up interview, revealed that the spaced retrieval technique led to fairly rapid learning and long-term retention of a face–name pair, and both sets of patient–care giver participants reported successful use of the technique at home during the study period and after 6 months (I can provide additional details on the procedures and outcomes; see last page of this chapter for correpondence address).

Modifications That Work

The study described previously illustrates how several methodological modifications suggested by researchers and clinicians (Kahana et al., 1988; West & Tomer, 1989) can enhance the utility and effectiveness of memory skills training programs in the applied setting. The specific modifications that I employed included individually designed training programs, the use of care givers as part of the research team, the use of homework assignments, and long-term follow-up (Riley, 1990). Each of these additions to or alterations in the methods of relevant research will be discussed in relation to their use by future practitioners and investigators.

Memory skills training programs often include a variety of special procedures in addition to the basic mnemonic training (Hill et al., 1990; Zarit et al., 1981), and some researchers have recently called for the individualized assessment of study participants as a means of enhancing the effectiveness of intervention programs (Yesavage et al., 1990; West & Tomer, 1989). Riley (1990) used neuropsychological test data as well as data collected for the purpose of the spaced retrieval study to develop this kind of individualized training system, while still following the published procedures on the use of the technique (Camp, 1989).

Practicing clinicians should be in a good position to capitalize on their knowledge of and access to patients who can serve as research participants. Another example of modifications to training programs involve the effects of the individual's mood on memory performance. Yesavage and his colleagues (see Yesavage & Jacobs, 1984; Yesavage et al., 1990) have recommended the use of relaxation training as a part of their programs for highly anxious individuals. Both participants in my study (Riley, 1990) reported that anxiety played a role in their daily life attempts to learn and remember information. In addition to teaching the mnemonic strategy, relaxation training with home practice sessions was included in the study design.

Thus, clinicians who develop interventions based on the published works may be in a good position to choose those special procedures that best fit their patients' needs, thereby testing the empirical procedures under optimal conditions when the training procedures are an exact match with the participants' characteristics.

Generalizability and Maintenance of Skills Training

I have noted that little data exist on the generalizability and long-term maintenance of memory skills training programs. However, practitioners can address these issues in their clinical intervention studies, which in turn should spur other researchers to test practitioners' procedures in large-scale studies. Involvement of care givers in the training process and the use of homework assignments that included both care givers and patients (Riley, 1990) allowed for an examination of the practical utility of the spaced retrieval technique over a relatively long period of time (7 months). These procedures also reduced the amount of time that the participants had to spend in the investigator's office, making it easier for them to add the study to their schedules.

The use of homework and the involvement of the care giver throughout the four weekly training sessions as well as the 1- and 6-month follow-up sessions seemed particularly valuable to the participants' successful use of the spaced retrieval technique (Riley, 1990). Both individuals were able to learn and retain over a 7-week period one face–name pair, using this technique. In addition, both participants and their care givers used the strategy at home (as evidenced by daily or weekly logs) to learn and remember meaningful and important pieces of information, such as appointments or the location of a household key. Others have suggested (Hill et al., 1990; West, 1990) that the strategies used in training studies or interventions be applicable to daily life and usable by older adults on their own. Again, the practitioner who has a personal relationship with prospective study participants can work to increase the practical utility of the training program.

Finally, the follow-up sessions conducted in this study (Riley, 1990) that have been recommended by many researchers (Baltes et al., 1989; West, 1990) were probably made more feasible as a result of my clinical relationship with both of the patients and their care givers, as well as by the fact that all of the participants were quite invested in contributing something to knowledge about memory impairment and Alzheimer's dementia. The use of clinical populations by practitioners in field trials of laboratory-based memory skills training programs may therefore overcome two problems commonly seen in experimental studies: low motivation on the part of participants to use the strategies on their own or to take part in long-term follow-up sessions. The individualized assessment of patients and intensive involvement of care givers should prove to be extremely helpful in creating successful intervention programs that have their roots in laboratory-based designs and procedures.

Conclusions

The area of everyday memory and aging provides a natural bridge between experimental investigators and practitioners. As this field develops and more work is done in the related area of AAMI and the dementias, the clinical implementation of theoretical knowledge in the form of viable and cost-effective intervention programs for older adults should also progress. The further development of an exciting and important field of research will be enhanced by the active participation of clinicians who can share their expertise and knowledge of their older clients' special characteristics and needs. This kind of systematic and constructive dialogue between professionals can help this field reach its fullest potential.

Note. Additional information can be obtained from Kathryn Perez Riley, Department of Psychiatry, Marshall University School of Medicine, Huntington. WV 25755-9760.

References

Baltes, P.B., Sowarka, D., & Kliegl, R. (1989). Cognitive training research on fluid intelligence in old age. What can older adults achieve by themselves? *Psychology and Aging, 4,* 217–221.

Camp, C.J. (1989). Facilitation of new learning in Alzheimer's disease. In G.C. Gilmore, P.J. Whitehouse & M.L. Wykle (Eds.), *Memory, aging and dementia: Theory, assessment and treatment* (pp. 212–225). New York: Springer Publishing.

Crook, T., Bartus, R.S., Ferris, S.H., Whitehouse, P., Cohen, G.D., & Gershon, S. (1986). Age-Associated Memory Impairment: Proposed diagnostic criteria and measures of clinical change—Report of a National Institute of Mental Health work group. *Developmental Neuropsychology, 2,* 261–276.

Crook, T., & Larrabee, G.J. (1988). Age-Associated Memory Impairment: Diagnostic criteria and treatment strategies. *Psychopharmacology Bulletin, 24,* 509–514.

Erickson, R.C., & Howeison, D. (1986). The clinician's perspective: Measuring change and treatment effectiveness. In L.W. Poon (Ed.), *Handbook for clinical memory assessment of older adults* (pp. 69–80). Washington, DC: American Psychological Association.

Hill, R.D., Evankovich, K.D., Sheikh, J.H., & Yesavage J.A. (1987). Imagery mnemonic training in a patient with primary degenerative dementia. *Psychology and Aging, 2,* 204–205.

Hill, R.D., Storandt, M., & Simeone, C. (1990). The effects of memory skills training and incentives on free recall in older learners. *Journal of Gerontology, 45,* 215–226.

Kahana, E., Kahana, B., & Riley, K.P. (1988). Contextual issues in qualitative studies of institutional settings for the aged. In G.D. Rowles & G. Reinhartz (Eds.), *Qualitative gerontology* (pp. 197–216). New York: Springer.

Landauer, T.K., & Bjork, R.A. (1978). Optimum rehersal patterns and name learning. In M.M. Gruneberg, P.E. Morris, & R.N. Sykes (Eds.), *Practical aspects of memory* (pp. 625–632). New York: Academic Press.

Poon, L.W., Fozard, J.L., & Treat, N. (1978). From clinical and research findings on memory to intervention programs. *Experimental Aging Research, 4,* 235–253.

Poon, L.W., Gurland, B.J., Eisdorfer, C., Crook, T., Thompson, L.W., Kaszniak, A.W., & David, K.L. (1986). Integration of experimental and clinical precepts in memory assessment: A tribute to George Talland. In L.W. Poon (Ed.), *Handbook for clinical memory assessment of older adults* (pp. 3–10). Washington, DC: American Psychological Association.

Riley, K.P. (1989). Psychological interventions in Alzheimer's Disease. In G.C. Gilmore, P.J. Whitehouse & M.L. Wykle (Eds.), *Memory, aging and dementia: Theory, assessment and treatment* (pp. 199–211). New York: Springer.

Riley, K.P. (1990). *The application of a memory maintenance program with demented elderly and their caregivers.* Paper presented at the Cognitive Aging Conference, Atlanta.

Rowles, G.D., & Reinhartz, G. (Eds.). (1988). *Qualitative gerontology.* New York: Springer.

Scogin, F., Storandt, M., & Lott, L. (1985). Memory skills training, memory complaints, and depression in older adults. *Journal of Gerontology, 40,* 562–568.

Sheikh, J.I., Hill, R.D. & Yesavage, J.A. (1986). Long-term efficacy of cognitive training for Age-Associated Memory Impairment: A six month follow-up study. *Developmental Neuropsychology, 2,* 413–421.

West, R.L. (1986). Everyday memory and aging. *Developmental Neuropsychology, 2,* 323–344.

West, R.L. (1990). Planning practical memory training for the aged. In L.W. Poon, D.C. Rubin, & B.C. Wilson (Eds.), *Everyday cognition in adulthood and late life* (pp. 573–597). Cambridge, England: Cambridge University Press.

West, R.L., & Tomer, A. (1989). Everyday memory problems of healthy older adults: Characteristics of a successful intervention. In G.C. Gilmore, P.J. Whitehouse, & M.L. Wykle (Eds.), *Memory, aging and dementia: Theory, assessment and treatment* (pp. 74–98). New York: Springer.

Willis, S. (1987). Cognitive training and everyday competence. In K.W. Schaie & C. Eisdorfer (Eds.), *Annual review of gerontology and geriatrics* (Vol. 7, pp. 159–188). New York: Springer.

Yesavage, J.A., & Jacob, R. (1984). Effects of relaxation and mnemonics on memory, attention and anxiety in the elderly. *Experimental Aging Research, 10,* 211–214.

Yesavage, J.A., & Rose, T.L. (1984). Semantic elaboration and the method of loci: A new trip for older learners. *Experimental Aging Research, 10,* 155–159.

Yesavage, J.A., Sheikh, J.I., Friedman, L., & Tanke, E. (1990). Learning mnemonics: Roles of aging and subtle cognitive impairment. *Psychology and Aging, 5,* 133–137.

Zarit, S.N., Cole, K.D., & Guider, R.L. (1981). Memory training strategies and subjective complaints of memory in the aged. *The Gerontologist, 21,* 158–164.

13
The Interface Between Psychometric Abilities and Everyday Cognitive Functioning

BERT HAYSLIP, JR. AND ROBIN M. MALOY

Ascribing to a decrement with compensation model of intellectual aging, Baltes and Willis have demonstrated that general fluid ability (Gf) performance can be enhanced via the direct provision of solution rules (see Baltes & Willis, 1982). These interventions were specifically designed to impact the component skills defining Gf in aged persons. Other issues notwithstanding (e.g., new vs. old skills acquisition, practice, anxiety reduction as alternative means by which to enhance Gf), a persistent concern in the Gf training literature has been the narrowness of training effects (Hayslip, 1989a, 1989b). In this light, nearly all the Gf training studies to date have reported performance gains that were limited to the ability markers they were designed to impact (Hayslip, 1989b).

Related to this breadth of training issue are concerns about the transfer of training to measures of performance that may be less threatening and have more face validity to the older person. Compared to the Gf-training tasks themselves, such measures may reflect more directly the everyday cognitive tasks confronting many older adults (see Hoyer, 1987). This sensitivity to the contextual, ecological nature of human abilities has been underscored by Sternberg (1985) in his discussion of implicit versus explicit theories of intelligence. Whereas explicit (e.g., psychometric) theories often ignore the real-world context in which intelligence is exercised, implicit (e.g., people's notions regarding what intelligence is) approaches centralize the role of context and use tasks with ecological validity (Sternberg, 1985). In this light, exploring the linkage between both fluid and general crystallized ability (Gc) and everyday cognition can serve to bridge these two very different approaches to human abilities.

Willis and Schaie (1986) have demonstrated stronger relationships between Gf and ETS Basic Reading Skills test (Educational Testing Service, 1977) performance than for Gc and the ETS scale in aged persons (see also Marsiske & Willis, 1988), while Cornelius and Caspi (1987) found that both Gf and Gc predicted performance on an everyday problem-solving inventory. Despite the shortcomings of the ETS scale, that is, its limited memory demands, asocial content, emphasis on a "right" answer (see Willis & Schaie, 1986), and lack of functional validity with aged persons (see Hayslip, 1989b; Scheidt, 1981), it can serve as a very preliminary starting point for assessing everyday intelligence in late adulthood.

To date, we know of no published training research that has demonstrated transfer to an approximate measure of everyday intelligence like the ETS scale. Willis (1987), in her discussion of these issues, clearly describes factor analytic data linking the psychometric and everyday abilities domains, but no training data are presented. This chapter reports the results of several of our studies investigating the relationship between fluid ability performance and everyday (ETS Basic Reading Skill) cognition, as well as the impact of induction training on ETS Basic Reading Skill performance.

Phase 1: Interrelationships Between Psychometric Abilities and Everyday Cognition

In a descriptive study of the interrelationships among psychometric intelligence and ETS performance, we administered measures of crystallized (vocabulary, abstruse analogies) and fluid (matrices, letter series, common analogies) abilities to 102 healthy community-residing older adults (M age = 69.09, SD = 7.49; M education = 5.97, SD = 2.05, range = 2–17, where 1 = less than grade school and 17 = postdoctoral study). Participants also completed the ETS Basic Reading Skills test (Educational Testing Service, 1977) employing a 35-min time limit. This test assesses performance on a variety of paper-and-pencil tasks (e.g., reading maps, filling out forms, understanding charts and schedules; understanding labels; reading technical documents; paragraph, ads, and news text comprehension). Intercorrelations between each of the eight subscales of the ETS Basic Skills test and the ETS total score exceeded +.70, except for that involving reading labels (r = .61).

Correlations (see Table 13.1) between each of these subscales and the preceding measures of Gf/Gc favored indicators of fluid ability (average r = .32, p < .01). The highest correlation was between letter series and understanding technical documents. Correlations with measures of Gc were somewhat lower (average r = .22, p < .05), with the highest being between vocabulary and filling out forms.

In a supplementary stepwise regression analysis, we used measures of Gf and Gc, self-rated health, and age and level of education to predict ETS performance. This analysis generally confirmed our findings (see Table 13.2). Age was the best predictor of ETS total scores. For paragraph comprehension, understanding ads, and reading technical documents, letter series (Gf) best (p < .01) predicted performance. Letter series also predicted ETS total scores. For understanding labels, vocabulary (Gc) best

TABLE 13.1. Correlations between ability measures and ETS performance.[a]

ETS Scale		Ability measure			
	Vocabulary[b]	Abstruse analogies[b]	Common analogies[c]	Matrices[c]	Letter series[c]
Understanding labels	.31**	.21*	.22*	.33**	.40**
Reading maps	.08	.17*	.15	.25**	.21*
Understanding charts/schedules	.11	−.07	.19*	.12	.25**
Paragraph comprehension	.34**	.16	.22*	.28**	.46**
Filling out forms	.37**	.32**	.35**	.34**	.45**
Understanding ads	.15	.16	.19*	.37**	.42**
Understanding technical documents	.29**	.24**	.32**	.31**	.47**
News text comprehension	.33**	.24**	.36**	.26**	.42**
Total score	.35**	.24**	.34**	.35**	.51**

ETS, Educational Testing Service.
[a] $N = 102$.
[b] Gc, general crystallized ability.
[c] Gf, general fluid ability.
* $p < .05$, ** $p < .01$.

TABLE 13.2. Regression analyses of ETS scores.

Dependent variable	Predictors[a]	F[b]	B[c]	b[d]	R²[e]
Understanding labels	Vocabulary	8.70**	.31	.13	.24
	Common analogies	7.78**	.29	.14	
Reading maps	Matrices	6.96**	.25	.04	.10
	Health	6.65**	.24	.15	
Understanding charts/ schedules	Health	21.65**	.47	.43	.18
Paragraph comprehension	Letter series	27.04**	.22	.51	.34
	Age	4.92*	−.05	−.22	
Filling out forms	—	—	—	—	—
Understanding ads	Letter series	25.30**	.15	.46	.21
Understanding technical documents	Letter series	22.65**	.16	.57	.30
News text comprehension	Common analogies	24.18**	.43	.58	.33
ETS total score	Letter series	6.91**	1.18	.31	.44
	Age	28.09**	−.77	−.42	
	Vocabulary	8.82**	1.45	.25	

ETS, Educational Testing Service.
[a] Stepwise regression method.
[b] F value for B.
[c] unstandardized regression coefficient (B).
[d] standardized regression coefficient (b).
[e] adjusted R^2.
$*p < .05$, $**p < .01$.

predicted ($p < .01$) performance and served as a tertiary predictor of ETS total scores. Matrices (Gf) best predicted map-reading scores ($p < .01$), while common analogies (Gf) best predicted ($p < .01$) understanding news text and secondarily predicted understanding labels. Age secondarily predicted paragraph comprehension, while health best predicted understanding charts/schedules, and secondarily predicted map reading.

The psychometric ability measures and ETS total scores were then subjected to a principal axis factoring procedure, with a subsequent varimax rotation to a terminal solution (see Table 13.3). This analysis suggested that ETS total scores load more heavily on a fluid-type factor, though Table 13.3 also suggests some shared variance between Gc and ETS total scores.

In sum, these data are consistent with those reported by Willis and Schaie (1986) illustrating a somewhat stronger relationship between ETS Basic Reading Skills performance and fluid abilities than between ETS scores and crystallized skills, though such relations did vary by ETS subscale in both studies.

TABLE 13.3. Normative data and factor structure of Gf-Gc and ETS scales.[a]

Measure	Mean	SD	Range	Factor 1 (Gf)[b]	Factor 2 (Gc)[c]
Vocabulary	11.30	2.36	2–15	.201	.784
Abstruse analogies	7.09	1.88	1–12	.289	.457
Common analogies	7.61	2.01	2–11	.516	.472
Matrices	6.94	2.93	1–11	.654	.189
Letter series	9.14	3.67	0–15	.781	.285
ETS total score	50.34	13.55	15–65	.474	.299

ETS, Educational Testing Service.
[a] $N = 102$.
[b] Accounts for 49.8% of common variance.
[c] Accounts for 14.8% of common variance.

Phase 2: The Impact of Gf Intervention on Everyday Cognition

Based on the preceding analyses, we designed a more restricted intervention study to explore the relationship between psychometric abilities and ETS performance in a cause and effect manner.

Thirty community-residing older volunteers (M age = 74.2, range = 63–87 years) served as subjects for the intervention study. The majority were retired women and were either married or widowed. Most persons (80%) saw their health as at least good relative to their age peers. All but three individuals had at least a high school education ($M = 4.91$, $SD = 1.73$, range = 1–10, where 1 = less than grade school and 10 = complete postdoctoral study). Sixteen were randomly assigned to the Adult Development and Enrichmant Project (ADEPT) (Baltes & Willis, 1982) induction training, while 14 were randomly assigned to a no-contact control condition.

Individuals were pretested and subsequently posttested (alternate forms) one week after training with a battery of measures assessing crystallized (vocabulary, abstruse analogies) and fluid (letter series, matrices) ability (see Hayslip, 1989a). In addition, we administered the ETS (1977) Basic Reading Skills test (alternate forms) at both pretest and posttest. All ETS subscales were significantly (r's > .60, $p < .01$) related to total ETS scores. With the exception of a 35-min time limit for the ETS measure, no ability measures were administered under timed conditions.

When we examined the preceding data with 2 (group) × 2 (testing, i.e., pretest–posttest occasions) analyses of variance (ANOVAs; see Table 13.4), we found significant group by testing effects for letter series ($F_{1,28} = 9.87$, $p < .01$) and for vocabulary ($F_{1,28} = 6.55$, $p < .02$). Follow-up simple effects analyses indicated that experimental subjects improved their letter series performance to a greater extent ($F_{1,15} = 51.07$, $p < .001$) than did controls ($F_{1,13} = 8.32$, $p < .02$), who evidenced a slight decline. Moreover, while pretest letter series scores did not differ between groups

TABLE 13.4. Observed and adjusted means for selected dependent variables.

| | Induction training ($n=16$) | | | | | No contact control ($n=14$) | | | | |
| | Pretest | | Posttest | | | Pretest | | Posttest | | |
Variable	M	SD	M	SD	Adjusted posttest[a]	M	SD	M	SD	Adjusted posttest[a]
Letter series	7.00	3.20	10.62	2.03	10.50*	6.64	3.10	6.43	5.15	6.54*
Vocabulary	11.18	1.60	11.31	2.46	12.09*	13.00	1.88	8.42	6.65	13.06*
Abstruse analogies	9.18	2.16	5.93	2.56	6.12	9.57	2.87	4.91	4.12	4.73
Matrices	5.75	2.29	7.37	1.85	7.15	4.50	3.69	5.00	3.94	5.22
ETS total score	48.37	13.27	44.18	11.65	37.97	34.05	22.29	31.07	25.36	37.28
ETS labels	5.43	.89	5.50	.73	5.05**	4.00	2.35	3.28	2.64	3.72**
ETS news text	2.06	2.46	1.18	1.75	.92***	1.28	2.55	1.29	2.19	1.55***
ETS maps	2.00	.00	1.93	.25	1.76	1.42	.85	1.21	.97	1.34
ETS charts	5.50	1.09	5.37	.88	5.01	4.42	2.47	3.71	2.92	4.08
ETS ads	6.75	1.12	6.31	1.53	5.69	5.14	3.41	4.35	3.38	4.97

ETS, Educational Testing Service.
[a] Pretest as covariate.
*$p<.01$, **$p<.05$, ***$p<.10$

$(F_{1,28} = .09, NS)$, at posttest, the experimental group's performance exceeded that of controls $(F_{1,28} = 7.95, p < .02)$.

For vocabulary, follow-up simple effects analyses indicated that whereas experimental subjects' scores remained stable $(F_{1,15} = 67, NS)$, controls' vocabulary performance declined $(F_{1,28} = 6.90, p < .02)$. Moreover, whereas pretest vocabulary scores were similar across groups $(F_{1,28} = 3.49, NS)$, at posttest the control group's performance was inferior to that of the experimental group $(F_{1,28} = 9.25, p < .01)$. For matrices, we obtained a nearly significant group main effect $(F_{1,28} = 3.97, p < .06)$, wherein experimental subjects' performance exceeded that of controls. Significant testing effects for all subjects were found for letter series $F_{1,28} = 7.79$, $p < .01$) and vocabulary $(F_{1,28} = 10.16, p < .01)$, where posttest scores were higher than pretest scores for letter series but not vocabulary.

In tests of the group main effect, overall ETS scores were higher for the induction-training group than for controls $(F_{1,28} = 4.25, p < .05)$; as were scores for labels $(F_{1,28} = 9.76, p < .01)$; maps $(F_{1,28} = 10.26, p < .01)$; charts $(F_{1,28} = 4.42, p < .05)$, and ads $(F_{1,28} = 4.29, p < .05)$. No testing effects or group by testing interactions were significant for ETS total scores or for any ETS subscale.

Supplementary one-way (group) analyses of covariance using the pretest as a covariate, yielded (see Table 13.4) main effects for training versus control conditions for ability performance. For the induction training group at posttest (adjusting for pretest), scores for letter series $(F_{1,27} = 11.17, p < .01)$ were higher, while for controls, adjusted posttest vocabulary scores were higher $(F_{1,27} = 6.79, p < .05)$. For the ETS Basic Reading skills measure, no training effects were found for total score. However, greater proficiency in understanding labels was found for induction subjects $(F_{1,27} = 4.49, p < .05)$, while a weak effect $(p < .09)$ favoring controls was found for understanding news text. While not statistically significant, most of the adjusted means for the ETS subscales did however, favor the induction training group. On the other hand, some evidence in study 2 indicates that, despite the positive relationship between ETS performance and Gf skills in study 1, ETS performance declined slightly for all subjects while Gf performance increased (see Table 13.4). This trend however, was not statistically significant.

Despite results suggesting some parallels between psychometric ability and everyday cognition, these findings do merit some discussion. It is surprising, in light of the purported experiential nature of the ETS subscales (and their correlation with Gc), *not* to observe practice effects for these variables. This strengthens the training effects found in this study, despite their attenuation when pretest scores are accounted for. While training on these everyday tasks may be more efficient (see Hayslip, 1989b; Willis, 1987), the present data nevertheless can be seen as evidence for Gf training effects' partial generalization beyond specific ability targets.

Also of interest in Table 13.4 is the fact that pretest levels of ETS scores were higher for trained subjects than for controls. When pretest scores were covaried, training effects on ETS performance were less substantial. Yet, the repeated measures ANOVA did not yield differential gains for controls, despite their lower pretest ETS scores. Moreover, the induction-training group maintained its advantage over controls at posttest for ETS performance.

The repeated measures ANOVA findings tend to support the notion of content (and perhaps process) specificity as a consideration in defining Gf–ETS scale relationships. Each may elicit similar heuristics, such as encoding, inference of a relationship between elements, mapping of higher order relations, reencoding, and comparison of this new relationship to a prototype (see Sternberg, 1985). The covariance analyses, however, are less encouraging; they support an explanation of Gf–ETS scale relationships in terms of the encapsulation (narrowing) of abilities in later life (Rybash, Hoyer, & Roodin, 1986), wherein a sweeping generalization of training effects to multiple domains would be unlikely.

In many respects then, these data can be used to support and reject the notion that the effects of an ability-specific cognitive intervention extend beyond those targets for which the program was designed. Depending on one's perspective, this may or may not be desirable. Our findings are even less definitive in providing a process-oriented basis for understanding the links between Gf/Gc and practical intelligence. Perhaps "think-aloud" procedures (e.g., Ericsson & Simon, 1984) might be valuable in this regard.

The experimental data should be viewed in the light of the small samples that precluded multivariate analyses and the lack of a long-term follow-up. Additionally, comparisons with a noncognitive intervention (e.g., stress inoculation) would be desirable, as would research with samples whose intellectual history is known (i.e., history of cognitive changes, occupational status). Despite these limitations, the experimental data suggest that for the most part, induction-training effects, while narrow in scope regarding ability performance, nevertheless do generalize to some ecologically relevant intellectual tasks, though these effects are weak.

Although these findings support an interpretation of a moderate degree of convergence between psychometric abilities and everyday intelligence, the two domains are by no means isomorphic. Moreover, these data do not address the questions of (a) whether older persons use similar problem-solving heuristics to solve Gf and ETS tasks, (b) what individual difference variables mediate performance on both sets of tasks, or (c) what degree of contextual or adaptive specificity exists with regard to determining psychometric ability–everyday cognition relationships. Our data do, however, substantiate the further exploration of everyday cognition in late adulthood, of which psychometric intelligence is but a component, albeit an important one. They also suggest that the differences between explicit and implicit theories of intelligence espoused by Sternberg (1985) may be more apparent than real.

References

Baltes, P.B., & Willis, S.L. (1982). Plasticity and enhancement of intellectual functioning in old age: Penn State's Adult Development and Enrichment Project (ADEPT). In F.I.M. Craik & S.E. Trehub (Eds.), *Aging and cognitive processes* (pp. 353–389). New York: Plenum.

Cornelius, S., & Caspi, A. (1987). Everyday problem solving in adulthood and old age. *Psychology and Aging, 2,* 144–153.

Educational Testing Service (1977). *Basic Skills Assessment Program.* Princeton, NJ.

Ericsson, K.A., & Simon, H. (1984). *Protocol analysis.* Cambridge, MA: Harvard University Press.

Hayslip, B. (1989a). Alternative mechanisms for improvements in fluid ability among the aged. *Psychology and Aging, 4,* 122–124.

Hayslip, B. (1989b). Issues in cognitive training research with the aged: A past with a future? *Educational Gerontology, 15,* 573–596.

Hoyer, W. (1987). Acquisition of knowledge and the decentralization of g in adult intellectual development. In C. Schooler & K.W. Schaie (Eds.), *Cognitive functioning and social structure over the life span* (pp. 120–141). Norwood, NJ: Ablex.

Marsiske, M., & Willis, S.L. (1988, August). *Description and prediction of age-related change in everyday task performance.* Paper presented at the annual convention of the American Psychological Association, Atlanta.

Rybash, J.M., Hoyer, W.J., & Roodin, P.A. (1986). *Adult cognition and aging.* New York: Pergamon Press.

Scheidt, R.J. (1981). Ecologically valid inquiry: Fait accompli? *Human Development, 23,* 225–228.

Sternberg, R.J. (1985). *Beyond IQ. A triarchic theory of human intelligence.* New York: University Press.

Willis, S.L. (1987). Cognitive training and everyday competence. In K.W. Schaie & C. Eisdorfer (Eds.), *Annual review of gerontology and geriatrics* (Vol. 7, pp. 159–188). New York: Springer.

Willis, S.L., & Schaie, K.W. (1986). Practical intelligence in later adulthood. In R. Sternberg & R. Wagner (Eds.), *Practical intelligence* (pp. 236–270). New York: Cambridge University Press.

Part 4
Issues and Illustrations of Everyday Memory Research

14
Spatial Skills, Memory, and Environmental Use in a Nursing Home Setting

KRISTEN K.A. NORRIS AND ISELI K. KRAUSS

Limited use of the environment by older adults may be related to a number of factors in addition to health and mobility problems. Memory skills are certainly necessary for knowing and negotiating the environment. Reduced basic cognitive skills, however, may also limit both environmental knowledge and use of that environment; and reduction of knowledge of the environment contributes to lower environmental use (Walsh, Krauss, & Regnier, 1981).

This complex relationship among cognitive skills, knowledge of the surroundings, and use of those surroundings may apply in one's immediate living quarters as well as in a larger neighborhood or community setting. Therefore, cognitive abilities and knowledge of the immediate environment may be just as important for residents of nursing homes as they are for community-dwelling older adults. The only difference in these cases is that the environment in question is limited—restricted to a few floors or wings and perhaps the grounds of a residential facility.

Some researchers have ventured into this research territory in attempts to determine the correlates of environmental use in older adults. Krauss (1989) and Evans, Smith, and Pezdek (1982) have shown that while there is overlap, older adults focus on different variables than do younger adults in their attempts to remember landmarks in a familiar neighborhood. Older adults are more likely than younger adults to attend to buildings with direct street access. Weber, Brown, and Weldon (1978) investigated older, mobile patients' knowledge of the nursing home in which they were living. They found that the residents were less able to identify photographs of locations within the nursing home than were young nonresidents who were unfamiliar with the nursing home. At the same time, Lawton (1977), Mac-Donald (1978), and McClannahan and Risley (1975) have shown that in a nursing home environment very little demand for either physical or social movement is placed on the residents who do not move voluntarily through their environment to the extent possible for them. These findings indicate age differences in memory for specific locations, movement throughout an environment, and knowledge of nursing home surroundings. However, the cause of such age differences and the behavioral correlates of the low levels of environmental knowledge in older hospitalized populations have not been identified.

Older adults have also been shown to perform more poorly than younger adults on a wide range of measures of spatial rotation ability (Berg, Hertzog, & Hunt, 1982; Gaylord & Marsh, 1975; Krauss, Quahagen, & Schaie, 1980), and while the literature is consistent in the general findings, relatively little has been reported on real-world spatial ability within the older population or the relationship between assessed spatial skills and real-world behavior (Kirasic, 1989).

One large-scale empirical study that did examine the contribution of basic spatial ability to environmental knowledge and to self-reports of use of the environment was reported by Walsh et al. in 1981. In that study, several measures of spatial ability were found to predict environmental knowledge in that those older adults who performed at a high level on tests of perspective taking, spatial rotation, and spatial memory demonstrated greater knowledge of their own neighborhoods. Neighborhood knowledge was measured by means of a free-hand map drawn by respondents, which was scored for extent of area covered, amount of information, accuracy and level of organization. A second measure of neighborhood knowledge was based on a landmark placement task in which respondents placed markers representing well-known landmarks on a sheet of paper, indicating relative distance and direction among the 10 landmarks. Walsh, et al. (1981) also found that environmental knowledge was related to the number of neighborhood services used by older adults and the frequency with which those services were used. Initial findings indicated that the indices of spatial ability should predict use of the neighborhood, but later analyses did not substantiate these early results.

Because of the Walsh et al. (1981) findings, we undertook the present study to see if these correlative patterns could be replicated with a nursing home population. There remained the possibility that the lower demand environment of the institution would reveal an underlying relationship between spatial skills and environmental use that was only suggested by the early results from the complex neighborhood environment. In addition, the general goal of increasing activity on the part of nursing home residents could be facilitated by knowledge of specific factors that contribute to that activity.

The methods to be employed in such research need to be appropriate for the population and the environment under consideration. Restrictions on nursing home residents are shaped by their environment as well as their individual conditions, which created the necessity for such a residence. Therefore, we suggest that both the cognitive skill and memory measures, and the behavioral measures need to be carefully tailored. Careful attention must then be paid to correspondence between the concepts of interest and their measures, to the reliability of the measures themselves, and to the situation-specific combination of these factors.

The present study extends the research of Weber et al. (1978) by looking for behavioral correlates of environmental knowledge in a nursing home population. The model relating environmental knowledge, use of the environment, and spatial ability proposed by Walsh et al. (1981) should generalize to a nursing home population. If the model were to be applicable in this setting, it should be possible to determine whether low knowledge of the nursing home environment is related to poor spatial ability, to low use of available facilities, to both, or to neither. Following these studies, we investigated three specific directional hypotheses: (a) individuals with good spatial ability scores would make fewer environmental knowledge errors; (b) those same individuals with good spatial ability scores would have high environmental use scores; and (c) individuals with fewer environmental knowledge errors would demonstrate high environmental use scores.

Methodology

Subjects

Twenty men living on two nursing home wards of a large metropolitan Veterans Administration (VA) Hospital volunteered to participate. They were selected using the criteria used and recommended by Weber et al. (1978), based on the recommendations of the nursing home staff. The criteria were general alertness, literacy, stability in physical condition, lack of any organic brain syndrome or related illness, and the ability to move safely and independently around the hospital and its grounds. We recruited only men because of the well-established gender-specific advantage in spatial abilities across age groups (Cohen, 1976; Krauss, 1987; McGee, 1982; Newcombe, 1982; Schaie, 1983) and a low availability of female patients in the VA Hospitals. The average age of the participants was 70.8 years with a range of 49 to 89 years, the average years of education was 11.7 with a range of 3 to 15 years, and they had resided on the ward on which they were tested for an average of 6.8 months, with a range of 1 to 23 months.

Materials

SPATIAL ABILITIES

The spatial abilities measures used were two subtests of the Krauss Card Tasks (Krauss, 1989; Krauss & Schaie, 1978). These tests were specially developed for use with elderly persons who are not familiar with common paper-and-pencil measures or who may have difficulty manipulating or re-

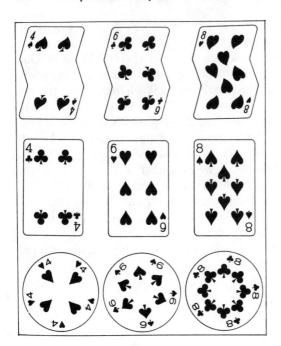

FIGURE 14.1.

sponding to paper-and-pencil test materials. The Krauss Card Tasks were constructed with combinations of standard, round, and zig-zag shaped playing cards (see Figure 14.1). No writing was involved for the participants because the investigator recorded the responses as they were given throughout the tasks.

In the spatial rotation task, the participant was shown a fixed rectangular matrix of nine cards, as shown in Figure 14.1, and given an identical set of nine separate cards to manipulate. The participant was then asked to imagine that he had rotated the entire matrix of cards around in his mind so that another side of it, indicated by a red pointer placed by the investigator, was in front of him. Then he was asked to arrange his cards in the way they would look if the matrix were so rotated. Four rotations (180°, 90°, 270° and 143°) of two matrices each, correctly arranged, yielded eight rotations. Each correct rotation received a point for a total of eight points possible on the rotation task. The reported reliability coefficient on this task was .75, and it had good correlational validity with similar factors from the Primary Mental Abilities Test (Krauss, 1989).

In the memory for a spatial configuration subtest of the Krauss Card Tasks, the participant looked at a third fixed matrix of nine cards also similar to Figure 14.1. In this task, he was asked specifically to remember the placement of each card individually as well as in relation to the other cards. When he felt he knew the placement of each of the nine cards, the matrix was removed from view, and he was asked to recreate it with an identical set of nine separate cards. This task is scored from 0 to 8 points, which are gained for numbers of patterns of suit, shape, and face value remembered, and for the cards' relationships correctly recreated. The reported reliability coefficient on this task was .83, and it had good correlational validity with similar factors from the Primary Mental Abilities Test (Krauss, 1989).

ENVIRONMENTAL KNOWLEDGE

We determined environmental knowledge using two simplifications of techniques used by Walsh et al. (1981). The first used seven full-color photographs taken of major behavior settings (Barker, 1968), commonly identified by the same names (e.g. day room, nurses station, main hallway, etc.) on each ward as indicated by the staff on the ward. The photographs were taken using a Minolta SRT 101, 35mm SLR camera with Kodak Kodacolor 400 speed film, color balanced for fluorescent lighting with a HOYA filter. All pictured locations were commonly accessible to residents and were reported to be frequently occupied by the mobile patients. The fifteen 5 × 7 in. color pictures were mounted on 8 × 10 in. beige cardboard. To ensure agreement on the names of the behavior settings a set of printed cards was created; 3 × 5 in. white index cards printed with large black block letters gave the common name of each location. This made the identification portion a task of matching the correct name to the photograph being presented. All of the printed name cards were placed face-up on the table in front of the participant throughout the environmental knowledge investigation. The number of pictured areas incorrectly identified by the names on the cards yielded an error score.

The second measure of environmental knowledge used an 8 1/2 × 11 in. unlabeled Xerox copy of the floor plan of the ward, which was shown to each participant. The men were then asked to indicate the location of each of the major behavior settings named on the 3 × 5 in. cards. The responses were recorded directly on the map by the investigator. Later, a measurement was taken of the map-equivalent walking distance between the location indicated by the participant and the correct location. The total centimeters of these measures yielded another error score.

ENVIRONMENTAL USE

Environmental use was measured by the participants' keeping a diary that provided information on how many places on and off the ward they visited over 1 week's time. The simple totals of places visited on and off the ward were the scores, thus producing on-the-ward and off-the-ward measures. Encouragement and writing assistance in keeping the diary was given to the participants individually throughout the diary week.

TABLE 14.1. Means and standard deviations of raw scores for each of the six measures.

Measure	Mean	Standard deviation
Spatial abilities		
Spatial rotation tasks	4.04	2.83
Memory for a spatial configuration	4.80	2.99
Environmental knowledge		
Picture identification errors	3.65	2.11
Map placement errors (in centimenters)	36.85	53.09
Environmental use (during 1 week)		
Places visited on-the-ward	15.45	7.13
Places visited off-the-ward	12.85	10.72

PROCEDURE

Following collection of demographic data, the spatial abilities and environmental knowledge measures were administered. No time measures were taken during any portion of the interview and tasks. This was explained to each participant, and some requested repeated assurances that time was clearly not a factor. The diary was explained and given to each participant at the end of the measurement session. The participants were also told that the nurses knew about the diary and its purpose. The investigator assured participants that she would be available for questions and assistance throughout the week.

Results

Raw Scores

The means and standard deviations for the raw scores for each of the six measures are reported in Table 14.1.

SPATIAL ABILITIES

The scores on the two spatial ability measures of the card tasks are well below the noninstitutionalized elderly standard of rotation: $M = 4.04$, $SD = 2.83$; memory: $M = 4.80$, $SD = 2.99$ as reported by Krauss and Schaie (1978). This difference is consistent with comparisons between community-active and institutionalized elderly on a wide variety of cognitive tasks (Chap & Sinnott, 1978).

ENVIRONMENTAL KNOWLEDGE

The error scores on the two environmental knowledge measures indicate consistency with other findings on similar measures. The means on these types of tasks reported by Weber et al. (1978) are similar to those reported here, and the direction of differences between tasks in the two studies is parallel.

ENVIRONMENTAL USE

Both the numbers of specified places visited and the frequencies of those visits were available from the diaries. Walsh et al. (1981) reported both in their study of community elderly. However, the numbers of places visited correlated so highly with the frequencies ($r = .98$, $p < .001$) that reporting them both here would be redundant. Because we assumed that locations on the ward would be much easier to visit than those off the ward, they are reported separately. While the standard deviations of the two counts were quite different, the difference between the two means was not significant.

Raw scores of the spatial and knowledge tasks were standardized ($M = 0.0$, $SD = 1.0$) and combined into single scores. The raw scores were then combined within each of the three variables measured. This was done to obtain single indicators of each variable with wide enough ranges to demonstrate any possible correlations in consideration of the extremely small sample size ($n = 20$). The simple total of the number of places visited both on and off the ward became the single environmental use score.

Correlations

The intercorrelations of all measures with each other and the demographic variables of age, years of education, length of residence on the ward, and self-reported health on the day of testing are presented in Table 14.2.

Of the three major variables, only environmental knowledge errors correlated significantly with age ($r = .498$, $p \le .05$). None of the other demographic variables, including length of residence on the ward, significantly correlated with any of the major variables in question. The major hypothesized correlations are presented in Figure 14.2.

The correlation of spatial abilities with environmental use ($r = .43$, $p \le .05$), predicted by the one-tailed hypothesis, was significant, as was the correlation of environmental knowledge errors with environmental use ($r = -.38$, $p \le .05$). The correlation between spatial abilities and environmental knowledge errors was $r = -.36$ ($p \le .06$). Although this correlation was not significant, it does suggest a trend.

When environmental use was broken down by visits on-the-ward and off-the-ward, it became evident that the significance of these findings was entirely accounted for by off-the-ward visits. This evidence is presented in Figure 14.3.

Environmental knowledge errors correlated significantly with off-the-ward environmental use ($r = -.46$, $p \le .05$) and with total spatial abilities ($r = .41$, $p \le .05$), whereas the correlations between on-the-ward use and spatial abilities ($r = .19$) were near zero and insignificant ($p \le 3.05$). This

TABLE 14.2. Intercorrelations of all measures with age, years of education, length of residence on the ward and self-reported health on the day of testing.

Measures and variables	2	3	4	5	6	7	8	9	10	11	12	13
Spatial abilities												
1. Total	.81**	.80**	-.36	-.21	-.41*	.43**	.19	.41*	-.13	.21	-.02	-.24
2. Rotation	—	.29	-.34	-.24	-.34	.29	.09	.30	-.24	.30	.07	.17
3. Memory		—	-.24	-.09	-.32	.41*	.23	.36*	.02	.03	.05	-.56**
Environmental knowledge												
4. Total			—	.84**	.84**	-.30	-.02	-.46*	.50*	-.06	-.08	-.13
5. Picture identification				—	.42*	-.29	.03	-.38*	.50*	-.17	-.11	-.13
6. Map placement					—	-.34	-.06	-.39**	.34	.08	-.05	.08
Environmental use												
7. Total						—	.61**	.85**	-.11	-.22	.06	-.11
8. On-the-ward							—	.10	.21	-.19	.25	-.05
9. Off-the-ward								—	-.29	-.14	-.09	-.10
Demographic variables												
10. Age									—	-.23	-.32	-.11
11. Years of education										—	.16	.32
12. Length of residence											—	-.03
13. Self-reported health												—

*$p < .05$, **$p < .01$.

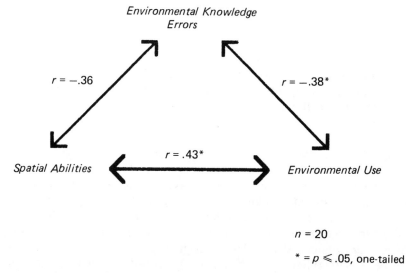

FIGURE 14.2. Three major hypothesized correlations in relationship to each other.

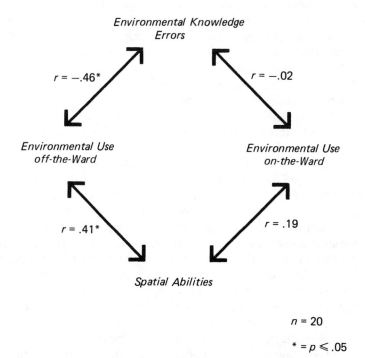

FIGURE 14.3. Environmental use broken down by off-the-ward and on-the-ward of residence use, correlated with total environmental knowledge errors and spatial abilities scores.

indicates that spatial abilities and environmental knowledge only partially predicted total environmental use, including all institutionally imposed movement, such as being pushed into the dining room for meals or the day room when the patient's room is being cleaned. Spatial abilities and environmental knowledge, however, were strongly related to noninstitutionally determined environmental use such as individually initiated trips to the recreation hall, patio, or canteen.

Discussion

As shown in the results, there was a positive relationship between spatial abilities and environmental knowledge, though not as strong as originally expected. Strong positive relationships were evident between these two kinds of spatial competence and the adaptive behavior of self-initiated off-the-ward environmental use. These results support the extension of the Walsh et al. (1981) findings to the nursing home setting. Such an extension is also supported by the strong similarities between these results and those of similar parts of other investigations (Weber et al., 1978).

With this extension demonstrated, it is possible to consider a nursing home environment as an appropriate realm for testing the fundamental person–environment processes as called for by Altman, Lawton, and Wohlwill (1984). The controllable low-press environment, housing the relatively less spatially competent, provides an ideal opportunity to attempt to select and/or train competence levels and vary press levels in a non-laboratory "real-world" environment. Outcomes of such investigations could be further detailed by observing possible changes in socially adaptive behaviors and affective states before, during, and after movement on and off the ward of residence.

These results demonstrate an extension to the nursing home setting, of a pattern of related competence and adaptation that has been established in many other settings. The existence of a correlation between a large number of daily travels and accuracy of knowledge of the environment in which one travels is well established (Evans, 1980). Thereby, the correlation between environmental knowledge and use variables were accurately predicted by the third hypothesis. In this study, however, the distinctive results between on-the-ward and off-the-ward of residence need to be emphasized. An outstanding observation was the fact that those patients who went to the most places *off*-the-ward were the ones who could most accurately identify and locate behavior settings *on*-the-ward.

Previous studies of nursing home patient behaviors have focused primarily on activities on the ward of residence (Bruce, 1981; Herman, 1981; MacDonald, 1978; McClannahan & Risley, 1975; Weber et al., 1978). In these and most other similar studies, trips away from the ward of residence were either not mentioned or specifically excluded from any data reported. This distinction appears to be very important in terms of its relationship to activity, participation, and competence levels of the individuals involved.

Because the total environmental use measure included the number of places on the ward, it was contaminated by the institutional routine required of all residents. To eat, all mobile patients must go to the dining room; to be bathed, they must go to the showers; and at least once a day, they must leave their rooms during cleaning and bed making. These movements are not determined by the patient but by the institution. In some cases, it is possible that these movements do not represent any awareness of the overall plan of the environment or any active use of it but, rather, passive compliance with it.

On the other hand, patients must actively seek out the opportunity to leave the ward. They need to use their environmental knowledge to leave and return to the ward. The significant relationship between spatial abilities and environmental use off-the-ward indicates that this knowledge may well be a determining factor in these patients' abilities to participate in a wide range of activities. It is clear in this sample that both spatial abilities and off-the-ward activities divided the competent active from the less competent inactive.

The self-reported diary was a relatively untried technique in studying residents of a nursing home. The extremely high correlation between numbers of places reported in the diaries and the number of times those places were visited is evidence of the consistency with which entries were made in the diaries. There was also an overall impression of agreement between the staff's and the subjects' perceptions of both frequency and variety of activities. Therefore, it is concluded that though the self-reported diary may be time-consuming for both the participant and the investigator, it is a useful technique in accounting for individual use of the nursing home environment.

The correlations of the demographic variables—age, education, length of residence on the ward, and self-reported health on the day of testing—with the major variables merely demonstrate the distinction between the institutionalized elderly and the active elderly. It should be noted that all of these demographic variables have demonstrated effects on general spatial abilities and environmental knowledge and use in the noninstitutionalized elderly (Awad, McCormick, Ohta, & Krauss, 1979). These same variables have also been correlated with overall performance on the Krauss Card Tasks also in noninstitutionalized elderly subjects (Krauss & Norris, 1980). The institutionalized population, however, maintains these effects only in terms of one variable, that of age. Age correlates with environmental knowledge in this and other such samples in the same direction as in the noninstitutionalized elderly. The older the patient, the fewer places he or she can identify. This cross-sectional age effect has been previously attributed to increased selective screening out of environmental cues with age (Walsh et al., 198t; Weber et al., 1978).

The size of this sample is the most clearly evident limiting factor in terms Of generalizing from these results. This study must be viewed as a preliminary indicator of the usefulness of these concepts with the institutionalized elderly only. It cannot be taken to indicate broadly applicable results without expansion and replication. Therefore, the next necessary phase of this line of research should be a replication and expansion. The results of such extensions would determine if the next suggested phase of research would be warranted.

The next logical phase in this line of work would then be to institute a training program at each point in the model. Pretraining and posttraining measures of each variable would serve at least three functions. Training in one area could be established with accompanying improvement in another; thereby, a causal direction could be established. Investigation of these complex cognitive and behavioral relationships outside the laboratory presents several difficulties. There is little precedent for investigations linking specific cognitive skills and environmental behavior in the real world (Altman et al., 1984; Walsh et al., 1981). Yet, the utility of such research is not in question. As Altman et al. (1984) state, "the potential is great and we look forward to increasing study of fundamental person–environment processes in relationship to the elderly" (p. 9).

Two major possibilities are in line with an overall goal of improvement of the quality of nursing home life. There is the possibility of the improvement of both cognitive skills and use of the physical environment of the institution. If training in any of these areas did improve performance in another, it would eliminate a need for multiple training programs. Finally, by revealing a specific person–environment interaction, the possibility exists of being able to balance an institutionalized individual's competence with his or her level of environmental press. Working toward such an ideal would be an attempt at cautiously challenging individuals so that their activity levels might be improved and could potentially be maintained overtime. These types of programs would represent an application of intervention to improve competence and, in turn, to expand adaptive behaviors and potentially. increase positive affect through increased environmental use. As a result, expanded adaptive abilities and behaviors could possibly expand potential compensation for the increasing decrements experienced by the institutionalized elderly.

Acknowledgments. The authors are indebted to Walter Riege and to the staff of the Memory Research Unit and the nursing staff of the Sepulveda Veterans Hospital for their generous assistance throughout the project. Support for this research was provided by NIH Grant AG04110 to the second author.

References

Altman, I., Lawton, M.P., & Wohlwill, J.F. (Eds.). (1984). *Elderly people and the environment.* New York: Plenum Press.

Awad, Z.A., McCormick, D.J., Ohta., R., & Krauss, I.K. (1979, September). *Neighborhood knowledge of the elderly: Psychological and environmental correlates.* Paper presented at the annual meeting of the Gerontological Society, Washington, DC.

Barker, R.C. (1968). *Ecological psychology.* Palo Alto, CA: Stanford University Press.

Berg, L., Hertzog, C., & Hunt, E. (1982). Age differences in the speed of mental rotation. *Developmental Psychology, 18,* 95–107.

Bruce, P.R. (1981, August). *Cognitive maps of elderly nursing home residents.* Paper presented at the 89th annual convention of the American Psychological Association, Los Angeles.

Chap, J.R., & Sinnott, J.D. (1978). Performance of institutional and community active old people on concrete and formal Piagetian tasks. *International Journal of Aging and Human Development, 8,* 269–278.

Cohen, D. (1976). Usefulness of the group-comparison method to demonstrate sex differences in spatial orientation and spatial visualization in older men and women. *Perceptual and Motor Skills, 43,* 338–390.

Evans, G.W. (1980). Environmental cognition. *Psychological Bulletin, 88,* 269–287.

Evans, G.W., Smith, C., & Pezdek, K. (1982). Cognitive maps and urban form. *Journal of the American Planning Association, 45,* 232–244.

Gaylord, S.A., & Marsh, G.R. (1975). Age differences in the speed of a spatial cognitive process. *Journal of Gerontology, 30,* 674–678.

Herman, J.F. (1981, April). The assessment of spatial cognition in elderly persons: A synthesis of laboratory and field experimentation. In *Spatial cognition in older adults: From lab to life.* Symposium presented at the meeting of the Society for Research in Child Development, Los Angeles.

Kirasic, K.C. (1989). Acquisition and utilization of spatial information by elderly adults: Implications for day-to-day situations. In L.W. Poon & B.A. Wilson (Eds.), *Everyday cognition in adulthood and late life* (pp. 265–283). Cambridge: Cambridge University Press.

Krauss, I.K. (1987, May). *Age, sex, and processing components of spatial rotations.* Paper presented at the first Cognitive Aging Conference, Atlanta.

Krauss, I.K. (1989). Testing cognitive skills with playing cards. In J.D. Sinnott (Ed.), *Everyday problem solving: Theory and applications* (pp. 234–240). New York: Praeger.

Krauss, I.K., & Norris, K.K.A. (1980, September). *Individual difference contributions to test–retest reliability in tests of cognitive skills.* Paper presented at the annual meeting of the Gerontological Society, San Diego, CA.

Krauss, I.K., Quayhagen, M., & Schaie, K.W. (1980). Spatial rotation in the elderly: Performance factors. *Journal of Gerontology, 35,* 199–206.

Krauss, I.K, & Schaie, K.W. (1978, August). *Five novel tasks for the assessment of cognitive abilities in older adults.* Paper presented at the 11th triennial meeting of the International Congress of Gerontology, Tokyo.

Lawton, M.P. (1977). The impact of the environment on aging and behavior. In J.E. Birren & K.W. Schaie (Eds.), *Handbook of the psychology of aging* (pp. 276–301). New York: Van Nostrand Reinhold.

MacDonald, M.L. (1978). Environmental programming for the socially isolated aging. *Gerontologist, 18,* 350–354.

McClannahan, L.R., & Risley, T.R. (1975). Design of living environments for nursing home recreational activities. *Journal of Applied Behavior Analysis, 8,* 261–268.

McGee, M.G. (1982). Spatial abilities: The influence of genetic factors. In M.M. Totegal (Ed.), *Spatial abilities: Developmental and physiological foundations* (pp. 199–222). New York: Academic Press.

Newcombe, N. (1982). Sex-related differences in spatial ability: Problems and gaps in current approaches. In M.M. Totegal (Ed.), *Spatial abilities: Developmental and physiological foundations* (pp. 223–250). New York: Academic Press.

Schaie, K.W. (1983). The Seattle longitudinal study: A 21 year exploration of psychometric intelligence in adulthood. In K.W. Schaie (Ed.), *Longitudinal studies of adult psychological development* (pp. 64–135). New York: Guilford Press.

Walsh, D.A., Krauss, I.K., & Regnier, V.A. (1981). Spatial ability, environmental knowledge, and environmental use: The elderly. In L.S. Liben, A.H. Patterson, & N. Newcombe (Eds.), *Spatial representation and behavior across the life span* (pp. 321–357). New York: Academic Press.

Weber, R.J., Brown, L.T., & Weldon, J.K. (1978). Cognitive maps of environmental knowledge and preference in nursing home patients. *Experimental Aging Research, 4,* 157–174.

15
Knowledge Factors in Everyday Visual Perception

WILLIAM J. HOYER AND JOHN M. RYBASH

The ability to use aquired knowledge to support performance in complex memory or perception tasks is an important characteristic of human cognition. Although many aspects of memory and perception show decline with advancing age, older adults frequently exhibit preserved or even expert performance in selected everyday domains. The main purpose of this chapter is to offer an explanation of everyday cognition that emphasizes knowledge factors and the component processes that enable (and constrain) the performance of older adults in familiar or everyday visual cognitive tasks. We argue that the availability of task-relevant knowledge facilitates performance by improving the efficiency of information extraction at the level of objects (or percepts). We suggest that the effortlessness of everyday visual perception, regardless of age, is related to the reduced demands of object-level extraction and to the reduced demands of interference associated with familiar processing domains. To support this claim, we refer to recent studies by Clancy and Hoyer (1988, 1990) showing that older experts differ from same-age nonexperts mainly in terms of the efficiency of domain-specific object-level extraction processes; as discussed in this chapter, nonexperts who had little or no special knowledge of the types of items that make up the selected domain showed a pattern of age-related deficits in item-level detection and extraction processes, and experts showed no age-related declines in the processing of relevant information within the selected domain. Based on these findings and related work, we suggest that task demands are reduced in everyday perceptual tasks and that the efficiency of age-sensitive extraction processes is enhanced, when observers have ready access to prior knowledge of object-level visual information.

Points of Departure

How is it that there are so few noticeable deficits in the ways in which older adults carry out everyday tasks involving memory and perception? The question has meaning because there are clear and large discrepancies between the findings of laboratory studies of memory and perceptual aging and real-world observations of everyday cognitive performance (e.g., Charness, 1989; Charness & Bosman, 1990; Salthouse, 1990). In contrast to the findings of many laboratory-based reports indicating decline for many aspects of memory and perception, the results of many naturalistic studies suggest substantial maintenance of visual cognitive function in many types of everyday tasks, across age (e.g., see Cohen, 1988). Although some ecologically oriented investigators argue that we should dismiss or de-emphasize the results of laboratory studies, on grounds that the procedures and materials of these studies give an exaggerated picture of age-related deficit, the study of age-related changes in everyday cognition must take into account the fact that there are real and reliable age-related declines in many of the basic processes of memory and perception. Although it is proper to critique the methods of some laboratory-type studies on the basis of artificiality and/or method bias favoring the performance of younger individuals, some cognitive aging phenomena are best studied under the controlled conditions provided by the laboratory (e.g., Bahrick, 1989). In recent years, a relatively clear picture of the nature of memory and perceptual aging has emerged from laboratory-type studies (e.g., for recent reviews, see Hultsch & Dixon, 1990; Light, 1990). It is also important, however, to consider data showing that the individual's prior knowledge, experience, and task history, as well as a range of context-related influences, serve to substantially reduce the processing demands of selected tasks, and consequently, the magnitude of reported age deficits.

Many researchers have already pointed out the value of ecological validity when examining memory aging. It is well established that research and theory in cognitive aging *should* take into account the analysis of contextual and ecological factors that serve to constrain or enhance performance. Despite the general appeal of this position, however, researchers have not given much attention to the factors that contribute to the differences between everyday and laboratory studies. Our point is that the differences between the results of laboratory studies and everyday investigations are due in part to the extent to which prior knowledge serves to attenuate the general-purpose processing demands of cognitive performance. Everyday visual cognitive tasks may be relatively nondemanding of general-purpose cognitive resources, and real declines in memory and visual information processing performance may be evident in laboratory studies because task conditions are more demanding (e.g., rapid presentation of unfamiliar and complex stimulus information). Research participants have relatively little domain-relevant knowledge to apply to the materials or content of the task. This interpretation is in line with the general view that age decrements will be observed in any type of cognitive task (laboratory or real-life) if the task requires a substantial amount of general-purpose processing resources, and if the individual does not have some amount of task-relevant knowledge that serves to alter or attenuate task demands (e.g., Salthouse, 1988).

Aging and Knowledge Use

The findings of two recent studies by Clancy and Hoyer (1988, 1990) suggest that one source of the discrepancy between skilled performance and standard laboratory assessments of visual perceptual aging has to do with the influence of knowledge on object-level information extraction processes. In the first study, Clancy and Hoyer (1988) found that middle-aged and older skilled subjects were less affected by dual-task demands compared with age-matched controls in a domain-specific visual recognition task. The skilled subjects were medical laboratory technologists having between 5 and 20 years of "everyday" experience in analyzing Gram's-stain micrographic displays. The domain-specific task involved visual recognition and matching of targets with probe items within photomicrographic displays. Age deficits were found for the medical technologists and age-matched control subjects in a comparable domain-general visual recognition task.

These results are consistent with the view that age-related declines in general-purpose processing resources occur with aging and that these limitations are spared for experienced individuals when performing the skilled task. That is, compared to controls, skilled observers may use different (or fewer) processing components to perform the same task. A general interpretation of these findings is that age-normal deficits in performance were not observed because there was less demand on the age-limited processes of item recognition, target–nontarget comparisons, search and localization, and/or other normally age-sensitive processes. In addition, there are several possible interpretations of these findings that are more specific. For example, it can be suggested that if skilled observers know what to *see* or *look for* in familiar displays, then compared to less skilled observers, less processing time (and/or resources) is required for handling nonsalient information. Compared to age-matched controls, skilled subjects may be less susceptible to distractor information in skilled domains. Perhaps skilled observers were better able to effectively "see through" noise in the skilled domain. Prior experience with specific kinds of information may also affect the observer's criterion for accepting partial stimulus information as evidence for stimulus identification.

In a second study of knowledge factors in skilled visual information processing, Clancy and Hoyer (1990) examined the effects of domain-specific semantic priming on visual recognition processes using a target-probe matching paradigm. Young adult and middle-aged medical technologists and age-matched controls were given a name of a cell type (e.g., eosinophils, staphylococcus), a target item, and then a one-item or a three-item probe display. The task was to verify whether or not the probe display contained an exact version of the bacteria item shown as the target for that trial. Relative to the targets, prime words were valid, invalid, or neutral ("specimen"), and they preceded target objects by 500 ms. Reaction time data revealed priming benefits but no costs for the medical technologists, for both age groups. For the nonskilled participants, a main effect of age and interactions involving age with display size and probe (negative vs. positive) were obtained. Middle-aged controls were slower to respond than were younger adult controls, especially with the larger displays and with negative probes (i.e., when the target was not present in the display). As expected, there was no evidence of priming for the control subjects. Results suggested that skilled observers, regardless of age, can effectively use word primes to facilitate visual object verification within a skilled domain.

Toward a Model of Aging and Everyday Perception

Everyday visual perception involves efficient encoding of object-level featural information and access to the meaning of visual information at a representational level. We now consider how age-related and knowledge-related interindividual and intraindividual differences affect the efficiency of object-level composition. Skilled older people probably do not have fast and slow hard-wired processing modules that correspond to particular domains. It is more likely that the processing demands of extracting information differ, depending on the observer's domain-relevant foreknowledge. Assuming that general-purpose processing resources are more limited with aging, the effects of such limitations will be most apparent when the perceptual information in complex displays is not easily selected. We suggest that individuals readily organize visual information in familiar arrays based on prior knowledge, which serves to minimize processing demands, and/or to minimize distractor interference.

At least two types of mechanisms might account for how prior knowledge serves to reduce age-sensitive task demands in visual object perception. We suggest that knowledge has its effects on visual information processing mainly in terms of object-level feature integration (and/or decomposition) processes, and in terms of priming effects at the level of meaning.

According to Duncan and Humphreys (1989), mechanisms of object-level feature integration determine the efficiency of visual search and perceptual organization; these mechanisms affect the ability to confine attention to critical information (i.e., selective attention). According to Farah (1989), Tulving and Schacter (1990), and others, the mechanisms of pre-semantic access serve to determine or clarify the meaning or interpretation of high-level visual information (e.g., as reflected by measures of semantic categorization or object naming). Many writers have pointed out that semantic knowledge has a strong, top–down influence on perceptual analysis (e.g., Tulving & Schacter, 1990). According to top–down interactive models (e.g., McClelland & Rumelhart, 1981), foreknowledge of the semantic properties of objects affect both semantic processing and perceptual processing. Most of the current models of semantic priming suggest that continued processing of visual information involves network activation that enables access to verbal labels and related semantic information (e.g., Neely, 1990; Ratcliff & McCoon, 1988). Semantic knowledge may increase the likelihood (or response bias) of identifying or naming an object in a familiar domain, without affecting the sensitivity of detection or extraction processes (see Farah, 1989). For example, in more familiar domains, individuals might be more prepared to infer object-level identification based on incomplete information.

Compared to the amount of recent work on semantic priming, considerably less research has examined the effects of foreknowledge on object-level extraction and feature-integration processes. Several investigators have argued that low-level featural information is relatively inert and rapidly transformed into more stable morphological codes that correspond to object representations (see Hoyer, 1990; Humphreys & Bruce, 1989; McClelland & Rumelhart, 1981). The elementary features of objects are readily constrained by a rich assortment of perceptual organizational factors. Featural elements, such as color or shading, contour, and line segments, readily combine into an object-level representation or percept. Many researchers have suggested that this level of visual computation is obligatory and relatively automatic (attention free), but we add that foreknowledge can directly affect *how* or *which* object parts and features are transformed into high-level (e.g., object-level) groupings. Witness that the prior specific visual knowledge of experts (e.g., medical technologists, radiologists) allows and constrains transformation of the available stimulus information into recognizable, domain-meaningful perceptual units (e.g., Clancy & Hoyer, 1990; Lesgold, et al., 1988; Myles-Worsley, Johnston, & Simons, 1988). For individuals who have no special knowledge of the domain or who cannot immediately retrieve domain-relevant knowledge, grouping or feature integration processes involved in creating objects or perceptual units depend on Gestalt-type general principles of perceptual organization and stimulus geometry.

Perceptual features and parts that make up everyday objects can certainly be grouped or organized in many different ways, depending on general principles of perceptual organization and sufficient prior experience with the object domain. One of the principles of Gestalt perception states that "a strong form coheres and resists disintegration by analysis into parts or by fusion with another form" (Boring, 1942, p. 253). It is well-known that selective attention to features (line segments) is difficult when such features are grouped into unitary shapes and that divided attention across shapes is easy or automatic, compared to ungrouped conditions (e.g., Humphreys, Quinlan, & Riddoch, 1989; Julesz & Bergen, 1983; Prinzmetal, Presti, & Posner, 1986). It is also relatively well established that the selective attentional mechanisms that are involved in feature integration and parsing are age-sensitive (e.g., Farkas & Hoyer, 1980; Madden, 1990; Plude & Doussard-Roosevelt, 1989; Plude & Hoyer, 1986).

Summary and Conclusions

Laboratory-based and naturalistic studies of memory and perception indicate a complex pattern of gains and losses in particular functions. Frequently, the results of naturalistic studies suggest the robustness of many aspects of everyday performance during the adult years. Perhaps one of the most challenging and most persistent problems for investigators of cognitive aging is to describe and explain unique patterns of age-related individual differences in performance during the adult years. The main point of this chapter is to call attention to the role of knowledge factors in memory and visual information processing performance in everyday situations. Current models of memory and visual perception are largely content neutral and do not address or account for the role of experience or knowledge in everyday performance. Treisman's (e.g., Treisman & Gelade, 1980; Treisman & Gormican, 1988) feature-integration theory of preattentive and attentive processing, for example, includes little or no mention of how the processes of feature detection, integration, and decomposition are affected by experience and/or age. Similarly, current models of aging and visual cognitive function are overly simplistic, in that they attempt to account for aging in terms of general slowing across mechanisms and tasks. These models underspecify the sources of interindividual differences and intraindividual differences across domains or tasks. We suggest that experienced-based, task-specific proficiencies involving object-level extraction may enable older adults to efficiently manage familiar visual processing tasks, even ones that are quite complex or demanding and that yield age-related deficits in the absence of task-relevant prior knowledge.

Acknowledgments. Preparation of this chapter was supported by National Institute on Aging grant AG06041.

References

Bahrick, H.P. (1989). The laboratory and ecology: Supplementary sources of data for memory research. In L.W. Poon, D.C. Rubin, & B.A. Wilson (Eds.), *Everyday cognition in adulthood and late life* (pp. 73–83). New York: Cambridge University Press.

Boring, E.G. (1942). *Sensation and Perception in the history of experimental psychology.* New York: Appleton-Century-Crofts.

Charness, N. (1989). Age and expertise: Responding to Talland's challenge. In L.W. Poon, D.C. Rubin, & B.A. Wilson (Eds.), *Everyday cognition in adulthood and late life* (pp. 437–456). New York: Cambridge University Press.

Charness, N., & Bosman, E.A. (1990). Expertise and aging: Life in the lab. In T.M. Hess (Ed.), *Aging and cognition: Knowledge organization and utilization* (pp. 343–386). Amsterdam: Elsevier.

Clancy, S.M., & Hoyer, W.J. (1988). Effects of age and skill on domain-specific search. In V.L. Patel & G.J. Groen (Eds.), *Proceedings of the tenth conference of the Cognitive Science Society* (pp. 398–404). Hillsdale, NJ: Erlbaum.

Clancy, S.M., & Hoyer, W.J. (1990, April). *Age and skill in priming*. Paper presented at the Cognitive Aging Conference, Atlanta.

Cohen, G. (1988). Memory and aging: Toward an explanation. In M.M. Gruneberg, P.E. Morris, & R.N. Sykes (Eds.), *Practical aspects of memory: Current research and issues* (pp. 78–83). Chichester: Wiley.

Duncan, J., & Humphreys, G.W. (1989). Visual search and stimulus similarity. *Psychological Review, 96,* 433–458.

Farah, M.J. (1989). Semantic and perceptual priming: How similar are the underlying mechanisms? *Journal of Experimental Psychology: Human Perception and Performance, 15,* 188–194.

Farkas, M.S., & Hoyer, W.J. (1980). Processing consequences of perceptual grouping in selective attention. *Journal of Gerontology, 35,* 207–216.

Hoyer, W.J. (1990). Levels of knowledge utilization in visual information processing. In T.M. Hess (Ed.), *Aging and cognition: Knowledge organization and utilization* (pp. 387–409). Amsterdam: Elsevier.

Hultsch, D.L., & Dixon, R.A. (1990). Learning and memory in aging. In J.E. Birren & K.W. Schaie (Eds.), *Handbook of the psychology of aging* (3rd ed., pp. 258–274). New York: Academic Press.

Humphreys, G.W., & Bruce, V. (1989). *Visual cognition: Computational, experimental, and neuropsychological perspectives*. Hillsdale, NJ: Erlbaum.

Humphreys, G.W., Quinlan, P.T., & Riddoch, M.J. (1989). Grouping processes in visual search: Effects with single- and combined-feature targets. *Journal of Experimental Psychology, 118,* 258–279.

Julesz, B., & Bergen, J.R. (1983). Textons, the fundamental elements in preattentive vision and perception of texture. *Bell Systems Technology, 62,* 1619–1646.

Lesgold, A., Rubinson, H., Feltovich, P., Glaser, R., Klopfer, D., & Wang, Y. (1988). Expertise in a complex skill: Diagnosing X-ray pictures. In M. Chi, R. Glaser, & M. Farr (Eds.), *The nature of expertise* (pp. 311–342). Hillsdale, NJ: Erlbaum.

Light, L.L. (1990). Interactions between memory and language in old age. In J.E. Birren & K.W. Schaie (Eds.), *Handbook of the psychology of aging* (3rd ed., pp. 275–290). New York: Academic Press.

Madden, D.J. (1990). Adult age differences in attentional selectivity and capacity. *European Journal of Cognitive Psychology, 2,* 229–252.

McClelland, J.L., & Rumelhart, D.E. (1981). An interactive model of context effects in letter perception: I. An account of basic findings. *Psychological Review, 88,* 375–407.

Myles-Worsley, M., Johnston, W.A., & Simons, M.A. (1988). The influence of expertise on X-ray image processing. *Journal of Experimental Psychology: Learning, Memory, and Cognition, 14,* 553–557.

Neely, J.H. (1990). Semantic priming effects in visual word recognition: A selective review of current findings and theories. In D. Besner & G. Humphreys (Eds.), *Basic processes in reading: Visual word recognition* (pp. 1–73). Hillsdale, NJ: Erlbaum.

Plude, D.J., & Doussard-Roosevelt, J.A. (1989). Aging, selective attention, and feature integration. *Psychology and Aging, 4,* 98–105.

Plude, D.J., & Hoyer, W.J. (1986). Aging and the selectivity of visual information processing. *Psychology and Aging, 1,* 1–9.

Prinzmetal, W., Presti, D.E., & Posner, M.I. (1986). Does attention affect visual feature integration? *Journal of Experimental Psychology: Human Perception and Performance, 12,* 361–369.

Ratcliff, R., & McKoon, G. (1988). A retrieval theory of priming in memory. *Psychological Review, 95,* 385–408.

Salthouse, T.A. (1988). Resource-reduction interpretations of cognitive aging. *Developmental Review, 8,* 238–272.

Salthouse, T.A. (1990). Cognitive competence and expertise in aging. In J.E. Birren & K.W. Schaie (Eds.), *Handbook of the psychology of aging* (3rd ed., pp. 310–319). New York: Academic Press.

Treisman, A., & Gelade, G. (1980). A feature integration theory of attention. *Cognitive Psychology, 12,* 97–136.

Treisman, A., & Gormican, S. (1988). Feature analysis in early vision: Evidence from search asymetries. *Psychological Review, 95,* 15–48.

Tulving, E., & Schacter, D.L. (1990). Priming in human memory. *Science, 247,* 301–306.

16
A Proposed Role for Affect in Everyday Memory

CAROL Y. YODER AND JEFFREY W. ELIAS

Research efforts described in many of these chapters underscore the importance of studying everyday cognitive abilities. With an ear to public demands for greater research applicability and accountability, many investigators are seeking to better understand memory under naturalistic circumstances (Cohen, 1989). Empirical study of real-life cognitive processes is complicated by confounds that occur as a result of the limitations or absence of experimental controls. Much of what we know about basic cognitive processes, however, comes from controlled laboratory experiments, and these controlled experiments may provide a blueprint for exploring everyday cognitive processes.

Although everyday cognitive activities include a variety of tasks, one mediating factor deserving special consideration is affect. In this chapter we will discuss several studies related to affect and everyday cognition in adults. The means by which affect is processed and retrieved within a memory system are discussed with special attention given to the unique nature of the study of affect within the confines of everyday memory.

Defining Affect

Although clear conceptual definitions of constructs are important for any research endeavor, researchers interested in affect will find its definition problematic. Affect is a widely used but ill-defined construct that typically refers to feelings, attitudes, and preferences that vary in intensity and duration. This is not to say that affect defies operational definition but rather that operational definitions are usually driven by theoretical perspectives. As a consequence, affect has been described in several ways.

Levanthal and Tomarken (1986) suggest that much of the confusion in the area of affect and emotion emerges "from an unwillingness to grant independent conceptual status to emotion" (p. 566), which is due in part to remnants of behaviorism and a cognitive set for experimenters to consider affect as arousal plus cognition. Levanthal and Tomarken's (1986) comments call attention to a historical past in experimental psychology (e.g., John B. Watson) when affect in the laboratory signaled a loss of experimental control and, by inference, a loss of personal control. Even cognitive researchers such as Piaget (1967) focused on knowledge of inanimate objects, rather than animate objects who invoke and display considerable affect. There is a legitimate question in the developmental literature regarding how we come to understand social objects. To achieve this understanding, researchers will have to turn to consideration of everyday situations and the affective components of social interaction. In the area of child development, a good source for discussion of these issues is Flavell and Ross (1982). A similar integrated discussion is not yet available in the area of adult development.

Lazarus (1984) tackled the definition of affect by considering it as a part of the concept of emotion and defined emotions as:

an organic mix of action impulses and bodily expressions, diverse positive or dysphoric (subjective) cognitive-affective states, and physiological disturbance. Although there are arguments about whether these physiological disturbances are diffuse or patterned, an emotion is not defined solely by behavior, subjective reports, or physiological changes; its identification requires all three components, since each one can be generated by conditions that do not necessarily elicit emotion. (p. 125)

Lazarus's (1984) definition focuses on the social nature of humans; that is, humans have agendas, some of which can be noted by observing behavior, which may or may not reflect a personal cognitive component, and some of which may be noted by measuring a physiological response that gives some indication of the nature and degree of arousal. We caution researchers interested in affect and memory to be careful to distinguish between situations involving social interaction and situations that focus on personal action or action toward inanimate objects.

The multivariate definition of affect urged by Lazarus (1984) is seldom found in the literature because the usual approach embraces a univariate methodology with a particular content area foci. For the purposes of this chapter, affect is considered to be the result of an idiographic synthesis of multiple sociocognitive inputs that influence the way information is learned and recalled. Our interpretation and evaluation of what we perceive and experience impacts information processing. This affective appraisal may evolve over time as one's skills and expertise change. As a consequence, a comprehensive look at everyday memory requires consideration of the relationship between cognition and affect across the life span.

Laboratory Blueprints

Several extensive reviews of the laboratory literature on affect and memory are available (Bower, 1981; Blaney, 1986; Niederehe, 1986). From these reviews it can be quickly understood that there are only a few basic experimental paradigms, with considerable variation within each paradigm. Laboratory blueprints such as mood dependent and mood-inductive manipulations (Blaney, 1986; Bower, 1981) have been prominent among the affect paradigms. Mood-dependent research focuses on the state of affect (state dependency) at the time of memory encoding and the effect of this state on storage and retrieval processes. What one remembers within a mood state is thought to be partially a function of learning and memory within that mood state on a previous occasion. The nature of the material and its affective valence may be irrelevant (Blaney, 1986). In a mood-congruent paradigm, mood and the to-be-remembered items are similar in affective value. Mood at exposure and mood at recall need not be similar for it to be considered a mood-congruent paradigm (Blaney, 1986), but similar moods at learning and recall should improve memory performance because of the combination of state dependency and mood congruence.

Testing randomly occurring moods or waiting for a specific mood to occur does not fit well with the experimental model. Thus, the mood-induction procedures are popular. They involve creating a mood through one of several procedures that include recitation of mood-inducing sentences (Velton, 1968), imaging personal experiences, hypnosis, music, and physical posturing. The effects of induced mood are then assessed via a variety of cognitive tasks (Blaney, 1986).

The mood-induction procedure can be contrasted with paradigms that provide information that differs in affective valence and/or strength. In these paradigms, the differing affective saliency of the stimuli is the primary manipulation (Erber, Herman, & Botwinick, 1980; Yesavage, Rose, & Bower, 1983). For example, a mood might be induced by the saliency of the stimuli, but the mood of the subject is less important than the affective nature of the information that is processed. Nevertheless, it has been demonstrated that subject mood adds to or detracts from the valence of stimuli (Eysenck, 1976).

Information recall is influenced to some extent by congruence between emotional states at the time of learning and retrieval. This effect has been found to be stronger with positive than negative moods (Blaney, 1986; Isen, 1984; Leight & Ellis, 1981). Apparently, it is easier to manipulate a positive mood state above a neutral point than it is to create a negative mood state much below a neutral point. As might be expected, negative mood states tend to impair learning and memory (cf. Leight & Ellis, 1981), and positive mood states tend to enhance memory (cf. Isen & Daubman, 1984). Such negative mood states should not necessarily be considered tantamount to clinical depression. The inherent ability to use organization as well as other strategies is not altered in negative mood states, but the effort expended to use such strategies may be reduced. Because the use of organizational strategies requires resource allocation and attention, a requirement for the use of such strategies is likely to be perceived as more effortful under conditions of negative mood or depression (Ellis, Thomas, & Rodriguez, 1984; Kennelly, Hayslip, & Richardson, 1985; Leight & Ellis, 1981;

Niederehe, 1986). This distinction in the use of organization is important, because severely depressed individuals fail to use organizational strategies with material to be remembered (Wells, 1979).

This is not to say that negative mood-induction states can be safely considered a part of a continuum with clinical depression at one end of that continuum. A true depression, as opposed to an induced negative mood state, is considered likely to shift the balance of affect toward the screening out of positive material and an enhancement of negative material (Blaney, 1986). The individual who is in a depressed mood state is not starting from a presumed neutral point. It has been suggested that attempts to induce negative mood congruence in depressed individuals can result in mood perpetuation (Blaney, 1986; Ingram, 1984). Not surprisingly, the degree of memory difficulty seems to increase with the severity of the induced depression (Gilligan & Bower, 1984).

Affect-Valence Paradigms and the Older Adult

The affect-valence paradigms have provided a different perspective on affect and memory than that suggested by the mood congruence and state-dependency paradigms. These effects have resulted in research that seems more immediately applicable to the understanding of everyday cognition. A brief review of this research, particularly as it pertains to aging, finds that affect seems to effect memory performance in similar fashion across the adult life span.

With respect to valence of stimuli, a question arises as to how well older adults retain their abilities to respond affectively to stimuli. Available evidence indicates that age differences are not present in this respect. After reviewing the literature on this topic, Schulz (1982) concluded that emotional responsivity is maintained throughout the life span and intensity does not decline with increasing age. Having had additional life experiences may promote multidimensional affective responses to stimuli as individuals discriminate the affective valence of stimuli and have different expectancies for potential outcomes. In illustration of Schulz's (1982) suggestion, Yoder and Elias (1987) found that when provided with pictorial scenarios of relatively common life events (e.g., experiencing car trouble, holiday preparation) older adults tended to describe and recall the events with more emotional elaboration of depicted actions and more discussion of potential outcomes. In this respect, the older adults indicated a much richer interpretation of the scenarios than the younger adults, who tended to elaborate less in recall of the events. Despite this richer interpretation by the older adults, younger individuals showed better recall of specific events.

Further evidence to support the idea that older adults tend to maintain emotional responsivity comes from Labouvie-Vief (1982) and Labouvie-

Vief, Devoe, and Bulka (1989). In the latter study, a cross-sectional sample of individuals between the ages of 10 and 77 were asked to describe situations that evoked certain emotions and their feelings in this situation. Ego level, verbal ability, and coping skills were assessed. Their findings indicate that one's understanding of emotions develops as cognitive complexity increases. Adults who were older or who exhibited greater cognitive complexity revealed better ways of coping with difficulties and also expressed their feelings in more sophisticated and individualized ways. Whereas ego level and verbal ability were strongly correlated with emotional understanding, ego level was a stronger predictor of emotional conceptualization than age. The relationship between age and emotional conceptualization was curvilinear: Adults in the middle years had higher levels of emotional understanding relative to young and older adults. The possibility was mentioned that older adults in the study might have represented a cohort that was raised to be more careful in the expression of emotions. Thus, the interpretation of affective valence may have cohort influences and affective stimulus–event valence has qualitative as well as quantitative dimensions.

Blanchard-Fields (1986) examined the reasoning abilities of adolescents and young and middle-aged adults by varying the emotional saliency of social dilemmas. Responses to these dilemmas were assigned numerical values based on assessments of reflective judgment; measures of formal operational reasoning, verbal ability, and ego development were also used to measure cognitive functioning. On the least emotionally salient dilemma, adolescents and young adults demonstrated similar levels of cognitive maturity on open-ended reasoning questions, whereas middle-aged adults demonstrated significantly higher levels. On the more emotionally salient dilemmas, adolescents showed lower levels of cognitive maturity on open-ended reasoning questions relative to nonemotional dilemmas and relative to young and middle-aged adults. This suggests that younger thinkers may have difficulty combining cognitive and affective factors. Middle-aged adults outperformed younger subjects on both the emotional and nonemotional dilemmas, although better reasoning was also moderately associated with higher ego levels, as determined by a sentence-completion task. Blanchard-Fields has commented that younger reasoners may not be as effective at integrating cognitive and affective information. That is, emotionally salient information may be more problematic and disruptive for individuals with less cognitive maturity.

A Paradigm Shift

The finding of greater elaboration of events by older adults (Blanchard-Fields, 1986; Yoder & Elias, 1987) is in direct contrast to verbal learning studies of memory that typically find older adults less likely to produce elaborative mediators in the recall of paired associate stimuli or word lists (Elias, Elias, & Elias, 1977; Kausler, 1982). In choosing a paired associate or word list task, one has control over the frequency with which stimuli might appear in an environment (word-frequency effects) and the ease with which associations or mediators might be formed (imagery and item concreteness). These are the kinds of tasks that have formed the basis for much of our knowledge about memory and memory systems, and they are not to be disparaged. The focus in such paradigms is on accuracy of recall, not accuracy of interpretation. Mood-induction research tends to use laboratory tasks such as paired associate learning, list learning, or perceptual organization. Research investigating stimulus affective valence is more likely to allow for elaboration and interpretation of events, particularly if the stimuli are presented within a story, event, or probable event format. Everyday memory follows the stimulus-affective-valence format. Thus, what we have traditionally learned about the probable reduction of memory elaboration processes with age does not seem applicable when memory involves recall of events that have affective valence and require interpretation.

Accuracy of recall of events does not indicate accuracy in interpretation. The training we receive as researchers tends to make us want to stress recall of events as the most important memory component of that event. As a consequence, accurate interpretation of events and possible outcomes of events has not been the typical focus of memory research and aging. When considering the role of affect in conjunction with everyday memory, one must consider the need for a paradigm shift. We need to know how accuracy of recall for an event interacts with interpretation of the event and how the affective valence of the event colors the interpretation.

Studies of courtroom testimony indicate that recall of events over time is quite hazy. Our recall of events from long-term memory is such that the explicit nature of an event is often confused in recall with the implied aspect of the events (Cohen, 1989). We fill in the gaps that appear over time with meaning rather than fact (Cohen, 1989). We have all seen enough media-depicted courtroom drama to know that witnesses are urged to recall events without providing a conclusion or interpretation. To a certain extent, that is impossible; to consider the affective valence of a stimulus or an event is to interpret its meaning and come to a conclusion about that stimulus or event. A careful consideration of factual recall must include a better understanding of affective factors, whether we preside in a courtroom or a cognitive laboratory.

Improving Memory via Affect

Several researchers have investigated the possibility of improving memory in individuals by providing information or stimuli that had more affective valence. A few of these researchers have included several adult age groups in their sample. Erber, Herman, and Botwinick (1980) manipulated incidental and intentional recall of word lists in young (mean age = 24) and old subjects (mean age = 69) by having them (a) check the words for specific letters, (b) check the lists for letters and prepare for recall, (c) read the lists for later recall, (d) check whether a word was pleasant or unpleasant, and (e) check pleasant or unpleasant and prepare for later recall.

Erber et al. (1980) found that the young performed better than the old across all conditions except with check-the-letter-only instructions. The semantic task of rating words for affective valence resulted in improved recall for both age groups relative to the letter-check condition. Rating affective valence was quite effective as an incidental instructional task. In both age groups, it was as effective in promoting recall as was direct instruction to recall. Rating for affective valence plus instructions for recall further improved performance for the young, but older adults did not receive extra benefit from valence plus direct-recall instructions. Because only the young benefited in both conditions requiring dual processes, the authors offered the suggestion that for older adults the combination of explicit instructions to recall plus the incidental rating task resulted in an increased cognitive load and divided attention.

The effectiveness of using affective valence to improve memory was also shown by Yesavage et al. (1983), who studied the everyday activity of face–name learning in a controlled experiment conducted with older adults only (mean age = 65.6). Subjects were asked to learn face–name pairs under instructional conditions that involved (a) forming an image between a prominent facial feature and the person's name, (b) forming the image and judging its pleasantness, and (c) concentrating on prominent facial features. Performance was best when imagery was accompanied by overt affective valence judgment, followed in order by imagery-alone instructions and prominent facial feature-alone instructions. In a 48-hr–delay condition, imagery plus valence judgment still improved memory relative to the imagery-alone and facial feature-alone instructions, but the latter two conditions did not differ. Hence, the affective component enhanced delayed recall performance. Presumably, the facial features were by themselves not sufficient in affective salience to promote enhanced retention if the judgment was not specified.

A further illustration of the efficacy of affective valence in enhancing recall can be found in the previously discussed study of Yoder and Elias (1987). In this study, young, middle-aged, and older adults were shown a series of eight-frame picture stories, which were designed to have either emotional or more neutral affective content (Yoder, 1983). Subjects were asked to rate the emotional impact of the stories as well as how typical the stories seemed in relation to their own experiences and culture. All the stories used had equivalent amounts of information, similar typicality ratings, and were judged to be somewhat typical. The affectively laden stories were remembered better than the more neutral stories, regardless of age, with both recall and recognition measures. As previously noted, the young remembered significantly more information than the middle-aged or older adults, but the magnitude of the effect for remembrance of stories with more emotional valence was the same for the young and old. Of particular interest, however, was the finding that type of content became more important over a 72-hr delayed recall period. Emotional material was retained far more completely over time than neutral information. There was no indication that this effect was more or less exaggerated for the middle-aged or older groups.

From these studies, it can be seen that affective salience provided in a variety of forms enhances performance and seems to slow the rate of forgetting in both young and old. There is little evidence from these few studies that affect improves memory performance differentially in young or old, only that recall and recognition tends to be enhanced when stimuli have greater affective valence.

Mechanisms of Affect

The effectiveness of affective valence as an aid to recall and recognition is an observation, not an explanation. How affect impacts memory is less clear than the fact that it can facilitate remembering in certain cases. One school of thought suggests that the mechanism of affect can best be described via network theory (Blaney, 1986). Network theory proposes that nodes or units in memory exist for purposes of representing emotion or affect. Each node is linked to an event in life that represents that particular affective node. Activation of the emotion nodes can result in a spreading of activation through memory structures to which the node is connected (Bower, 1981). This perspective on affect allows it to fit within depth of processing models (e.g., Erber et al., 1980), as well as cognitive priming models relying on the spreading activation concept.

The idea that affect might be part of a separate memory system has been argued by both Zajonc (1980) and Posner and Snyder (1975). After reviewing the social psychological literature related to impression formation, Zajonc (1980) concluded that affective reactions occurred early in perceptual and cognitive operations, were derived from a parallel, separate, and partly independent system, and that in contrast to cold cognitions, affective responses were effortless, inescapable, irrevocable, holistic, difficult to verbalize, but easy to communicate and understand.

Posner and Snyder (1975) based their conclusions on data gathered from an experiment designed to test the hypothesis that processing trait adjectives involves an automatic activation of affective meaning. Affective meaning was described as one of several positive semantic dimensions that can be quickly and habitually processed. In two separate experiments, subjects were presented sentences consisting of a proper name followed by one to four adjectives. The adjectives were either all positive, all negative, or a mixture of positive and negative traits. The results suggested that matched valences between cues and targets enhanced recall. In addition, reaction time for "match" decisions was affected by the positive or negative valence of the cue-matched sentence valence. These findings suggested that two separate systems were acting in parallel fashion and could facilitate or retard reaction time at the point of identification, depending on the degree of match or mismatch of the two systems. Two memory systems were proposed. One system was proposed for processing the list of trait adjectives. This system showed the expected serial search and retrieval function. The other system was one that integrated the value of the adjectives to result in one generalized affective impression. This system could be accessed as a contextual whole, and access time was reduced with more cues that matched the target.

The notions of automaticity, spreading activation, priming, separate processing, and compilation of affective valence outside of the usual circuits devoted to retrieval from short-term memory, all fit well with the data reviewed with respect to aging and affect. With the limited available literature, the effectiveness of affective salience as an aid to memory retrieval has been shown to be unaffected by the aging process.

The Posner and Snyder (1975) evidence for a different retrieval process for affective information also fits well with evidence from clinical case studies of sexual abuse where particularly traumatic memories, at one time suppressed, begin to come into consciousness. The retrieval of this information is selective rather than systematic or logical (Bass & Davis, 1988) and more sensory than episodic or contextual. Similar, but less dramatic observations have been made in individuals suffering from post-traumatic stress disorder. This form of retrieval of information is so unusual relative to the more consciously driven retrieval processes that individuals often express the feeling that they must be losing their mind.

Most discussions of memory systems suggest that similar information can be processed via different systems and that the same information can be encoded and retrieved differently via different memory systems. With affect, particularly when affective tone overwhelms all other information, affective valence may not only enhance retrieval of factual or episodic information but also may be processed and retrieved within its own memory system.

The Nature of Everyday Memory and Affect

Several texts in addition to this one have pointed out the difficult nature of measuring everyday memory processes (Cohen, 1989; Poon, Rubin, & Wilson, 1989) as opposed to the relatively discrete kinds of experiences offered in laboratory studies. If affect is distinct as a form of information within the domain of memory, the everyday concept is no less distinct.

Everyday memories are a flow of memories integrated into a series of past memories, as well as a set of potential future actions. Information is filtered as relevant or nonrelevant on a conscious and unconscious basis. Everyday memories can be evaluated on the day of the occurrence and everyday thereafter. Our interpretations and remembrances of old information can change as we process new information (Linton, 1982); what is important today may not be important a few weeks from now and vice versa (Linton, 1982). We deal not only with factual information but information integrated into knowledge and general concepts. Because everyday memory involves not only factual information but the affective response to that information in terms of action and evaluation of self and action, an individual differences perspective may be more applicable here than in other areas of memory investigation. Personality variables such as blunting, repression–sensitization (Kobasa, 1979), or neuroticism, extraversion, and openness (Costa, McCrae, & Norris, 1981) may be of particular interest. Psychophysiological measures of arousal–reactivity as well as paper and pencil tasks assessing subjective affective response or preference (e.g., emotional salience, defense mechanisms, cognitive style) may also prove useful.

To better understand how emotion influences cognitive abilities, we must employ additional everyday materials to study learning and memory. For example, cognitive processes should be studied more extensively in social situations, in typical institutional and business-type circumstances, and with everyday materials such as letters, mailings, newspapers, magazines, journals, media presentations, and telephone conversations. Other elicitors of affect may involve memories of individuals or events. While these stimuli may have different affective valences, they provide rich material for understanding cognitive processes that are well practiced over the years.

Given the complexity of both affect and everyday memory, investigators in this area will tend to want to statistically control and partial out variables that contribute extraneous noise. We have been trained that this is the way to get to the essence of a variable. Everyday memory and affect are both very different conceptually from other aspects of memory. We should be cautious in our attempts to partial out and control too many variables for fear that we might lose the real essence.

References

Bass, E., & Davis, L. (1988). *The courage to heal: A guide for women survivors of child sexual abuse.* New York: Harper & Row.

Blanchard-Fields, F. (1986). Reasoning on social dilemmas varying in emotional saliency: An adult developmental perspective. *Psychology and Aging, 1,* 325–333.

Blaney, P. (1986). Affect and memory: A review. *Psychological Bulletin, 99,* 229–246.

Bower, G. (1981). Mood and memory. *American Psychologist, 31,* 129–148.

Cohen, G. (1989). *Memory in the real world.* London: Erlbaum.

Costa, P.T., McCrae, R.R., & Norris, A.H. (1981). Personal adjustment to aging: Longitudinal prediction from neuroticism and extraversion. *Journal of Gerontology, 36,* 78–85.

Elias, M.F., Elias, J.W., & Elias, P.R. (1977). *Basic processes in adult developmental psychology.* St. Louis, Mo: C.V. Mosby.

Ellis, H.C., Thomas, R.L., & Rodriguez, I.A. (1984). Emotional mood states and memory: Elaborative encoding, semantic processing,a nd cognitive effort. *Journal of Experimental Psychology: Learning, Memory, and Cognition, 10,* 470–482.

Erber, J., Herman, T.G., & Botwinick, J. (1980). Age differences in memory as a function of depth of processing. *Experimental Aging Research, 6,* 341–348.

Eysenck, M. (1976). Arousal, learning, and memory. *Psychological Bulletin, 83,* 389–404.

Flavell, J.H., & Ross, L. (1982). *Social cognitive development.* New York: Cambridge University Press.

Gilligan, S., & Bower, G. (1984). Cognitive consequences of emotional arousal. In C. Izard, J. Kagan, & R. Zajonc (Eds.), *Emotions, cognition, and behavior* (pp. 547–588). New York: Cambridge University Press.

Isen, A.M. (1984). Toward understanding the role of affect in cognition. In R.S. Wyer & T.K. Srull (Eds.), *Handbook of social cognition* (pp. 179–236). Hillsdale, NJ: Erlbaum.

Isen, A.M., & Daubman, R.A. (1984). The influence of affect on categorization. *Journal of Personality and Social Psychology, 47,* 1206–1217.

Kausler, D.H. (1982). *Experimental psychology and human aging.* New York: John Wiley.

Kennelly, K., Hayslip, B., & Richardson, S. (1985). Depression and helplessness-induced cognitive deficits in the aged. *Experimental Aging Research, 11,* 169–173.

Kobasa, S.C. (1979). Stressful life events, personality, and health: An inquiry into hardiness. *Journal of Personality and Social Psychology, 37,* 1–11.

Labouvie-Vief, G. (1982). Dynamic development and mature autonomy. *Human Development, 25,* 161–191.

Labouvie-Vief, G., Devoe, M., & Bulka, D. (1989). Speaking about feelings: Conceptions of emotion across the life span. *Psychology and Aging, 4,* 425–437.

Lazarus, R.S. (1984). On the primacy of cognition. *American Psychologist, 39,* 124–129.

Leight, K.A., & Ellis, H.C. (1981). Emotional mood states, strategies, and state-dependency in memory. *Journal of Verbal Leaning and Verbal Behavior, 20,* 251–266.

Levanthal, H., & Tomarken, A.J. (1986). Emotion: Today's problems. *Annual Review of Psychology, 37,* 565–610.

Linton, M. (1982). Transformations of memory in everyday life. In U. Neisser (Ed.), *Memory observed. Remembering in natural contexts.* San Francisco: W.H. Freeman.

Niederehe, G. (1986). Depression and memory impairment in the aged. In L.W. Poon (Ed.), *Handbook for clinical memory assessment of older adults* (pp. 226–237). Washington, DC: American Psychological Association.

Piaget, J. (1967). The mental development of the child. In D. Elkind (Ed.), *Six psychological studies* (pp. 3–73). New York: Random House.

Poon, L.W., Rubin, D.C., & Wilson, B.A. (1989). *Everyday cognition in adulthood and late life*. New York: Cambridge University Press.

Posner, M.I., & Snyder, C.R. (1975). Attention and cognitive control. In R.L. Solso (Ed.), *Information processing and cognition: The Loyola symposium* (pp. 55–86). Hillsdale, NJ: Erlbaum.

Schulz, R. (1982). Emotionality and aging: A theoretical and emperical analysis. *Journal of Gerontology, 37*, 42–51.

Velton, E. (1968). A laboratory task for the induction of mood states. *Behavioral Research and Therapy, 6*, 473–482.

Wells, C.E. (1979). Pseudodementia. *American Journal of Psychiatry, 6*, 895–900.

Yesavage, J.A., Rose, T.L., & Bower, G.H. (1983). Interactive imagery and affective judgments improve face-name learning in the elderly. *Journal of Gerontology, 38*, 197–203.

Yoder, C.Y. (1983). *Emotionality, memory and aging: Assessing evaluative memory with imaginal story sequences*. Unpublished manuscript.

Yoder, C.Y., & Elias, J.W. (1987). Age, affect and memory for pictoral story sequences. *British Journal of Psychology, 78*, 545–549.

Zajonc, R.B. (1980). Feeling and thinking—Preferences need no inferences. *American Psychologist, 35*, 151–175.

17
Aging, Selective Attention, and Everyday Memory

DANA J. PLUDE AND LISA J. MURPHY

Having left your house, you suddenly wonder if you turned off the stove. It is quite likely that you cannot remember for certain having done so. As a precautionary measure, you return home only to find that the stove has indeed been shut off. Such a situation is often accompanied by some self-deprecating remark concerning faulty memory function.

In a different but related vein, you may have on occasion been upset by being unable to remember a new acquaintance's name. You know that you were introduced, but you simply cannot recall the person's name. The fact that the acquaintance recalls your name at a subsequent encounter adds fuel to your concern about seeming memory impairment.

These two vignettes represent the kind of "memory" complaints that are most commonly lodged by older adult audiences to whom we lecture on the topic of memory and aging. Before initiating the lectures, the members of the audience are requested to list common memory complaints on an index card. Of the several hundred responses accumulated to date, by far the highest percentage of complaints concern remembering facts, and within this domain, remembering people's names is the hands-down winner (comprising some 90% of the complaints). The second most common complaint involves remembering whether or not routine activities have been performed (comprising some 20% of the responses overall). We recognize that this sampling is far from representative of the kinds of memory complaints that may be lodged in a clinical setting, wherein the incidence of dementing diseases and other disorders of cognition is much larger and in which the degree of memory impairment has far greater significance for everyday functioning. Nevertheless, these data fairly represent the kinds of memory phenomena that are of interest (if not concern) to community-dwelling elderly adults.

The common thread in these experiences involves blaming memory for the inability to recall some information. However, it is worth asking if memory is the real (or only?) culprit.

In this chapter, we argue that failing to attend selectively to some source of information lies at the core of many alleged "memory" failures. In outlining our argument, we review selected findings concerning aging and selective attention as well as recent developments in mainstream cognitive psychology concerning the role of selective attention in laboratory-based memory performance. We consider the role of selective attention in everyday life, with emphasis on the performance of and memory for various activities. We conclude by identifying initiatives for future research. Before embarking on these goals, we first define our conceptualization of selective attention.

Attention is a multidimensional construct as witnessed by a variety of indicators. For example, a survey of the 13 published volumes of the series entitled *Attention and Performance* indicates a span of topics ranging from sensory detection to text comprehension. Similarly, Parasuraman and Davies's (1984) text entitled *Varieties of Attention* comprised no fewer than eight chapters, each devoted to a different aspect of attention. The impressive diversity of attention defies a single encompassing definition. Perhaps that is why William James (1892) observed that "we all know what attention is" and went on to discuss various aspects of attention in his classic text that introduced psychology in America near the turn of the century. Despite its diversity, attention can be conceptualized as comprising three fundamental dimensions: alertness, capacity, and selectivity (e.g., Posner & Boise, 1971). The alertness dimension concerns the ability to maintain concentration over time, such as in a vigilance task in which an observer monitors some repetitive event to detect an infrequent target event (e.g., Parasuraman, 1984). The capacity dimension is analogous to the energy available to sustain an electric appliance, such as a computer, with decreasing capacity (an electrical "brown out"), yielding progressively poorer performance (e.g., Kahneman, 1973). Finally, the selective dimension of attention concerns the ability to restrict information processing to a relevant source (or sources) of information while ignoring or filtering out irrelevant sources (e.g., Johnston & Dark, 1986). Clearly, these dimensions are interdependent; however, the focus of this chapter centers on the selective aspect of attention (for an overview of age effects in all three dimensions see Plude & Doussard-Roosevelt, 1990). Further, we consider only the selective processing of environmental information, thus excluding that aspect of attention that focuses on internal processes (e.g., thoughts, ideas, emotions) as well as other aspects of attention relating to the other dimensions discussed previously.

Having identified selectivity as the relevant dimension of attention, it is important to consider its role in everyday life. Selective attention is critical for performing optimally in a wide variety of situations such as driving an automobile and operating precision equipment. Even the simple act of listening to a friend's conversation requires selective attention insofar as that message must be discriminated from the host of other acoustic signals in the environment. In addition to its involvement in performing various everyday activities, selective attention also plays a key role in everyday memory. The ability to recall some desired fact presupposes that the fact is stored in memory. Now, although some facts may be encoded into memory "automatically"—that is, without conscious awareness or selective processing—more often, purposeful memories, those that we intend to remember at some later time, require selective attention to be encoded for successful retrieval later. We return to this point in the following discussion. For now, suffice it to say that selective attention plays an important role in everyday life, and there is reason to believe that its significance in this arena increases with increasing adulthood age.

Aging and Selective Attention

The assessment of selective attention involves comparing patterns of performance tradeoffs in various conditions that place different demands on selective processing. Considerable cognitive aging research has been devoted to this enterprise, (e.g., Plude & Doussard-Roosevelt, 1990) with the magnitude of age effects depending on an impressive variety of factors, all of which concern the complexity of the task being performed in conjunction with the level of skill and/or practice of the individual. In a nutshell, it is commonly found that age decrements in performance increase proportionally with the complexity of the task being performed. We have demonstrated this pattern of age effects in various studies involving "visual search," in which an individual searches for a specific target (usually an alphanumeric character) in a visual display that varies in the number of nontargets (other characters), with performance assessed on both speed and accuracy of target identification (see Plude & Hoyer, 1985, for review). In such a task, age decrements increase with increasing emphasis on selective attention (e.g., Plude & Doussard-Roosevelt, 1989). This outcome is often visualized in a graph that plots the performance of older adults (typically in their 60s) against the performance of young adults (typically in their 20s) with the relationship being described in large part by a linear function with a slope somewhere in the vicinity of 1.5 to 2.0 (e.g., Cerella, 1985, 1990; Salthouse, 1985). Figure 17.1 depicts such a relationship, which was obtained in our recent investigation of aging and divided attention (Plude, Murphy, & Gabriel-Byrne, 1989). In this study, we found that task complexity rather than the requirement to divide attention (vs. focus it) was the key determinant of age decrement. Thus, as the task imposes greater demand on the performance of young adults (i.e., increments in response time along the abscissa), the elderly exhibit a proportionally greater demand on performance (i.e., increments in response time along the ordinate). This outcome agreed with others in the cognitive aging literature (e.g., McDowd & Craik, 1988; Salthouse, Rogan, & Prill, 1984) and emphasizes the centrality of task complexity in determining the presence and magnitude of age decrement. This so-called complexity effect

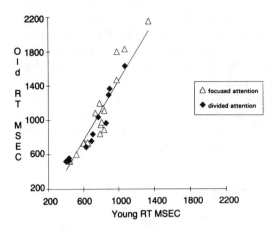

FIGURE   17.1. Age-related complexity effects under focused (open triangles) and divided (solid diamonds) attention. (RT, reaction time. *Note.* Data originally reported in Plude et al., 1989.)

(Birren, 1965) has been accounted for in a variety of ways among which is an argument based on impaired selective attention (e.g., Hoyer & Plude, 1980, 1982).

As noted, task complexity is but one side of the issue. The other side concerns the skill or expertise of the individual performing the task (see Chapter 15, this volume). As an example of this contribution, it has been shown that consistent practice in a visual search task reduces or eliminates age decrements in performance (e.g., Madden & Nebes, 1980; Plude & Hoyer, 1981). More generally, performance in skilled domains, such as typing (Salthouse, 1990) and chess (Charness, 1985), shows relatively little age impairment compared with performance in nonskilled domains. The acquisition of skill depends in large part on consistent practice, which reduces the demand on selective attention, thereby attenuating age decrements in performance. Recent evidence suggests, however, that aging may compromise certain aspects of the consistent practice effect such that after extensive practice age decrements remain (see Fisk, McGee, & Giambra, 1988). This may indicate that the ability to acquire expert levels of skill is impaired in later life. Nevertheless, it appears that previously acquired skill remains intact well into the late adulthood years.

Selective Attention and Everyday Memory

At the outset, we must acknowledge that research concerning the role of selective attention in everyday life is scarce. Despite Schonfield's (1974) elegant call for increased effort at the interface between laboratory and real-life settings, there remains a paucity of empirical research devoted to ecologically realistic situations. A clear exception to this is the recent work by Reason (1979, 1983, 1984), Harris (1983), and others (see Harris & Morris, 1983, for review) on the topic of absentmindedness and memory for actions and intentions, which has rekindled some of James's (1892) earlier work on the attention–memory link. The common thread between the present linkage and these others is that attention is given a central role in the memory process. Indeed, selective attention can be conceived of as ✶ executive control in the memory system, determining which inputs receive priority and which are ignored. Selection is a necessary (albeit insufficient) condition for successful memory storage and (later) retrieval (see Hasher & Zacks, 1988, for a related conceptualization emphasizing the role of inhibitory control in modulating memory performance).

The conceptualization of selective attention as executive control relates to the model of memory introduced by Baddeley and associates (e.g., Baddeley, 1976; Baddeley & Hitch, 1974) in which the active part of memory consists of two slave systems (an articulatory loop and a visual-spatial scratch pad) dedicated to an executive control process that oversees the flow of information through the slave systems and other, relatively static components of the memory system (e.g., long-term memory). Although other models of memory also contain a control process of one sort or another (e.g., Atkinson & Shiffrin, 1968; Reason, 1984; Wingfield & Stein, 1989), Baddeley's captures the essence of an intentional, consciously allocated, limited capacity process for selectively processing environmental inputs.

The notion that executive control relates to memory for everyday activities has been investigated by Reason and his associates (Reason, 1979, 1983, 1984; Reason & Lucas, 1983). Reason has argued that attentional control is a key determinant of memory performance, playing a central role in absentmindedness and "slips of action." Action slips occur when an unintended action is performed in lieu of an intended one, such as, for example, going upstairs into one's bedroom rather than into the bathroom to fetch a desired item. According to Reason, the momentary lapse in control allows a routinized action to run itself off in response to some evoking stimulus in the environment. Carrying this logic further, it can be reasoned that memory for actions that are performed automatically should be poor as a result of the withdrawal of executive control from their execution. So, for example, memory for turning off the stove, an action that may be performed automatically, should be quite poor, as exemplified in one of the vignettes introduced previously.

In all, the benefit of automatic performance is clear cut: Information processing is expedient and effortless. However, there is a cost of automatic performance as well. Habitual acts are resistant to modification and as such may interfere with performance when the automatized activities are no longer appropriate, as in the action slips described by Reason (1983). Thus, automatization is a mixed blessing with regard to everyday performance.

The same conclusion applies to automatization with regard to everyday memory: It is a mixed blessing. In one introductory vignette, a stove was rechecked because the act of turning it off was not remembered. Laboratory-based research has shown that memory for automatic performance is poorer than memory for effortful performance (e.g., Fisk & Schneider, 1984). Thus, the cost of automatization is a decreased memory for habitual acts that have been performed. Of course, the benefit of automatization has to do with the economy of habitual acts: They needn't be remembered (consciously) in order to be performed. One way to account for the different patterns of recall for automatic versus effortful activities appeals to a "levels of processing" approach to memory (Craik & Lockhart, 1972; Craik & Tulving, 1975). In brief, this approach envisions memory as a by-product of the analysis performed on information encountered in the environment. A shallow level of analysis, that is, attending to physical features of a stimulus, yields an ephemeral memory trace, whereas a deep (semantic) level of analysis, that is, attending to the meaning of a stimulus, yields a durable memory trace. Automatic processing requires little if any attention to any aspect of processing and thus would be expected to yield fragile memory traces. Imposing a demand on selective attention, as required under effortful processing, would be expected to prompt a meaningful level of analysis that yields stable and enduring memory traces. Precious little empirical research has examined age effects in memory for automatic versus effortful activities (but see Kausler's, 1985, review of memory for conversations). Considerable research has been devoted to age effects within the levels of processing framework (see, e.g., Craik & Byrd, 1982; Craik & Simon, 1980). In general, it has been found that elderly adults tend to engage a shallower level of analysis compared with younger adults, which impairs the older adult's performance in laboratory-based memory tasks. It is noteworthy that matching the level of analysis with the level of retrieval cues enhances the older adult's ability to recall information but does not eradicate the age deficit in memory test performance (e.g., Smith, 1980).

In summary, we assume that executive control can be allotted in a continuous manner to input. That is, some inputs require the full capacity of the executive control to coordinate their progress through the information processing system, whereas other inputs require relatively little (if any) of the executive control's capacity for their processing. Although such processing has usually been dichotomized as constituting either effortful or automatic processing, respectively, (e.g., Hasher & Zacks, 1979; Schneider & Shiffrin, 1977) it is probably more accurate to conceive of a continuum of processing with effortful and automatic processing falling at the endpoints (e.g., Kahneman, 1973). The importance of this assumption for the attention–memory link is apparent in considering the fate of inputs that are processed with relatively little attentional control compared with those that are processed with attentional effort. James (1892) recognized this aspect of attention in commenting that "habit diminishes the conscious attention with which our acts are performed" (p. 139). Given that attentional control is necessary for encoding inputs into memory, the extent to which such control is withdrawn from to-be-remembered information will be a strong determinant of subsequent retrieval success or failure, regardless of age.

The present conceptualization of the attention–memory link implicates an age-related selective attention deficit as a significant deterrent to effective explicit memory function. In this vein, interventions designed to ameliorate selective attention deficits in the elderly should produce particular dividends for improving explicit memory (whether in or out of the laboratory), and we turn to such considerations in the closing section.

Concluding Remarks

As is the case in the mainstream cognitive literature, cognitive aging research on selective attention (see Plude, 1990) and on explicit memory for facts and actions (see Kausler, 1985) has taken quite separate paths. Despite this divergence, there is a tendency in recent times to integrate the two bodies of research (e.g., Backman, 1989; Plude, in press) in order to yield a comprehensive picture of cognitive aging. These two independent lines of investigation implicate age decrements in executive control as playing a central role in the alleged memory difficulties of elderly adults. Moreover, Graf, Tuokko, and Gallie (1990) recently argued with similar logic in accounting for the memory and performance deficits associated with Alzheimer's disease. Their main thesis was that attentional dysfunctions accompanying this and other forms of dementia provide a parsimonious explanation of a wide variety of deficits in demented elderly adults. Thus, even in the absence of the much- needed experimental work, there is sufficient face validity for pursuing further the role of selective attention in everyday memory and aging.

Various directions for future research suggest themselves for establishing and clarifying the role of selective attention in everyday life. First, with respect to human performance, much work clearly needs to be done to bridge the gap between the laboratory and real life. To take only a single example, it seems that selective attention is a critical component to assess in evaluating age increments in accidents in the home, while driving, and on the job. Sterns, Barrett, and Alexander (1985) have cogently summarized the nature of age changes in these settings, and their review suggests several avenues for assessing the role of selective attention. Similarly, in considering the role of selective attention in everyday memory, a variety of research initiatives has been suggested. Again, taking only a single example, it seems that selective attention is a critical component of remembering a wide variety of to-be-recalled contents (activities, events, persons, etc.), and Kausler's (1985) review of ecologically realistic research on aging and episodic memory suggests numerous paths for future research efforts.

We have not touched on what may be the most obvious avenue for future work involving aging, selective attention, and everyday life, namely, mechanisms by which selective attention decrements can be compensated to enhance memory and performance. The acquisition of skill broaches the topic, but there is need for developing and evaluating other interventions as well. How might we optimize the older adult's memory of habitual acts and recent acquaintances? Two suggestions derive from our review of selective attention research (see also Plude, in press). To remember having performed an automatized act, the actor should endeavor to de-automatize it. One means by which to accomplish this quite simply is to speak aloud when commiting the act: "I am turning off the stove now." This forces attention to be devoted to the performance of the task, increasing the likelihood that it will be recalled later on. On meeting a new acquaintence, Cermak's (1976) four recommendations should be followed: (a) pay attention, (b) repeat the name, (c) elaborate on the name, and (d) test yourself in the absence of the target person. Each of these steps involves devoting some attention to the act of remembering the new acquaintance. The first step clearly implicates selective attention by emphasizing the importance of attending to the relevant aspect of the environment, that is, the person's name. Both of these recommendations hinge on a common theme: It must be attended to be remembered.

Acknowledgment. Preparation of this chapter was supported by NIA Grant R01-AG08060 to DJP.

References

Atkinson, R.C., & Shiffrin, R.M. (1968). Human memory: A proposed system and its control processes. In K.W. Spence & J.T. Spence (Eds.), *Advances in the Psychology of learning and motivation research and theory* (Vol. 2, pp. 89–195). New York: Academic Press.

Backman, L. (1989). Varieties of memory compensation by older adults in episodic remembering. In L.W. Poon, D.C. Rubin, & B.A. Wilson (Eds.), *Everyday cognition in adulthood and later life* (pp. 509–544). Cambridge: Cambridge University Press.

Baddely, A. (1976). *The psychology of memory.* New York: Basic Books.

Baddeley, A., & Hitch, G. (1974). Working memory. In G.H. Bower (Ed.), *The psychology of learning and motivation* (Vol. 8, pp. 47–90). New York: Academic Press.

Birren, J.E. (1965). Age changes in speed of behavior: Its central nature and physiological correlates. In A.T. Welford & J.E. Birren (Eds.), *Behavior, aging and the nervous system* (pp. 191–216). Springfield, IL: Charles C. Thomas.

Cerella, J. (1985). Information processing rates in the elderly. *Psychological Bulletin, 98,* 67–83.

Cerella, J. (1990). Aging and information processing rate. In J.E. Birren & K.W. Schaie (Eds.), *Handbook of the psychology of aging* (3rd ed., pp. 201–221). New York: Academic Press.

Cermak, L.S. (1976). *Improving memory.* New York: McGraw-Hill.

Charness, N. (1985). Aging and problem-solving performance. In N. Charness (Ed.), *Aging and human Performance* (pp. 225–259). London: Wiley.

Craik, F.I.M, & Byrd, M. (1982). Aging and cognitive deficits: The role of attentional resources. In F.I.M. Craik & S.E. Trehub (Eds.), *Aging and cognitive Processes* (pp. 191–211). New York: Plenum.

Craik, F.I.M., & Lockhart, R.S. (1972). Levels of processing: A framework for memory research. *Journal of Verbal Learning and Verbal Behavior, 11,* 671–684.

Craik, F.I.M., & Simon, E. (1980). Age differences in memory: The roles of attention and depth of processing. In L.W. Poon, J.L. Fozard, L.S. Cermak, D. Arenberg, & L.W. Thompson (Eds.), *New directions in memory and aging* (pp. 95–112). Hillsdale, NJ: Erlbaum.

Craik, F.I.M., & Tulving, E. (1975). Depth of processing and the retention of words in episodic memory. *Journal of Experimental Psychology: General, 104,* 268–294.

Fisk, A.D., McGee, N.D., & Giambra, L. (1988). The influence of age on consistent and varied semantic-category search performance. *Psychology and Aging, 3,* 323–333.

Fisk, A.D., & Schneider, W. (1984). Memory as a function of attention, level of processing, and automatization. *Journal of Experimental Psychology: Learning, Memory, and Cognition, 10,* 181–197.

Graf, P., Tuokko, H., & Gallie, K. (1990). Attentional deficits in Alzheimer's disease and related dementias. In J.E. Enns (Ed.), *The development of attention: Research and theory* (pp. 527–544). Amsterdam: Elsevier Science Publishers (North-Holland).

Harris, J.E. (1983). Remembering to do things: A forgotten topic. In J.E. Harris & P.E. Morris (Eds.), *Everyday memory, actions, and absent mindedness* (pp. 71–92). London: Academic Press.

Harris, J.E., & Morris, P.E. (1983). *Everyday memory, actions, and absent mindedness.* London: Academic Press.

Hasher, L., & Zacks, R.T. (1979). Automatic and effortful processes in memory. *Journal of Experimental Psychology: General, 108,* 356–388.

Hasher, L., & Zacks, R.T. (1988). Working memory, comprehension, and aging: A review and a new view. In G.H. Bower (Ed.), *The psychology of learning and motivation* (Vol. 22, pp. 193–225). New York: Academic Press.

Hoyer, W.J., & Plude, D.J. (1980). Attentional and perceptual processes in the study of cognitive aging. In L.W. Poon (Ed.), *Aging in the 1980's: Psychological issues* (pp. 227–238). Washington, DC: American Psychological Association.

Hoyer, W.J., & Plude, D.J. (1982). Aging and the allocation of attentional resources in visual information processing. In R. Sekuler, D. Rline, & K. Dismukes (Eds.), *Aging and human visual function* (pp. 245–263). New York: Alan R. Liss.

James, W. (1892). *Psychology, briefer course.* New York: Henry Holt.

Johnston, W.A., & Dark, V.J. (1986). Selective attention. *Annual Review of Psychology, 37,* 43–75.

Kahneman, D. (1973). *Attention and effort.* Hillsdale, NJ: Erlbaum.

Kausler, D.H. (1985). Episodic memory: Memorizing performance. In N. Charness (Ed.), *Aging and human Performance* (pp. 102–141). London: Wiley.

Madden, D.J., & Nebes, R.D. (1980). Aging and the development of automaticity in visual search. *Developmental Psychology, 16,* 377–384.

McDowd, J.M., & Craik, F.I.M. (1988). Effects of aging and task difficulty on divided attention performance. *Journal of Experimental Psychology: Human Perception and Performance, 14,* 267–280.

Parasuraman, R. (1984). Sustained attention in detection and discrimination. In R. Parasuraman & D.R. Davies (Eds.), *Varieties of attention* (pp. 243–271). Orlando, FL: Academic Press.

Parasuraman, R., & Davies, D.R. (Eds.) (1984). *Varieties of attention* (pp. 243–271). Orlando, FL: Academic Press.

Plude, D.J. (1990). Aging, feature integration, and visual selective attention. In J.E. Enns (Ed.), *The development of attention: Research and theory* (pp. 467–487). Amsterdam: Elsevier Science Publishers (North-Holland).

Plude, D.J. (in press). Attention and memory improvement. In D. Herrmann, H. Weingartner, A. Searleman, & C. McEvoy (Eds.), *Memory Improvement: Implications for memory theory.* New York: Springer-Verlag.

Plude, D.J., & Doussard-Roosevelt, J.A. (1989). Aging, selective attention, and feature integration. *Psychology & Aging, 1,* 4–10.

Plude, D.J., & Doussard-Roosevelt, J.A. (1990). Aging and attention: Selectivity, capacity, and arousal. In E.A. Lovelace (Ed.), *Aging and cognition: Mental processes, self awareness, and interventions* (pp. 97–133). Amsterdam: Elsevier Science Publishers (North-Holland).

Plude, D.J., & Hoyer, W.J. (1981). Adult age differences in visual search as a function of stimulus mapping and information load. *Journal of Gerontology, 36,* 598–604.

Plude, D.J., & Hoyer, W.J. (1985). Attention and performance: Identifying and localizing age deficits. In N. Charness (Ed.), *Aging and human performance* (pp. 47–99). London: Wiley.

Plude, D.J., Murphy, L.J., & Gabriel-Byrne, J. (1989, August). *Aging, divided attention, and visual search.* Paper presented at the meeting of the American Psychological Association, New Orleans.

Posner, M.I., & Boise, S.J. (1971). Components of attention. *Psychological Review, 78,* 391–408.

Reason, J. (1979). Actions not as planned: The price of automatization. In G. Underwood & R. Stevens (Eds.), *Aspects of consciousness* (Vol. 1, pp. 67–89). London: Academic Press.

Reason, J. (1983). Absent-mindedness and cognitive control. In J.E. Harris & P.E. Morris (Eds.), *Everyday memory, actions, and absent-mindedness* (pp. 113–132). London: Academic Press.

Reason, J. (1984). Lapses of attention in everyday life. In R. Parasuraman & D.R. Davies (Eds.), *Varieties of attention* (pp. 515–549). New York: Academic Press.

Reason, J., & Lucas, D. (1983). Using cognitive diaries to investigate naturally occurring memory blocks. In J.E. Harris & P.E. Morris (Eds.), *Everyday memory, actions, and absent-mindedness* (pp. 53–70). London: Academic Press.

Salthouse, T.A. (1985). Speed of behavior and its implications for cognition. In J.E. Birren & K.W. Schaie (Eds.), *Handbook of the Psychology of aging,* (2nd ed., pp. 400–426). New York: Van Nostrand Reinhold.

Salthouse, T.A. (1990). Cognitive competence and expertise in aging. In J.E. Birren & R.W. Schaie (Eds.), *Handbook of the psychology of aging* (3rd ed., pp. 310–319). New York: Academic Press.

Salthouse, T.A., Rogan, J.D., & Prill, K. (1984). Division of attention: Age differences on a visually presented memory task. *Memory & Cognition, 12,* 613–620.

Schneider, W., & Shiffrin, R.M. (1977). Controlled and automatic human information processing: I. Detection, search, and attention. *Psychological Review, 84,* 1–66.

Schonfield, D. (1974). Translations in gerontology—From lab to life: Utilizing information. *American Psychologist, 29,* 796–801.

Smith, A.D. (1980). Age differences in encoding, storage, and retrieval. In L.W. Poon, J.L. Fozard, L.S. Cermak, D. Arenberg, & L.W. Thompson (Eds.), *New directions in memory and aging* (pp. 23–45). Hillsdale, NJ: Erlbaum.

Sterns, H.L., Barrett, G.V., & Alexander, R.A. (1985). Accidents and the aging individual. In J.E. Birren & K.W. Schaie (Eds.), *Handbook of the psychology of aging* (2nd ed., pp. 703–724). New York: Van Nostrand Reinhold.

Wingfield, A., & Stine, L. (1989). Modeling memory processes: Research and theory on memory and aging. In G.C. Gilmore, P.J. Whitehouse, & M.L. Wykle (Eds.), *Memory, aging, and dementia* (pp. 4–40). New York: Springer.

18
Eyewitness Memory and Aging Research: A Case Study in Everyday Memory

CAROLYN ADAMS-PRICE AND MARION PERLMUTTER

Relatively recently, memory researchers have become sensitive to the specificity of memory operations. According to Jenkins (1979), for example, memory performance depends on stimulus, task, and person variables. Because stimulus, task, and subject variables used in laboratory studies may fail to resemble the variables that exist in everyday memory situations, some researchers have questioned the applicability of findings from laboratory studies for understanding everyday memory. Over the last decade or two, concern about this issue has motivated a substantial amount of research on everyday memory.

Some traditional memory theorists have criticized everyday memory research (e.g., Banaji & Crowder, 1989), claiming that everyday memory studies have generated inconclusive results and have failed to contribute new hypotheses about memory. In this chapter, we review eyewitness memory research. We believe this research serves as a good case study of the value of investigations of everyday memory. It has yielded some consistent findings and has generated some new hypotheses about memory. Moreover, and relevant to the present volume, we believe that findings from eyewitness memory research shed important light on practical and theoretical issues concerning aging and memory.

Eyewitness Memory Research in a Historical Perspective

Eyewitness memory research differs from most studies of memory in that it often has been motivated by social or political concerns. Early writings on eyewitness memory were primarily concerned with practical problems, especially legal problems. However, they usually had strong theoretical underpinnings. Whipple (1911) and Yarmey (1985) credit Binet with the first scientific studies of eyewitness memory. Binet found that the testimony of child eyewitnesses could be influenced by suggestive questions. Stern (1939), in Germany, also studied the suggestibility of eyewitnesses.

For his 1910 report (described by Loh, 1981), Stern had subjects describe from memory pictures and events they had witnessed and remembered with certainty. He described many of the same kinds of imaginative intrusions and embellishments to verbal reports later described by Bartlett (1932), which suggests that his model of memory may have been a precursor to Bartlett's reconstructive model.

Muensterberg's (1908) book, *On the Witness Stand*, illuminated the legal problems in relying on eyewitness memory. He took a position strongly critical of the court's reliance on often unreliable eyewitness testimony, which was in return sharply rebuked by the legal profession (Loh, 1981). Significantly, Muensterberg's activist stand on eyewitness memory is similar to the stand taken by recent eyewitness memory researchers, which is still countered by some legal professionals (e.g., Lane, 1984).

A reemergence of the psychology of eyewitness memory began in the early 1970s, ostensibly as a part of psychologists' efforts to make psychology "socially relevant" (Loh, 1981). Two of the most influential researchers in this area, Loftus and Buckhout (e.g., Buckhout, 1974; Loftus, 1975, 1983), focused much of their efforts on convincing the legal establishment of the dangers of eyewitness identifications. Buckhout (1974) listed 10 sources of unreliability in eyewitness identifications, including both tangible variables, such as lighting and the length of time of an observation, and psychological variables, such as stress and the tendency to "fill in" details. Buckhout was also one of the first modern psychologists to resurrect Bartlett's (1932) reconstructive model of memory.

Loftus has articulated the reconstructive model even further. Her work (e.g., Cole & Loftus, 1979; Gentner & Loftus, 1979, Loftus, 1975, 1979; Loftus & Palmer, 1973) has been particularly concerned with the degree to which misleading questions can influence memory of witnessed events, a practical issue. Phrased in theoretical terms, Loftus has found that people have a strong tendency to integrate information presented in different modalities, a task that is inherently reconstructive. Thus, it seems that eyewitness memory research began as a means to address practical problems, but the research can address theoretical questions as well.

In the late 1970s and 1980s, eyewitness memory research focused on questions of legal significance and particularly the factors associated with the accuracy of eyewitness identifications. Much research was spurred by a 1972 Supreme Court decision. In *Neil v. Biggers*, the court decided that it did not matter if police stations used suggestive eyewitness identification procedures, as long as the identification was accurate, which they believed was determinable. Since then, judges' instructions to juries have encouraged the belief that the accuracy of the identification could be determined from the accuracy of details and eyewitness confidence (e.g., Lane, 1984; Wells & Murray, 1983). In light of *Neil v. Biggers*, eyewitness memory researchers focused largely on the relationships between the accuracy of identifications and confidence and between memory for details and accurate identifications. Much of the rest of this chapter will be used to describe research and theory generated on these two topics.

Eyewitness Memory and Age

Recent eyewitness memory research has focused on a newly fashionable topic: the eyewitness memory ability of children. A number of special journal issues and conferences have examined the eyewitness memory of children (e.g., Goodman, 1984). The current interest in children's testimony reflects a national concern with child sexual abuse as a political issue. Indeed, many of the issues being addressed by researchers in eyewitness memory in childhood are directly related to questions about child sexual abuse. These issues include the ability of children to distinguish between fantasy and reality and children's resistance to misleading questions. Identification accuracy, which is often not a question in child sexual abuse cases, is hardly researched with children.

One contrast between child eyewitness memory research and adult eyewitness memory research is its goal. Child eyewitness memory research seems intent on measuring and bolstering the competence of young rememberers; whereas adult eyewitness memory seems focused on the fallibility of adult rememberers.

Compared to children's eyewitness memory ability, the eyewitness memory ability of older adults has been relatively uninvestigated. This paucity of information about the eyewitness memory of older adults is somewhat surprising, considering the huge amount of research conducted on memory in older persons.

The most likely explanation for the dearth of research in this area is that no specific social issue has appeared to spur on the research. We believe, however, that there are good theoretical and practical reasons to examine eyewitness memory and aging. One reason is the general stereotype about the memory ability of older persons and its likely implications in the legal arena. Older people are often stereotyped as forgetful, which certainly could work against them in court. Yarmey (1985) found that older persons are considered by jurors to be poor eyewitnesses but are considered by police officers and judges to be good witnesses. One explanation for these discrepant views of the elderly as witnesses may be that jurors are concerned about the memory ability of older witnesses, which they consider faulty, whereas judges and police officers are more concerned with the honesty of older witnesses, which they consider to be beyond reproach.

In addition to the general stereotype of the elderly as poor rememberers, other aspects of their memory performance may make them appear to be poor witnesses. For example, some researchers have suggested that the elderly have poorer memory for details than the young and that they are less confident than the young about their memory performance (e.g., Labouvie-Vief, 1980), although neither pattern has been consistently found. If these characterizations are accurate in eyewitness contexts, they could make the elderly appear to be particularly poor eyewitnesses, even in the absence of stereotyping (Yarmey, 1985).

At least six studies of eyewitness memory and aging have appeared in journals or edited books, of which most have examined identification accuracy. Yarmey and associates have conducted three of these studies (Yarmey, 1985; Yarmey, Jones, & Rashid, 1984; Yarmey & Kent, 1980). Yarmey and Kent initially found no age differences in identification accuracy, but in the later studies, they found reduced accuracy for elderly subjects (aged 60 and up) compared to college students. List (1986) showed younger and older adults a videotaped scenario of a shoplifting event. She found that older subjects were less able to identify young suspects than were young subjects but were better able to identify old suspects. O'Rourke, Penrod, Cutler, and Stuve (1989) showed subjects in six age groups from 18 to 72 years of age a videotaped robbery. They found a modest age-related decline in identification accuracy that did not interact with weapon presence, disguise of the criminal, or violence of the crime. Adams-Price (1988, 1989a, 1989b) studied eyewitness memory of three age groups (20–35, 40–55, and 60–75 years) from a wide range of educational backgrounds, none of whom were enrolled students. She found that age was a negative predictor of the accuracy of identifying six characters from two videotaped robberies, but not the best predictor (which was education, also in a negative direction). Thus, most studies show a modest age-related decline in identification accuracy, confounded by the fact that older subjects usually are asked to identify suspects from an age group other than their own.

Eyewitness Accuracy and Confidence

The relationship between accurate eyewitness identifications and confidence is theoretically interesting to memory researchers in general, and aging researchers in particular. The ability to assess one's own memory performance may be an important component of the ability to control it. Significant confidence–accuracy correlations have been found for some forms of memory but not for others. Research on feeling-of-knowing (e.g., Brown & McNeill, 1966) has long suggested that people can distinguish between those instances during which they can remember a piece of information and those instances that force them to guess.

Other measures of the correspondence between memory ability and memory self-report have been more mixed. Herrmann (1982) reviewed all of the major questionnaire and diary self-assessments of everyday memory ability. He found that most memory self-assessments do not correlate with objective measures of memory, except for some modest correlations between very specific and easily observable memory skills and self-assessments of those skills. Berry, West, and Dennehy (1989) have come to similar conclusions. They have suggested that general memory beliefs predict item-specific predictions, which in turn predict item performance. The accuracy and confidence measures employed in eyewitness identification experiments are highly specific and observable. Thus, modest but significant correlations should be expected if identification confidence is similar to other item-specific memory assessments.

Eyewitness memory researchers have come up with interesting insights about the relationship between memory accuracy and confidence. They have found that confidence is affected by variables other than accuracy. Confidence is likely to improve with time, while accuracy stays the same or declines. Wells, Ferguson, and Lindsay (1981) found that repetition of testimony, from the police station to the courtroom, increases confidence but not accuracy. Leippe (1980) suggested that choosing a suspect from a lineup makes an eyewitness more confident the next time he or she has to identify that suspect which is due to increased familiarity and cognitive dissonance.

Eyewitness memory researchers also have found a modest but somewhat predictable relationship between confidence and accuracy. Deffenbacher (1980) suggested that the correlation between the confidence and the accuracy of an eyewitness tends to be significant and positive when the perpetrator is seen under optimal viewing conditions and tends to be non-significant or negative when the perpetrator is seen under poor viewing conditions. He called this the "optimality hypothesis." Evidence for the optimality hypothesis has been found by Adams-Price (1988; 1989b) and Bothwell, Brigham, and Deffenbacher (1986). Some reseachers have suggested that optimality works because eyewitnesses have a general sense of their memory accuracy relative to others but that overall confidence does not change much when task difficulty increases (Deffenbacher, 1980; Bothwell et al., 1986). Adams-Price (1988, 1989b), however, found significant within-subject decreases in confidence levels when subjects tried to identify hard-to-see perpetrators. This finding suggests that confidence levels are not simply fixed traits.

Cognitive aging researchers have long been interested in the relationship between memory accuracy and confidence. Cognitive aging researchers are interested in determining if age changes in memory performance are reflected in age change in beliefs about one's own memory and in turn if those beliefs affect (adversely or otherwise) future memory performance (i.e., Berry, 1989; Cavanaugh, 1989; Perlmutter, 1978). Some researchers have suggested that accuracy–confidence correlations should be higher for the elderly than for the young, perhaps because the elderly are more aware of the fact that their memory is fallible. Lachman and Lachman (1980) and Zelinski, Gilewski, and Thompson (1980) found that the elderly were better than the young at distinguishing between accurate and inaccurate memories. Cavanaugh (1989) reviewed studies of predictions of accuracy (i.e., confidence estimates) and actual accuracy and reported that studies show that older people tend to overestimate their accuracy on memory tasks, except when the tasks are very familiar and when the confidence estimate comes after the task rather than before it. These results suggest, consistent with the optimality hypothesis, that older people do not adjust their confidence levels adequately when task difficulty is unclear.

Thus, the observed relationship between eyewitness confidence and accuracy in elderly subjects is interesting for several reasons. One reason is because it is not known if the factors that affect the confidence–accuracy correlation in the young affect the old similarly. Another reason is that the relationship might take several possible patterns. Given the complicated findings for other confidence–accuracy relationships in the elderly and the young, we could find higher or lower correlations for the elderly. Elderly eyewitnesses might be overly confident and have lower correlations over-all, which would suggest to the theorist that their memory monitoring was impaired. To the legal expert, it would suggest that their testimony would be falsely optimistic. By contrast, the relative familiarity of the eyewitness task might result in higher confidence–accuracy correlations for the elder-ly, which would mean that their testimony was particularly useful. Last, the relationship between accuracy and confidence for the old might be consis-tent with the optimality hypothesis.

The few studies of eyewitness confidence and accuracy in aging have produced mixed results. Yarmey and associates (Yarmey et al., 1984; Yar-mey & Kent, 1980) reported positive confidence–accuracy correlations for older subjects and negative confidence–correlations for young subjects but only for valid lineups (i.e., lineups with the perpetrator present). O'Rourke, Penrod, Cutler, and Stuve (1989) used preidentification and postidentification confidence assessments with subjects in four adult age groups. They found no age differences in confidence, nor did they report any age differences in the confidence–accuracy correlations. They did re-port, consistent with Cavanaugh's (1989) observations, that postidentifica-tion confidence is more strongly correlated with identification accuracy than is preidentification confidence.

Adams-Price (1988, 1989b) tested the optimality hypothesis in three adult age groups. She examined the relationship between the identification of characters of varying degrees of visibility in a filmed crime scene and confidence in those specific identifications. Although confidence decreased with task difficulty, the confidence–accuracy correlations were only signif-icant and positive for the easiest identifications. She observed no age dif-ferences in confidence or in the confidence–accuracy correlations, and the pattern of correlations was consistent with the optimality hypothesis for all three age groups.

This research suggests no major differences between young and old in the relationship between confidence and accuracy in eyewitness identifications. It also suggests that older people, like younger people, have some sense of their memory ability but that this sense may be distorted in ambiguous or difficult memory situations. We also suggest, however, that confidence is poorly measured in most eyewitness experiments, in that a single confidence estimate may not reflect jurors' judgments of witness confidence in the courtroom. The confidence perceived by a juror is likely affected by the eyewitness's "item" confidence but probably also is affected by general aspects of his or her personal demeanor, such as body language, articulation, and appearance. Kassin (1985) found that subjects who were made aware of the cues they emitted while making eyewitness identifications (e.g., facial expressions and hesitancy) had higher correlations between accuracy and confidence than subjects who were not made aware. Awareness of the confidence cues they emitted may have made their confidence assessments more honest and thoughtful.

Recall of Details Versus Main Points

As mentioned earlier, the accurate recall of details from a crime scene is considered by many jurors to be a good predictor of identification accuracy, despite the fact that researchers have failed to find any relationship between the two (Adams-Price, 1989a, 1989b; Buckhout, 1974; Christiaansen, Sweeney, & Ochalek, 1983; Cutler, Penrod, & Martens, 1987; Pigott & Brigham, 1985; Wells & Leippe, 1981; Yuille & Cutshall, 1986). Several studies on this issue have examined the relationship between memory for specific details and identification accuracy and found no relationship (Christiaansen et al., 1983; Pigott & Brigham, 1985). Some eyewitness researchers have suggested that persons who are good at recalling details may in fact be poor at recognizing criminals and vice versa (Adams-Price, 1989a; 1989b; Buckhout, 1974; Cutler et al., 1987; Wells & Leippe, 1981; Yuille & Cutshall, 1986). Buckhout (1974) suggested that detail recall and identification accuracy may not be related because attention to one factor takes away from attention to the other. In fact, Adams-Price (1989a; 1989b) found that education was positively related to verbal recall but negatively related to identification accuracy.

One problem with most of the research on memory for details and identification accuracy is the failure to differentiate systematically between details and main points. Wells and Leippe (1981) and Cutler et al. (1987) reported that the recall of details was unrelated to identification accuracy, but what they really meant was that the answers to specific questions about the crime scenes were unrelated to identification accuracy. They have not shown that free recall, or subjects' verbal description of the events, is unrelated to identification accuracy. By contrast, Yarmey (1985) reported data on free recall but did not differentiate between details or main points or report the relationship between total recall and identification accuracy.

Without a system for systematically differentiating between main points and details, it is impossible to clarify the nature of the relationship.

Researchers on prose recall have used story grammars to separate information recalled into details and main points (e.g., Kintsch, 1974; Kintsch & van Dijk, 1978; Mandler & Johnson, 1977). Most research on eyewitness memory has used live or filmed crime scenes as stimuli. One could argue that such stimuli are similar to stories in that the task of recalling them is reconstructive rather than reproductive and they contain more than one level of importance from "essential element of story" to "fine detail." Thus, eyewitness memory research could borrow a methodology from story grammar research to systematically distinguish between detail and gist. There is some precedence for this approach. Cavanaugh (1983, 1984) and Baggett (1979) have used story grammars to distinguish between main points and details in films.

A related controversy in cognitive aging is the ability of older persons to recall main points or details of stories. Some researchers have maintained that older people tend to recall main points but forget details (Labouvie-Vief, 1980; Labouvie-Vief & Schell, 1982; Zelinski et al., 1980). Cavanaugh (1984) found that highly verbal older persons recalled as many of the main points from films as younger persons but fewer of the details. By contrast, Meyer and Rice (1981) found that older subjects remembered *more* minor details than younger subjects. Other researchers have argued that older people are less able than the young to recall main points (e.g., Taub, 1979). Hultsch and Dixon (1984) have summarized the findings on aging and recall of main points versus details by suggesting that older individuals with high verbal ability tend to recall as many main points but not as many details as the young, whereas less verbally skilled older individuals tend to show the largest age differences on recall of main points. This suggests that eyewitness researchers interested in the recall of details from crime scenes should take into account verbal ability.

Schemas and Eyewitness Memory

An interesting perspective on the kind of detail remembered in eyewitness situations is afforded by studies looking at schemas and eyewitness memory. Neisser (1981) studied John Dean's memory for Watergate and found that in spite of systematic biases, Dean's memory was generally consistent with schematic representations of the events that transpired. List (1986) examined memory for schema-consistent and schema-inconsistent information from filmed shoplifting episodes. She found that for younger adults, schema-inconsistent information tended to be remembered better a few moments after viewing the videotapes, but by the next day, schema-consistent information was better remembered. By contrast, List found that older people remembered schema-consistent information better right from the start. This pattern is consistent with other research in cognitive aging, which suggests that older people are more dependent than are the young on their schematic representations of events (e.g., Hess, 1985; Hess, Donley, & Vandermaas, 1989).

Interestingly, the misleading questions paradigm discussed earlier also has relevance for schema theory, in that schema consistency may predict which misleading questions are most effective. Previous research has suggested that some kinds of questions are more likely to mislead than others (i.e., questions that use *the* rather than *a*) and that some information is more changeable than other information (i.e., minor details) (e.g., Loftus & Greene, 1980). To our knowledge, however, the hypothesis that schema-consistent misleading questions are more likely to produce changes in memory has not been tested. In addition, little is known about the suggestibility of elderly eyewitnesses. If older subjects are more schema dependent and schema consistency is related to suggestibility, then one would expect older persons to be more suggestible than the young. In her dissertation, Adams-Price (1989b) examined the suggestibility of young, middle-age, and older persons to leading and misleading questions. She found no consistent age difference in suggestibility. Some misleading questions had more effect on young subjects, and some had more effect on older subjects. Schema consistency may have something to do with this result.

Conclusions: Practical Versus Theoretical Implications

This chapter has examined some key issues in eyewitness memory that have implications for cognitive aging. One theme has been the relative influence of practical as opposed to theoretical issues. Eyewitness memory research, though clearly of theoretical relevance, often has been designed with concern for practical issues.

Accumulated eyewitness memory research certainly has implications of both theoretical and practical importance. Practically, eyewitness memory research suggests that most individuals do not have a "good memory" or a "poor memory" overall but may be better at different kinds of memory. Some witnesses may be good at recalling details, while others are good at recognizing faces. Still others exude confidence and look good on the witness stand.

Theoretically, eyewitness memory research suggests that recall is a blend of perceptions and knowledge. It also suggests a model for understanding people's limited ability to judge their own memory, the optimality hypothesis, which suggests that the relationship between accuracy and confidence disappears when task difficulty or ambiguity increases. Optimality may be applicable to many late-life memory tasks. To the extent that many memory tasks are less familiar or more ambiguous for older than for younger persons, the ability to assess performance may disappear sooner for the old than for the young. This may result in lower overall confidence and less strategic behavior on a variety of memory tasks.

Future research needs to address both practical and theoretical issues. Given that age declines are found on some eyewitness tasks, it would be useful to know how often older persons engage in memory tasks similar to eyewitness memory: for example, how often are they called in to make identifications or produce oral recall? We need to know more about the special problems faced by aging witnesses: for example, the conditions under which they are prone to be suggestible. Better theoretical formulations of suggestibility and confidence are also needed.

Finally, despite the pessimism of researchers such as Banaji and Crowder (1989), everyday memory research has a clear future. Eyewitness memory research has resulted in at least one new theory, the optimality hypothesis. Cognitive aging researchers would do well to look at eyewitness memory research for ideas and inspiration concerning the investigation of theoretical and practical issues in everyday memory research.

References

Adams-Price, C.E. (1988, October). *Eyewitness memory and aging: Accuracy and confidence in the identification of characters in crime scenes.* Paper presented at the annual meeting of the Gerontological Society of America, San Francisco.

Adams-Price, C.E. (1989a, August). *Eyewitness memory and aging: Predictors of accurate identification of characters seen in crime scenes.* Paper presented at the annual meeting of the American Psychological Association, New Orleans.

Adams-Price, C.E. (1989b). *Eyewitness memory and aging: Recall and recognition of persons and objects in a crime scene.* Unpublished doctoral dissertation, West Virginia University, Morgantown, WV.

Baggett, P. (1979). Structurally equivalent stories in movie and text and the effect of the medium on recall. *Journal of Verbal Learning and Verbal Behavior, 18,* 333–346.

Banaji, M.R., & Crowder, R.G. (1989). The bankruptcy of everyday memory. *American Psychologist, 46,* 1185–1193.

Bartlett, J.C. (1932). *Remembering: A study in experimental and social psychology.* Cambridge, England: Cambridge University Press.

Berry, J.M. (1989). Cognitive efficacy across the life-span: Introduction to the special series. *Developmental Psychology, 25,* 683–686.

Berry, J.M., West, R.L., & Dennehy, D.M. (1989). Reliability and validity of the metamemory self-efficacy questionnaire. *Developmental Psychology, 25,* 701–713.

Bothwell, R.K., Brigham, J.C., & Deffenbacher, K. (1986). Correlation of eyewitness accuracy and confidence: The optimality hypothesis revisited. *Journal of Applied Psychology, 72,* 691–695.

Brown, R., & McNeill, D. (1966). The "tip-of-the-tongue" phenomenon. *Journal of Verbal Learning and Verbal Behavior, 5,* 325–337.

Buckhout, R. (1974). Eyewitness testimony. *Scientific American, 231,* 23–32.

Cavanaugh, J.C. (1983). Comprehension and retention of television programs by 20- and 60-year olds. *Journal of Gerontology, 38,* 190–196.

Cavanaugh, J.C. (1984). Effects of presentation format on adults' retention of television programs. *Experimental Aging Research, 10,* 51–54.

Cavanaugh, J.C. (1989). The importance of awareness in memory aging. In L.W. Poon & D.C. Rubin (Eds.), *Everyday cognition in adulthood and late life* (pp. 416–436). New York: Cambridge University Press.

Christiaansen, R.E., Sweeney, J.D., & Ochalek, K. (1983). Influencing eyewitness descriptions. *Law and Human Behavior, 7,* 59–65.

Cole, W., & Loftus, R. (1979). Incorporating new information into memory. *American Journal of Psychology, 92,* 413–425.

Cutler, B.L., Penrod, S.D., & Martens, S.K. (1987). The reliability of eyewitness identification: The role of system and estimator variables. *Law and Human Behavior, 11,* 233–258.

Deffenbacher, K.A. (1980). Eyewitness accuracy and confidence: Can we infer anything about their relationship? *Law and Human Behavior, 4,* 243–260.

Gentner, D., & Loftus, E. (1979). Integration of visual and verbal information as evidenced by distortions in picture memory. *American Journal of Psychology, 92,* 363–375.

Goodman, G.S. (Ed.). (1984). The child eyewitness [Special issue]. *Journal of Social Issues, 40*(2).

Herrmann, D. (1982). Know thy memory: The use of questionnaires to assess and study memory. *Psychological Bulletin, 92,* 434–452.

Hess, T.M. (1985). Aging and context influences on recognition memory for typical and atypical script actions. *Developmental Psychology, 21,* 1139–1151.

Hess, T.M., Donley, J., & Vandermaas, M.O. (1989). Aging-related changes in the processing and retention of script information. *Experimental Aging Research, 15,* 89–96.

Hultsch, D.F., & Dixon, R.A. (1984). Memory for text materials in adulthood. In P.B. Baltes & O.G. Brim, Jr. (Eds.), *Life-span development and behavior* (Vol. 6, pp. 77–108). New York: Academic Press.

Jenkins, J.J. (1979). Four points to remember: A tetrahedral model of memory experiments. In L.S. Cermak & F.I.M. Craik (Eds.), *Levels in processing in human memory* (pp. 429–446). Hillsdale, NJ: Erlbaum.

Kassin, S. (1985). Eyewitness identification: Retrospective self-awareness and the accuracy-confidence correlation. *Journal of Personality and Social Psychology, 49,* 878–893.

Kintsch, W. (1974). *The representation of meaning in memory.* Hillsdale, NJ: Erlbaum.

Kintsch, W., & van Dijk, T. (1978). Toward a model of text comprehension and production. *Psychological Review, 85,* 363–394.

Labouvie-Vief, G. (1980). Adaptive dimensions of adult cognition. In N. Datan & N. Lohmann (Eds.), *Transitions of aging* (pp. 3–26). New York: Academic Press.

Labouvie-Vief, G., & Schell, D.A. (1982). Learning and memory in later life. In B.B. Wolman (Ed.), *Handbook of developmental psychology* (pp. 828–846). Englewood Cliffs, NJ: Prentice-Hall.

Lachman, J.L., & Lachman, R. (1980). Age and the actualization of world knowledge. In L.W. Poon, J.L. Fozard, L.S. Cermak, D. Arenberg, & L.W. Thompson (Eds.), *New directions in memory and aging* (pp. 285–308). Hillsdale, NJ: Erlbaum.

Lane, M.J. (1984). Eyewitness identification: Should psychologists be permitted in the courtroom? *Journal of Criminal Law and Criminology, 75*, 1321–1365.

Leippe, M.R. (1980). Effects of integrative and memorial cognitive processes on the correspondence between eyewitness accuracy and confidence. *Law and Human Behavior, 4*, 261–274.

List, J. (1986). Age and schematic differences in the reliability of eyewitness testimony. *Developmental Psychology, 22*, 50–57.

Loftus, E.F. (1975). Leading questions and the eyewitness report. *Cognitive Psychology, 7*, 560–572.

Loftus, E.F. (1979). *Eyewitness testimony*. Cambridge, MA: Harvard University Press.

Loftus, E.F. (1983). Silence is not golden. *American Psychologist, 38*, 564–572.

Loftus, E.F., & Greene, E. (1980). Warning: Even memory for faces may be contagious. *Law and Human Behavior, 4*, 323–334.

Loftus, E.F., & Palmer, J.C. (1973). Reconstruction of automobile destruction: An example of the interaction between language and memory. *Journal of Verbal Learning and Verbal Behavior, 13*, 585–589.

Loh, W.D. (1981). Psycholegal research: Past and present. *Michigan Law Review, 79*, 659–707.

Mandler, J.M., & Johnson, N.S. (1977). Remembrance of things parsed: Story structure and recall. *Cognitive Psychology, 9*, 111–151.

Meyer, B.J.F., & Rice, G.E. (1981). Information recalled from prose by young, middle, and old adults. *Experimental Aging Research, 7*, 253–268.

Muensterberg, H. (1908). *On the witness stand: Essays on the psychology of crime*. New York: Clark Boardman.

Neil v. Biggers, 409 U.S. 188 (1972).

Neisser, U. (1981). John Dean's memory: A case study. *Cognition, 9*, 1–22.

O'Rourke, T., Penrod, S., Cutler, B. & Stuve, T. (1989). The external validity of eyewitness identification research across age groups. *Law and Human Behavior, 13*, 385–395.

Perlmutter, M. (1978). What is memory aging the aging of? *Developmental Psychology, 914*, 330–345.

Pigott, M., & Brigham, J. (1985). The relationship between accuracy of prior description and facial recognition. *Journal of Applied Psychology, 70*, 547–555.

Stern, W. (1939). The psychology of testimony. *Journal of Abnormal and Social Psychology, 34*, 3–30.

Taub, H.A. (1979). Comprehension and memory of prose by young and old adults. *Experimental Aging Research, 5*, 3–13.

Wells, G.L., & Leippe, M.R. (1981). How do triers of fact infer the accuracy of eyewitness identifications? Using memory for peripheral detail can be misleading. *Journal of Applied Psychology, 64*, 440–448.

Wells, G.L., & Murray, D.M. (1983). What can psychology say about the *Neil v. Biggers* criteria for judging eyewitness accuracy? *Journal of Applied Psychology, 68*, 347–362.

Whipple, G.M. (1911). The psychology of testimony. *Psychological Bulletin, 8*, 307–309.

Yarmey, A.D. (1985). Accuracy and credibility of the elderly witness. *Canadian Journal on Aging, 3,* 79–89.

Yarmey, A.D., Jones, H.P., & Rashid, S. (1984). Eyewitness memory of elderly and young adults. In D. Mueller, D. Blackman, & A. Chapman (Eds.), *Psychology and Law* (pp. 215–228). Chichester, England: John Wiley.

Yarmey, A.D., & Kent, J. (1980). Eyewitness identification by elderly and young adults. *Law and Human Behavior, 4,* 123–137.

Yuille, J.C., & Cutshall, J.L. (1986). A case study of eyewitness memory of a crime. *Journal of Applied Psychology, 71,* 291–301.

Zelinksi, E.M., Gilewski, M.J., & Thompson, L.W. (1980). Do laboratory tests relate to self-assessment of memory ability in the young and old? In L.W. Poon, J.L. Fozard, L.S. Cermak, D. Arenberg, & L.W. Thompson (Eds.), *New directions in memory and aging* (pp. 519–544). Hillsdale, NJ: Erlbaum.

19
Cooperative Action and Reconstructing the Personal Past as Functions of Autobiographical Remembering

JOHN A. MEACHAM

My intention in this chapter is to initiate a survey of the functions of autobiographical remembering and, on the basis of that survey, to make some recommendations for researchers. One approach to providing such a survey would be to review and acknowledge the contributions of other writers to our understanding of this topic (e.g., Cohler, 1982; Fitzgerald, 1988; Fitzgerald & Lawrence, 1984; Hyland & Ackerman, 1988; Pillemer & White, 1989; Rubin, 1986), attempting to organize their insights into a coherent framework, one that might generate new approaches and insights into the topic. Such an approach, however, is open to the false assumption that what is presently believed about autobiographical remembering should be believed and furthermore that our present beliefs should not be challenged. What is needed, therefore, is to approach the phenomenon of autobiographical remembering from a neutral standpoint outside that of the existing literature.

I have chosen as this neutral standpoint a framework set forth by Habermas (1971). Habermas has set as his goal the construction of a theory of society that is inherently emancipatory, that is, a theory directed toward the securing of freedom from forces of domination. In a powerful critique of the major social science theories of society, Habermas (1971) suggests that human activity can be understood in terms of three fundamental and intrinsically human interests. Employing these three interests as strategies for interpreting our life experiences will direct our attention to the full range of functions of autobiographical remembering.

The Technical Interest

A first of these fundamental interests, according to Habermas (1971), is an interest in predicting and controlling events in the natural environment. The procedures of inquiry that support this interest involve such notions as measurement, control over observations through experimental manipulation, and lawlike statements about the covariance of events, which, together with descriptions of initial conditions, can be taken as predictions about processes and events in the natural environment. This first human interest, which Habermas refers to as the technical interest, unfolds in the medium of work or instrumental action. The science associated with the technical interest is an empirical analytic science.

Investigations of autobiographical remembering, particularly in the past decade, reflect primarily an expression of this technical interest. A glance through the rapidly increasing literature on autobiographical remembering reveals that researchers are concerned with such questions as the incidence, substance, or pattern of autobiographical memories, the veridicality of autobiographical memories—that is, the degree to which these memories correspond with actual environmental events—and the extent to which the organization of autobiographical memories can be modeled, so that researchers will be able to predict their occurrence under a variety of prompting conditions (e.g., Fitzgerald, 1988; Hyland & Ackerman, 1988; Pillemer & White, 1989; Rubin, 1986).

A concrete illustration of the technical interest can be provided by drawing on the results of the following exercise. What four events and dates would one set forth as the most significant in the history of the United States? Constructing such a chronology is similar to what we do when we engage in autobiographical remembering. That is, out of the multitude of diverse events in our lives, we select a few as meaningful and significant, and these few then become the framework around which we construct the narrative of our lives. To facilitate constructing this brief history of the United States, limit the exercise to four dates drawn from the following list:

1776, 1848, 1861 to 1865, 1865, 1914 to 1918, 1920,
1941 to 1945, 1954, 1964, 1965, 1966, 1972

Most readers, certainly those who have been schooled in the United States, will have little difficulty selecting four meaningful and significant dates.

Based on a similar exercise with American university students conducted by Riegel (1973), the most likely set of dates to have been selected is the following: 1776, 1861 to 1865, 1914 to 1918, and 1941 to 1945. In the history of the United States, these dates correspond to the American Revolution, the Civil War, and World Wars I and II. Riegal notes that the view of history as a series of wars does not necessarily describe history as it really happened but instead represents the students' construction of a particular view of the historical past. The example is an apt parallel to what takes place in the course of autobiographical remembering, namely, the selection of memories for recollection in the context of a particular view of one's personal past.

Both historians investigating our societal memory and researchers into autobiographical remembering are likely to raise similar questions, questions that reflect the technical interest in prediction and control: Is the correct date of the American Revolution 1776 and not, perhaps, 1775 or 1787? What are the procedures by which we can strengthen the correspondence between our constructed history and our autobiograpical remembering, on the one hand, and the actual sequence of events in the past, on the other? Given that one date from this group has been recalled, let's say, 1776, what is the likelihood that other dates from the same group will subsequently be recalled? Under what conditions might dates referring not to warfare but to other themes in societal history or in one's personal history, such as the arts, sciences, education, and social progress or education, family, and career, be selected?

The Practical Interest

The second of the three fundamental interests, according to Habermas (1971), is an interest in successful interpersonal relations within which persons strive to establish and maintain an intersubjective understanding—a shared meaning—that can be the foundation for cooperative actions. Habermas has termed this second interest the practical interest, to refer to humans' interest in successful social action, which in turn depends on shared meanings, intentions, values, reasons, and so forth. This second interest reveals itself in the medium of interpersonal communication. The science (the procedures of inquiry) associated with the practical interest is a historical and hermeneutic or interpretive science.

The Interpersonal in Autobiographical Remembering

This second interest, the practical or interpersonal interest, manifests itself in autobiographical remembering in two major respects: How autobiographical remembering serves as the foundation for cooperative action will be discussed in a subsequent section. First, however, I will argue that it is inappropriate to conceive of autobiographical remembering as exclusively auto-remembering or self-remembering. Instead, autobiographical remembering is interpersonal and social not merely in its developmental origins but indeed throughout life. Pillemer and White (1989, pp. 328–331) conclude their review of the recall of childhood events by emphasizing the social construction of personal memory, drawing on the work of Vygotsky as well as contemporary researchers. They point to the 3rd year of life as a time when children must develop an understanding of memory sharing and an awareness of the social functions of remembering, noting that the age at which children begin to engage in conversations with others about their pasts immediately precedes the earliest autobiographical memories for most adults. Even in late adulthood, according to data presented by Marshall (1974), reminiscing takes place within the presence of, and often with the active support and assistance of, other persons.

The strongest argument for the interpersonal basis of autobiographical remembering, however, is methodological: without entering into dialogue with others about my memories, I am unable to determine whether the interpretive framework for my memories is valid. As an isolated individual, I must experience my life course *longitudinally*. The events of the times in which I live and of my own personal life proceed one after another in the same unalterable sequence as the passing moments of my own felt existence. Indeed, the utter synchrony of these events with my experience of them makes it difficult even to describe how the two might be independent. As in any longitudinal research design, there is a confounding of effects attributable to specific historical events associated with the time of observation, on the one hand, and attributable to processes of development and aging, on the other.

Suppose that in comparing my present attitudes with what I recollect these to have been several years previously, I perceive that my attitudes have changed so that I am now more conservative. On the one hand, I might attribute these changes to my immersion within a society that, for a variety of social, economic, and political reasons, has drifted toward the right, carrying me along with it. On the other hand, I might attribute the changes in my attitudes to the maturing of my own personality and outlook on life, as I have become more realistic and grown beyond the idealism of my adolescence and young adulthood. If I remain isolated, I have no hope of disentangling these two potential explanations (time of observation and developmental processes) for the changes in attitude that I find in the autobiographical recollections of my life course.

SAME-AGED FRIENDS

A first step toward disentangling the times through which I have lived from my own psychological development as competing explanations might be to turn to a close friend, likely someone of the same age who has necessarily lived through the same times, and ask whether he or she has observed similar changes in attitude when comparing recollections from earlier in the life course with how he or she feels now. For example, if we were both age 50 in 1990, we might consider how our attitudes have changed as we matured from age 40 to age 50 between 1980 and 1990. This might be a fruitful strategy of inquiry if I discover differences between the attitude changes within my friend and within myself, that is, if my friend has become more liberal while during the same period I have become more conservative. I could then reject the notion that my own change in attitude was merely a reflection of my drifting toward the right along with the rest of society. Instead, I would now lean toward the view that my change in atti-

TABLE 19.1. Age, cohort, and time of measurement.

Cohort	Time of measurement			
	1960	1970	1980	1990
1920	40	50	60	70
1930	30	40	50	60
1940	20	30	40	50
1950	10	20	30	40
1960	0	10	20	30

tude was a consequence of processes intrinsic to my own life-style and personality development. In general, however, this strategy of inquiry is faulty, for as close friends it is likely that the other person and I share many attitudes and assumptions about the life course as well as a similar history of becoming more conservative. If we are both more conservative now than we recollect having been 10 years previously, we cannot, even working together, distinguish the changing times from our changing personalities as possible explanations. Rather than leaving its occurrence to chance, I must build a *difference* into my research design to gain a valid understanding of my autobiographical recollections.

DIFFERENT-AGED FRIENDS

One difference quite easy to take advantage of is that I know people of a variety of ages. Thus, I can vary age in my strategy of inquiry while holding constant the times through which all these people have lived. For example, I might ask a 70-year-old (perhaps my parent) to consider whether he or she has become more conservative or liberal from age 60 to 70 between 1980 and 1990, as well as ask a 30-year-old (perhaps my child) whether he or she has become more conservative or liberal during the same period. Such a strategy indeed conforms to one of the complex research designs employed by developmental psychologists, the *cross-sequential* design (Schaie, 1977) (see Table 19.1). If I find differences in how our attitudes have changed, then I would be inclined to attribute these differences not to the times in which we have lived but to developmental processes occurring uniquely within each of us. If I find similarities in how our attitudes have changed despite our different ages, then I would likely look to the influence of societal changes as an explanation. But I must be cautious in drawing conclusions from such a design, for persons of different ages represent different cohorts (birth years) who have lived through differing lengths of history and sequences of events before the 1980–1990 period in question. I can't know, for example, whether my 70-year-old friend might have become more conservative between ages 40 and 50 (between 1960 and 1970) and subsequently remained conservative. In a cross-sequential design, age effects are confounded with interactions of cohort and time of measurement effects.

DISTANT FRIENDS

An opposite strategy might be to hold age constant but to introduce difference into the research design by making comparisons with persons who have lived through quite different social and historical times. The logic of such a strategy appears sound, but the strategy is likely to be too cumbersome to be of much help in interpretation of everyday autobiographical recollections. For example, in an effort to understand whether my conservativism has come about mainly because of political and economic changes in my society in the 1980s or because of psychological changes in my own development during the same time, I might visit another society in which the direction of political and economic changes has been from conservative to liberal and engage in a comparison of recollections with several 50-year-olds. Or I might go to the library and survey a number of autobiographies and diaries of persons from a wide range of societies and historical periods and consider how their attitudes might have changed in the decade of their 40s. If I find differences in the direction of attitude change, then I could attribute these to differences among the societies and historical periods; if I find similarities, then I could attribute these to a commonality of psychological changes during middle adulthood. This strategy of inquiry would be more successful the greater the range of societies and historical periods that might be compared.

Fortunately, individuals engaged in autobiographical remembering do have as a convenient resource friends of a variety of ages, especially older friends who might be asked to recollect how they felt about the changes they perceived in themselves at earlier ages and in earlier times. For example, as a 50-year-old interested in how I might have changed from age 40 (in 1980) to age 50 (in 1990), I might ask a 70-year-old how to consider how he or she changed from age 40 (in 1960) to age 50 (in 1970). In such a comparison, termed a *cohort-sequential* design, age has been held constant, while differences in time of measurement have been introduced into the research design. If differences are found in how the 70-year-old and I changed during the decade of our 40s, then I would attribute these changes to the influence of the time in which we lived, rather than to some common developmental process. On the other hand, if similarities are found—we both became conservative at this age—then I would attribute this change to a common age-related psychological process. There are, however, some disadvantages with this strategy of inquiry. I cannot be certain that now, in 1990, my 70-year-old friend is recalling feelings and attitudes from ages 40 and 50 as he or she in fact experienced them at that time; my friend is 20 years distant from the feelings that I am experiencing right now. A further disadvantage to this cohort-sequential design is that time of measurement effects are confounded with the interaction of age and cohort.

Many Friends

All of the strategies of inquiry described thus far for providing interpretations of our autobiographical recollections have drawbacks. As these research strategies were described, I implied that each design might be employed on only one occasion. Fortunately, we engage in autobiographical remembering throughout our lives, so that what we as individuals actually do might be thought of as a sequence and repetititon of all the strategies outlined here. When we desire to disentangle social and historical influences from psychological development as possible explanations, we can compare our autobiographical memories with those of other persons who are drawn from a cross-section of ages. This strategy of inquiry corresponds to the time-sequential research design. On each of several occasions, the researcher observes or measures persons representing a cross-section of possible ages. For example, I might at age 30 in 1970 compare my recollections with those of 50-, 40-, and 20-year-olds, at age 40 in 1980 with 60-, 50-, and 30-year-olds; and at age 50 in 1990 with 70-, 60-, and 40-year-olds (see Table 19.1).

This time-sequential design is in fact the design most often used by developmental researchers for avoiding the confounding inherent within the simple longitudinal design of effects attributable to time of measurement with those attributable to psychological development. If I find that my autobiographical recollections differ from those of persons of other ages, then I am inclined to attribute my recollections to my own psychological development; if I find that our recollections are similar, then it becomes more likely that social, economic, and political influences have been at work. In summary, no matter what approaches I might pursue to establish an unambiguous interpretation of autobiographical memories from my personal past, I remain dependent on negotiating the meaning of these recollections with other persons of a broad range of ages and experiences.

Autobiographical Remembering and Cooperative Action

A primary function of autobiographical remembering, quite consistent with the practical or interpersonal interest (Habermas, 1971), is to provide a foundation for interpersonal and cooperative action. Boden and Bielby (1983), for example, provide data showing how strangers draw heavily on autobiographical recollections to establish a shared sense of meaning in anticipation of mutual problem solving. Elsewhere (Meacham, 1982), I have outlined how remembering processes, traditionally construed as intrapersonal, should instead be understood as subplans within superordinate, interpersonal contexts. The latter involve shared expectations and mutual understanding of intentions.

Consider the brief exercise from earlier in this chapter. Many readers might have selected as a meaningful sequence of four dates 1848, 1920, 1966, and 1972. The year 1848 marks the presentation at the Seneca Falls

Convention of the Declaration of Sentiments and Resolutions drafted by Elizabeth Cady Stanton, asserting the equality of women with men and calling for the right of women to vote. In 1920, women won the right to vote when the Nineteenth Amendment to the Constitution was passed. In 1966, the National Organization for Women was founded; 1972 marks the defeat of efforts to pass an Equal Rights Amendment to the Constitution. Each of these dates provides a context for attributing meaning and significance to all the others. This shared historical understanding serves not merely to motivate but also to give meaning to the actions of women as they work together to support various causes. In parallel fashion, the mutual construction of autobiographical memories that are not only appropriate to the personal past of each individual but also understandable among a community of persons provides the essential foundation for cooperative social actions.

The Emancipatory Interest

The third fundamental interest of humans, according to Habermas (1971), is an interest in securing freedom from forces and conditions of distorted communication and oppression along with achievement of an awareness by men and women of their place in history. That humans have this interest, along with the technical and practical interests, stems from their capacity to act rationally and self-consciously so as to change the course of their own history. This third interest, which Habermas has termed the emancipatory interest, unfolds in the medium of power, that is, asymmetrical relations of constraint and dependency. The science associated with the emancipatory interest is critical science, that is, methodical self-reflection.

The emancipatory interest is not merely one of helping people to cope with problems that have devastated their lives, as the profession of clinical psychology might claim to do. Instead, it is an interest in recognizing the impact of social structures and in changing those social structures. The emancipatory interest becomes evident in history when oppressed peoples achieve a conscious understanding that their current status within society has not always been that way. For example, racism comes to be understood not as timeless but as a mere historical construction. In the 1600s blacks enjoyed equal rights with whites, including the right to vote, in many of the areas that were to become the United States; it was not until the early 1700s that legislation creating the structure of racism was enacted (Bennett, 1970; Rothenberg, 1988, p. 179). The emancipatory interest is also evident when people understand that what was done in the past can be undone through the progress of social movements and when people understand that the freedoms that are enjoyed today are not timeless but have been won and must be maintained through hard struggle.

For blacks in the United States, a sequence of four dates expressing an emancipatory interest might include 1865, 1954, 1964, and 1965. The first date marks the passage of the Thirteenth Amendment to the Constitution, abolishing slavery throughout the United States. In 1954 the Supreme Court ruled, in the case of *Brown v. Board of Education,* that separate educational facilities are inherently unequal. But it was not until passage of the Civil Rights Act of 1964 and the Voting Rights Act of 1965 that discrimination in voting, public facilities, schools, courts, and employment was outlawed.

This simple exercise of constructing alternative sequences for a history of the United States illustrates two points relevant to an understanding of autobiographical remembering. First, as researchers, we should lower our expectations regarding the extent to which we will find regularity in the incidence, substance, and pattern of autobiographical remembering. Gender, race, ethnicity, religion, class, and so forth can have marked effects on how a group of people might construct its history—its societal autobiographical memories. And these same categories as well as many others, including our shared experiences as members of families, communities, professions, and so forth, play essential roles in determining the interpretive framework within which we weave the narrative of events and experiences in our personal lives. It will be a challenge for researchers into autobiographical remembering, most of whom represent a white, upper-middle class, educational elite, to recognize and provide an appropriate voice for the autobiographical memories of persons of different backgrounds.

Second, consideration of the emancipatory interest helps to identify an additional function of autobiographical remembering, namely, the freeing of the individual from forces of domination. These forces include not only those imposed from outside but also those constructed earlier in development by the individual himself or herself, for example, identities, outlooks on life, coping styles, and so forth. The emancipatory process for individuals parallels that for oppressed groups at the societal level and entails the achievement of a conscious understanding that one's current developmental plight was not preordained but reflects the outcome of actual events in one's past, that what was done in the past can be undone through continued struggle and personal development, and that the achievements of the present will be lost without continued vigilance and effort to maintain what was won in the past.

In sum, our understanding of autobiographical remembering should include an appreciation of the role that the reinterpretation of personal memories plays in the clinical or therapeutic process (Coleman, 1986; Perrotta & Meacham, 1981–1982). This reconstruction of the personal past can be as dramatic as the rejection of the 1776, 1861 to 1865, 1914 to 1918, and 1941 to 1945 sequence of warfare in favor of either of the other two historical sequences.

Working together with other persons, we have the capacity to find new interpretations for our autobiographical memories. This provides us with the possibility of enriching the events of our present lives as well as anticipating the future with hope and confidence. Erikson's (Erikson, Erikson, & Kivnick, 1986) conception of life review in late adulthood, as well as Cohler (1982) and Freeman (1984), provide elaborations of this theme.

Conclusion

My intention has been to initiate a survey of the functions of autobiographical remembering, using as a tool a framework set forth by Habermas (1971), who suggests that human activity can be understood in terms of three fundamental human interests. Investigations of autobiographical remembering, particularly in the past decade, reflect primarily an expression of the technical interest in maintaining a faithful record of the events and experiences of one's personal past. A comprehensive understanding will require consideration of the extent to which autobiographical remembering is an expression of all three fundamental interests.

The second interest, the practical or interpersonal interest, directs our attention to a primary function of autobiographical remembering, namely, to provide a foundation for *interpersonal or cooperative action*. Autobiographical remembering is not exclusively auto-remembering or self-remembering; it is also interpersonal and social. The strongest argument for the interpersonal basis of autobiographical remembering is methodological: Without entering into dialogue about my memories with other persons of a broad range of ages and experiences, I am unable to determine whether the interpretive framework for my memories is valid. Researchers into autobiographical remembering should investigate the phenomenon not as it occurs in isolated individuals but as an interpersonal and cooperative phenomenon.

The third interest, the emancipatory interest, directs our attention to an additional major function of autobiographical remembering, namely, the freeing of the individual from forces of domination, including identities, outlooks on life, and coping styles that are no longer adaptive for the individual. Pursuing the role that the *reconstruction of the personal past* can play in the clinical or therapeutic process promises to be a significant strategy for researchers into autobiographical remembering.

References

Bennett, L. (1970, August). The making of Black America, Part III. The road not taken. *Ebony, 10,* 71–77.

Boden, D., & Bielby, D.D. (1983). The past as resource: A conversational analysis of elderly talk. *Human Development, 26,* 308–319.

Cohler, B.J. (1982). Personal narrative and life course. In P.B. Baltes & O.G. Brim, Jr. (Eds.), *Life-span development and behavior* (pp. 87–104). New York: Academic Press.

Coleman, P.G. (1986). *Ageing and reminiscence processes: Social and clinical implications.* New York: Wiley.

Erikson, E.H., Erikson, J.M., & Kivnick, H.Q. (1986). *Vital involvement in old age.* New York: W.W. Norton.

Fitzgerald, J.M. (1988). Vivid memories and the reminiscence phenomenon. *Human Development, 31,* 261–270.

Fitzgerald, J.M., & Lawrence, R. (1984). Autobiographical memory across the life span. *Journal of Gerontology, 39,* 692–698.

Freeman, M. (1984). History, narrative, and life-span developmental knowledge. *Human Development, 27,* 1–19.

Habermas, J. (1971). *Knowledge and human interests.* Boston: Beacon Press.

Hyland, D.T., & Ackerman, A.M. (1988). Reminiscence and autobiographical memory in the study of the personal past. *Journal of Gerontology, 43,* P35–39.

Marshall, V.S. (1974, October). *The life review as a social process.* Paper presented at the meeting of the Gerontological Society, Portland, OR.

Meacham, J.A. (1982). A note on remembering to execute planned actions. *Journal of Applied Developmental Psychology, 3,* 121–133.

Perrotta, P., & Meacham, J.A. (1981–1982). Can a reminiscing intervention alter depression and self-esteem? *International Journal of Aging and Human Development, 14,* 23–30.

Pillemer, D.B., & White, S.H. (1989). Childhood events recalled by children and adults. In H.W. Reese (Ed.), *Advances in child development and behavior* (Vol. 21, pp. 167–189). New York: Academic Press.

Riegel, K.F. (1973).The recall of historical events. *Behavioral Science, 18,* 354–363.

Rothenberg, P.S. (1988). How it happened: The legal status of women and people of color in the United States. In P.S. Rothenberg (Ed.), *Racism and sexism: An integrated study* (pp. 177–184). New York: St. Martin's Press.

Rubin, D.C. (Ed.). (1986). *Autobiographical memory.* Cambridge England: Cambridge University Press.

Schaie, K.W. (1977). Quasi-experimental research designs in the psychology of aging. In J.E. Birren & K.W. Schaie (Eds.), *Handbook of the psychology of aging* (pp. 39–58). New York: Van Nostrand Reinhold.

20
Individual Differences in Everyday Memory Aging: Implications for Theory and Research

Deborah G. Ventis

There is a wicked inclination in most people to suppose an old man decayed in his intellects. If a young or middle-aged man, when leaving a company, does not recollect where he laid his hat, it is nothing; but if the same inattention is discovered in an old man, people will shrug up their shoulders, and say, 'His memory is going.'

Samuel Johnson

As an observer of everyday memory more than two centuries ago, Samuel Johnson recognized the folly of assuming that memory lapses reflect age-related declines. Such lapses may reflect stable individual differences (i.e., being more likely than others to forget things, regardless of your age), or accepting stereotypes concerning aging (a self-fulfilling prophecy that as you age you are more likely to forget things), rather than inevitable deterioration. Even when such forgetting is associated with age-related decline, it is clear that such changes occur in different individuals at different rates (see Krauss, 1980; Welford, 1985). Thus, the study of individual differences is crucial to our understanding of everyday memory aging.

Despite greater attention to individual variability by researchers of everyday memory (Cohen, 1989) and a growing emphasis on such differences by reviewers of research on memory aging (Hultsch & Dixon, 1990; Poon, 1985) there is still little research on individual performance differences on everyday tasks. The purpose of the present chapter is to review the available literature and discuss the implications of the study of individual differences for everyday memory aging.

Interindividual variation plays an important role in theoretical approaches to everyday memory aging, but much more research is needed. Although Hertzog (1985) emphasized the need for longitudinal research and the construction of structural equation models to examine individual differences in cognitive aging, Perlmutter (1988) notes that memory researchers treat both stable individual differences and transient states as error.

Another obstacle is the difficulty of measuring individual differences in everyday memory. Weinert, Schneider, and Knopf (1988), for example, observe that conclusions that greater interindividual variability occurs with age are affected by both the representativeness of the age samples and the nature of the tasks employed.

A brief overview of relevant theoretical models provides a framework for discussing individual differences in everyday memory aging. These models suggest that relationships among individual characteristics, task variables, and environmental variables are all important in understanding such differences and that perceived as well as actual differences must be considered.

Models of Everyday Memory Aging

Information Processing Models

Information-processing models of cognitive aging incorporate both individual variation and experiential factors as important components in explaining how cognitive abilities change with age. Two approaches to the study of expertise by Hoyer (1985) and Charness (1989) illustrate the usefulness of such models for an understanding of individual differences in everyday memory aging. Hoyer (1985) emphasizes the importance of both the efficiency of elementary information processing skills and the efficiency of the coordination of these elementary skills to understanding individual performance differences. Charness (1989) notes that, from an information processing perspective, both "hardware" (relatively invariant cognitive structures) and "software" (acquired experience) are possible sources of individual variation. He concludes that combining research on two individual difference variables—expertise and aging—will provide a better understanding of such differences than either alone.

Contextual Models

Contextual models of everyday memory aging emphasize the interaction between the individual and the social context in understanding both the direction and size of age differences (see Poon, 1985). Two such contextual theories relevant to the study of everyday memory aging are Perlmutter's (1988) model of memory development and Cavanaugh, Morton, and Tilse's (1989) model of everyday memory aging.

Perlmutter emphasizes that individual differences, transient subject states, and environmental context are all important components of memory. She speculates that generalizing across any of these variables may be as inadvisable as it is to generalize across levels of development.

Cavanaugh et al. (1989) stress developmental changes in self-evaluation. They suggest that the elderly may be more likely to have negative self-evaluations of their memories, in large part because of social stereotypes of inevitable decline in memory with age. Although they don't emphasize individual differences in self-evaluation, such differences may be an important variable in self-reports of memory.

Research on Individual Differences

Are some people more likely than others to experience age-related memory problems? Does such variability exist in both perceived and actual memory aging? What task and environmental factors influence such differences? Although memory researchers have paid relatively little attention to individual differences, the study of self-reported memory and of age-related slowing provide two examples of the importance of such differences in understanding everyday memory aging. Each illustrates the role of individual variation and problems with measuring this variation, as well as the important interrelationships among individual differences, task variables, and environmental variables.

Self-Reported Memory

Self-reports of memory performance are considered an important component of metamemory, and Johnson's example of forgetting the whereabouts of one's hat represents only one type of memory in which individuals report differences. Sehulster (1988) identifies three memory factors on which people perceive they differ in ability: memory for verbal material (names and other facts, jokes, trivia), memory for autobiographical and experiential material (childhood experiences, dreams, music, smells, etc.), and prospective memory (dates, whereabouts of personal items, e.g., one's hat).

Individuals may report high (H) or low (L) ability levels on any or all of these three factors, producing eight possible memory styles (HHH, HHL, HLH, HLL, LLL, LLH, LHL, LHH; see Sehulster, 1988, for a more detailed discussion of these). Although these styles have not been studied with respect to age-related changes, they obviously represent individual variation in self-evaluation. Given Sehulster's (1988) assertion that these self-reported memory styles are related to memory performance, age-related changes in memory style could be one mechanism through which negative stereotypes concerning memory aging are incorporated into the self-evaluations that Cavanaugh et al. (1989) suggest are so important. Although Hultsch, Hertzog, and Dixon's (1984) differential decline hypothesis, that ability interacts with age in producing declines in memory performance, has received little support (see Hultsch & Dixon, 1990), it is possible that age-related declines correlate with changes in self-assessment. If this is the case, longitudinal data are needed to see if changes in self-report precede or follow changes in performance.

MEASUREMENT ISSUES

It is not surprising that problems in the measurement of self-reported memory are receiving increasing attention. Cavanaugh et al. (1989) admit that because there is no objective way to assess the accuracy of self-evaluations, it may be difficult to study differences in self-assessments of memory.

In this vein, Nelson (1988) discusses the need for a procedure to yield stable individual differences in feeling of knowing, not only for research purposes but for diagnosis and intervention. He suggests the use of many more items than typically tested and the design of "standardized" meta-cognitive tasks as possible innovations. The development of new techniques like the Memory Self-Efficacy Questionnaire (Berry, West, & Dennehey, 1989), which separates self-ratings of skill from confidence levels, should be helpful in understanding the role of both developmental and interindividual variation in self-efficacy in everyday memory aging.

Measurement of self-reported decline in memory with age (as contrasted with stable differences in memory style) is also complicated by the fact that perceived age-related declines may be directly associated with pathology. Although a full discussion of pathological conditions associated with memory is beyond the scope of this chapter, it is noteworthy that Cutler and Grams (1988) found only 15% of their 55-year-old and over sample reported frequent trouble remembering things. Most often, such perceived difficulties were associated with increasing age and health problems; the authors speculate that psychological problems such as depression may be even more important than physical conditions in affecting self-reported memory. Indeed, Prescott (1990) found depression to be a better predictor of self-reported memory than either subjective or objective indicators of health status.

TASK AND ENVIRONMENTAL VARIABLES

Research on control beliefs illustrates the potential importance of task variables in understanding individual differences in self-reports of everyday memory performance. For example, Lachman, Steinberg, and Trotter (1987) concluded that control beliefs may influence some types of memory ability more than others after finding such beliefs only marginally related to memory performance on a task using shopping lists. In contrast, Dixon and Hultsch (1983), in a study of prose recall, concluded that age differences in control beliefs (such that older adults perceive less personal control over memory than younger people) were one of the best predictors of performance.

Although even less is known about how individual differences in control beliefs are related to task variables, such differences may provide an alternative explanation for the discrepant findings concerning the relationship between control beliefs and actual performance. In fact, Devolder, Brigham, and Pressley (1990) argue that the vast differences in affect, habit, and motivational beliefs found within age groups in their study of memory monitoring suggest that "more may be learned about adult meta-cognition and cognition by studying individual monitoring differences within ages and between tasks than by additional research on age differences per se" (p. 302).

The importance of considering environmental characteristics is highlighted by Abson and Rabbitt's (1988) assertion that self-ratings of cognitive efficiency can be made only by comparing one's competence to the performance of others or evaluating one's success in meeting daily demands. Changing environmental demands, therefore, should create changing self-ratings; individual differences in responsiveness to environmental demands as well as in the pattern of environmental changes experienced, will, similarly, affect self-ratings.

Age-Related Slowing

In contrast to self-reports that may or may not accurately reflect memory performance, everyday memory changes attributed to age-related slowing represent measurable performance declines. Salthouse (1985) estimates that older adults' reaction times are as much as twice as long as those of young adults.

Hertzog, Raskind, and Cannon (1986) speculate that individual differences in age-related slowing may account for age differences in information retrieval in semantic memory. Indeed, Hartley (1988) reports that individual differences, including speed measures, do become better predictors of memory for text performance as age increases. Rabbitt (1988), however, criticizes single-factor models of individual differences in memory based on information processing rate as too simplistic and emphasizes the need to consider social and experiential factors. As Schaie (1988) notes, there are probably few non-laboratory situations where such slowing actually interferes with functioning; he emphasizes the importance of individual differences in gauging the effects of any age-related behavior change.

Knopf, Körkel, Schneider, and Weinert's (1988) finding that even small amounts of prior knowledge were sufficient to produce significant increases in older people's prose recall suggests the importance of interindividual variation in expertise in moderating the effects of slowing. Similarly, Weinert, Schneider, and Knopf (1988) conclude that Knopf's (1987) finding that elderly persons with domain-specific knowledge performed significantly better than novices on memory tasks affirms that expertise is important in maintaining stability of memory performance with age. Thus, as information processing theorists predict, elderly individuals using an elaborated knowledge base can compensate for age-related declines such as slowing.

As in the example of self-reported memory, measurement problems as well as the role of task and environmental variables must be considered in assessing the importance of individual differences in age-related slowing to everyday memory aging.

MEASUREMENT ISSUES

Hultsch, Hertzog, and Dixon's (1990) finding that individual differences related to speed and working memory substantially account for age differences in memory performance on text and word recall undoubtedly has implications for everyday tasks as well. They stress that understanding age differences in memory performance on complex tasks requires measuring individual differences in resource abilities such as speed, preferably using longitudinal methods.

Methodological advances in neurophysiological techniques may also enhance our understanding of the role of individual differences in age-related memory declines such as slowing. For example, Gold's (1990) finding that individual differences in glucose tolerance are related to memory performance suggests that blood glucose tolerance tests may be useful in identifying which elderly have age-related memory loss. Although interindividual variations in glucose tolerance apparently affect memory storage rather than speed, Cerella (1990) argued that age-related slowing is more parsimoniously explained by central nervous system changes such as axonal degeneration and attenuation than by psychological task variables. If slowing is best explained by such changes, methodological advances in neurophysiology should be helpful in understanding individual differences.

TASK AND ENVIRONMENTAL VARIABLES

Individual differences in everyday memory aging are likely to be exaggerated by the extent that tasks increase in the need for self-initiated activities and/or decrease in the amount of environmental support (Craik, 1983). Ratner, Schell, Crimmins, Mittelman, and Baldinelli (1987) suggest that memory decline may be due to cognitive demands as much as to biological deterioration (such as slowing). In their study of prose recall, they found that noncollege young people perform very much like the elderly. Memory is adversely affected when organization is not provided by the learner; when this is the case, characteristics of the material to be remembered influence performance more heavily.

Although Weinert et al. (1988) assume that task characteristics contribute to variability in elderly individuals' memory performance (e.g., tasks requiring greater use of strategies are assumed to produce larger individual differences than tasks requiring less strategy use), Dempster's (1981) hypothesis that individual differences are better explained by nonstrategic factors—like speed of stimulus identification—is endorsed by Knopf et al. (1988), who found higher intraindividual consistency across memory tasks in old age. With respect to environmental influences, Bahrick (1984) notes that even if individuals excel in laboratory settings because of superior abilities, in the real world, social and motivational variables become more important.

Conclusion

Reviewing the literature on self-reported memory and age-related slowing from an individual differences perspective confirms that individual variation may be as important as age changes in understanding everyday memory aging. Recognizing the importance of individual differences may be a corollary of the proposition that "difference" is a better descriptor of cognitive aging than "deficit" (see Ventis, 1989 for a brief review of the deficit vs. difference distinction). Just as Schaie (1988) notes with respect to cognitive aging, generally, apparent age-related deficits in everyday memory may reflect individual differences rather than universal declines.

Whether or not such interindividual variations are the result of stable characteristics, the accumulation of different experiences across the life span, or age-related changes, they deserve greater attention in theoretical perspectives on everyday memory aging. They have important implications for intervention, as well. Given that many elderly individuals have overly negative self-efficacy beliefs, Hertzog, Hultsch, and Dixon (1989) endorse Zarit's (1982) suggestion that improving memory self-efficacy may be a worthwhile target of intervention, even if actual performance is not affected. Similarly, Cavanaugh et al. (1989) conclude that retraining individual's self-evaluations is more advantageous than training memory skills. There is evidence (Bergquist, Duke, & Davis, 1989), too, that providing a conceptual framework for understanding everyday memory problems and having elderly persons individualize their own interventions improves both memory performance and self-efficacy.

Returning to Samuel Johnson's example, we can conclude that older people are not *necessarily* more likely than younger ones to forget the whereabouts of their hats; if they do, individual differences may be very important in understanding why.

References

Abson, V., & Rabbitt, P. (1988). What do self-rating questionnaires tell us about changes in competence in old age?. In M.M. Gruneberg, P.E. Morris, & R.N. Sykes (Eds.), *Practical aspects of memory: Current research and issues: Vol. 2. Clinical and educational implications* (pp. 186–191). New York: Wiley.

Bahrick, H.P. (1984). Memory for people. In J.E. Harris & P.E. Morris (Eds.), *Everyday memory, actions and absent-mindedness* (pp. 19–34). New York: Academic Press.

Bergquist, T.F., Duke, L.W., & Davis, G. (1989, November) *Cognitive/behavioral interventions for age-related memory decline.* Paper presented at the meeting of the Gerontological Society of America, Minneapolis, MN.

Berry, J.M., West, R.L., & Dennehey, D.M. (1989). Reliability and validity of the Memory Self-Efficacy Questionnaire. *Developmental Psychology, 25,* 701–713.

Cavanaugh, J.C., Morton, K.R. & Tilse, C.S. (1989). A self-evaluation framework for understanding everyday memory aging. In J.D. Sinnott (Eds.), *Everyday problem solving: Theory and applications* (pp. 266–284). New York: Praeger.

Cerella, J. (1990). Aging and information-processing rate. In J.E. Birren & K.W. Schaie (Eds.), *Handbook of the psychology of aging* (3rd ed., pp. 201–221). San Diego: Academic Press.

Charness, N. (1989) Age and expertise: Responding to Talland's challenge. In L.W. Poon, D.C. Rubin, & B.C. Wilson (Eds.), *Everyday cognition in adulthood and late life* (pp. 437–456). New York: Cambridge University Press.

Cohen, G. (1989). *Memory in the real world.* Hillsdale, NJ: Erlbaum.

Craik, F.I.M. (1983). On the transfer of information from temporary to permanent storage. *Philosophical Transactions of the Royal Society of London, Series B, 302,* 341–359.

Cutler, S.J., & Grams, A.E. (1988). Correlates of self-reported everyday memory problems. *Journal of Gerontology: Social Sciences, 43,* S82–90.

Dempster, F.N. (1981). Memory span: Sources of individual and developmental differences. *Psychological Bulletin, 89,* 63–100.

Devolder, P.A., Brigham, M.C., & Pressley, M. (1990). Memory performance awareness in younger and older adults. *Psychology and Aging, 4,* 291–303.

Dixon, R.A., & Hultsch, D.F. (1983). Metamemory and memory for text relationships in adulthood: A cross-validation study. *Journal of Gerontology, 38,* 689–694.

Gold, P. (1990, June). *Regulation of memory storage in animals and humans: Implications for aging research.* Invited address, Second Annual Convention of the American Psychological Society, Dallas, TX.

Hartley, J.T. (1988). Aging and individual differences in memory for written discourse. In L.L. Light & D.M. Burke (Eds.), *Language, memory, and aging* (pp. 36–57). New York: Cambridge University Press.

Hertzog, C. (1985). An individual differences perspective: Implications for cognitive research in gerontology. *Research on Aging, 7,* 7–45.

Hertzog, C., Hultsch, D.F., & Dixon, R.A. (1989). Evidence for the convergent validity of two self-report metamemory questionnaires. *Developmental Psychology, 25,* 687–700.

Hertzog, C., Raskind, C.L., & Cannon, C.J. (1986). Age-related slowing in semantic information processing speed: An individual differences analysis. *Journal of Gerontology, 41,* 500–502.

Hoyer, W. (1985). Aging and the development of expert cognition. In T.M. Schlechter & M.P. Toglia (Eds.), *New directions in cognitive science* (pp. 69–87). Norwood, NJ: Ablex.

Hultsch, D.F., & Dixon, R.A. (1990). Learning and memory in aging. In J.E. Birren & K.W. Schaie (Eds.), *Handbook of the psychology of aging* (3rd ed., pp. 258–274). San Diego: Academic Press.

Hultsch, D.F., Hertzog, C., & Dixon, R.A. (1990). Ability correlates of memory performance in adulthood and aging. *Psychology and Aging, 5,* 356–358.

Hultsch, D.F., Hertzog, C., & Dixon, R.A. (1984). Text recall in adulthood: The role of intellectual abilities. *Developmental Psychology, 20,* 1193–1211.

Knopf, M. (1987). *Gedächtnis im Alter*. Berlin, Heidelberg, New York: Springer-Verlag.

Knopf, M., Körkel, J., Schneider, W., & Weinert, F.E. (1988). Human memory as a faculty versus human memory as a set of specific abilities: Evidence from a life-span approach. In F.E. Weinert & M. Perlmutter (Eds.), *Memory development: Universal changes and individual differences* (pp. 331–352). Hillsdale, NJ: Erlbaum.

Krauss, I.K. (1980). Between- and within-group comparison in aging research. In L.W. Poon (Ed.), *Aging in the 1980s: Psychological issues* (pp. 542–551). Washington, DC: American Psychological Association.

Lachman, M., Steinberg, E., & Trotter, S. (1987). Effects of control beliefs and attributions on memory self-assessments and performance. *Psychology and Aging, 2*, 266–271.

Nelson, T.O. (1988). Predictive accuracy of feeling of knowing across different criterion tasks and across different subject populations and individuals. In M.M. Gruneberg, P.E. Morris, & R.N. Sykes (Eds.), *Practical aspects of memory: Current research and issues: Vol. 1. Memory in everyday life* (pp. 190–196). New York: Wiley.

Perlmutter, M. (1988). Research on memory: Past, present, and future. In F.E. Weinert & M. Perlmutter (Eds.), *Memory development: Universal changes and individual differences* (pp. 353–380). Hillsdale, NJ: Erlbaum.

Poon, L.W. (1985). Differences in human memory with aging: Nature, causes, and clinical implications. In J.E. Birren & K.W. Schaie (Eds.), *Handbook of the psychology of aging* (2nd ed., pp. 427–462). New York: Van Nostrand Reinhold.

Prescott, C. (1990, April). *Self-reported memory as a function of clinical vs. everyday memory tasks*. Poster presented at the 12th West Virginia University Conference on Life-Span Developmental Psychology: Mechanisms of Everyday Cognition, Morgantown, WV.

Rabbitt, P. (1988). Does fast last? Is speed a basic factor determining individual differences in memory? In M.M. Gruneberg, P.E. Morris, & R.N. Sykes (Eds.), *Practical aspects of memory: Current research and issues: Vol. 2. Clinical and educational implications* (pp. 161–168). New York: Wiley.

Ratner, H.H., Schell, D.A., Crimmins, A., Mittelman, D., & Baldinelli, L. (1987). Changes in adults' prose recall: Aging or cognitive demands? *Developmental Psychology, 23*, 521–525.

Salthouse, T.A. (1985). Speed of behavior and its implications for cognition. In J.E. Birren & K.W. Schaie (Eds.), *Handbook of the psychology of aging* (2nd ed., pp. 400–426). New York: Van Nostrand Reinhold.

Schaie, K.W. (1988). Ageism in psychological research. *American Psychologist, 43*, 179–183.

Sehulster, J.B. (1988). Broader perspectives on everyday memory. In M.M. Gruneberg, P.E. Morris, & R.N. Sykes (Eds.), *Practical aspects of memory: Current research and issues: Vol. 1. Memory in everyday life* (pp. 323–328). New York: Wiley.

Ventis, D.G. (1989). Cognitive intervention: A review and implications for everyday problem solving. In J.D. Sinnott (Ed.), *Everyday Problem solving: Theory and applications* (pp. 285–299). New York: Praeger.

Weinert, F.E., Schneider, W., & Knopf, M. (1988). Individual differences in memory development across the life span. In P.B. Baltes, D.L. Featherman, & R.M.

Lerner (Eds.), *Life-span development and behavior* (pp. 40–86). Hillsdale, NJ: Erlbaum.

Welford, A.T. (1985). *Aging and human skill.* Oxford, England: Oxford University Press.

Zarit, S.H. (1982). Affective correlates of self-reports about memory of older people. *International Journal of Behavioral Geriatrics, 1,* 25–34.

Author Index

Abelson, R.F., 40, 42, 46–50, 52, 88–89, 94
Aberdeen, J.S., 105, 109
Abson, V., 9, 274
Ackerman, A.M., 259–260
Adams, C., 125–126, 129, 134–135
Adams-Price, C.E., x, 249–252, 254
Albert, M.O., 138
Alexander, R.A., 241
Allen, G.L., 67
Altman, I., 210, 212
Anderson, J.R., 97
Anderson, P.A., 40–42, 44–47, 51, 89–90, 95, 105
Andres, D., 140
Ansley, J., 177
Arbuckle, T., 140
Arlin, P., 124
Armon, C., 124
Arnold, D., 113
Atkinson, R.C., 239
Ausubel, D., 177
Awad, Z.A., 211

Backman, L., 241
Baddeley, A.D., 7, 104, 239
Baggett, P., 253
Bahrick, H.P., 5, 216, 275
Baker, C., 103
Baldinelli, L., 275
Baltes, P.B., 40, 51, 183–184, 186, 190, 194
Banaji, M.R., x, 6–7, 246, 255

Barclay, C.R., 29–30
Barker, R.C., 205
Baroni, M., 67
Barrett, G.V., 241
Bartlett, J.C., 247
Bartolucci, G., 103, 140
Bartus, R.T., 54–55
Bass, E., 231
Bayles, K.A., 138, 140
Becker, J., 159
Belbin, E., 174
Belbin, R.M., 174
Belmore, S., 113
Bennett, L., 266
Benton, A.L., 74–75
Berg, C.A., viii, 39, 42, 44, 46, 48, 51–52, 97–98
Berg, L., 202
Bergen, J.R., 219
Bergquist, T.F., 276
Bernard, R.M., 177
Berry, J.M., 4, 6, 11, 250, 273
Bielby, D.D., 265
Bieman-Copland, S., 40
Binet, A., 246
Birren, J.E., 51, 125, 174, 238
Bjork, R.A., 124–125, 162–165, 184
Black, J.B., 46
Blanchard-Fields, F., 227
Blaney, P., 224–226, 230
Blanken, G., 140
Boden, D., 265
Boise, S.J., 236
Boker, J.R., 177

Bolton, C.R., 174, 176
Boone, D.R., 138
Boring, E.G., 219
Bosman, E., 177–179
Boswell, D.A., 126
Bothwell, R.K., 250
Botwinick, J., 6, 175–176, 216, 225, 229
Bower, G.H., 6, 46, 224–226, 230
Breedin, S.D., 105
Brewer, M.B., 88
Brigham, J.C., 250, 252
Brigham, M.C., 273
Bronfenbrenner, U., 17
Brookfield, S., 175–176
Brown, A.L., 129
Brown, E.R., 54
Brown, L.T., 201
Brown, R., 249
Bruce, D., v
Bruce, P.R., 15, 69–70, 210
Bruce, V., 219
Bruning, R., 177
Bryant, K.J., 70
Buckhout, R., 247, 252
Bulka, D., 125, 227
Burke, D.M., ix, 4–5, 7, 27, 113, 140,
   148
Burkey, F.T., 175
Buschke, H., 56–57
Butters, N., 155–156, 158–159
Butterworth, B., 102, 115, 118
Byrd, M., 240

Camp, C.J., ix, 161, 164–170, 183–185
Campbell, S.O., 125
Cannito, M.P., 140
Cannon, C.J., 274
Caplan, D., 103
Caporael, L.R., 103, 116, 149
Carp, A., 23, 25
Carp, R.M., 23, 25
Carpenter, P.A., 104
Caspi, A., 190
Cavanaugh, J.C., 22, 25–26, 67,
   250–251, 253, 271–273, 276
Ceci, S.J., 17, 48, 87
Cerella, J., 237, 275
Cermak, L.S., 242
Chaffin, R., 4, 9

Chap, R.R., 206
Charles, D.C., 173
Charness, N., 8, 19, 40, 68–69,
   177–179, 216, 238, 271
Chase, W.G., 88
Cherry, K.E., 8, 15
Cheung, H., 141, 145, 150
Chi, M., 48
Chi, M.T.H., 87–88
Chiese, H.L., 87
Chinen, A.B., 127–128
Chomsky, N., 115
Christiaansen, R.E., 252
Clancy, S.M., 215, 217, 219
Clark, H.H., 114
Clark, T., 55
Cockburn, J., 7
Cohen, D., 203
Cohen, G., 116, 118, 216, 223, 228,
   231, 270
Cohen, G.D., 54
Cohen, S.H., 3, 17
Cohler, B.J., 259, 268
Colby, A., 135
Cole, J., 128
Cole, K.D., 184
Cole, W., 247
Coleman, P.G., 267
Collin, C., 7
Commons, M.L., 124
Cooper, W.E., 116
Corkin, S., 157
Cornelius, S., 190
Costa, P.T., 232
Coupland, J., 140
Coupland, N., 140
Craik, F.I.M., 101, 104, 156, 162, 237,
   240, 275
Cranton, P.A., 174, 176
Crimmins, A., 275
Cronbach, A., 144
Crook, T.H., viii, 4–7, 9–10, 15, 54–62,
   183
Cross, K.P., 174
Crowder, R.G., v, 6–7, 246, 255
Culbertson, G.H., 103, 116
Cullum, C.M., 155–156
Cunningham, W.R., 54–55
Curtiss, S., 138

Cutler, B.L., 249, 251–252
Cutler, S.J., 273
Cutshall, J.L., 252

Daneman, M., 104
Dark, V.J., 236
Darwin, C., 22
Daubman, R.A., 225
Davies, D.R., 236
Davis, G., 276
Davis, L., 231
Davison, M.L., 124
De Cooke, P.A., 29–31
Deffenbacher, K.A., 250
DeLange, N., 70
Delis, D.C., 54
Dempster, F.N., 275
Denman, S.B., 54
Dennely, D.M., 4, 250, 273
Denney, N.W., 125, 134
De Voe, M., 125, 227
Devolder, P.A., 273
DeWit, G.A., 125
Diaz, D.L., 13
Diefenderfer, K., 177
Dittman, J., 140
Dittmann-Kohli, F., 40
Dixon, R.A., 4, 40, 104, 108, 134, 216, 253, 270, 272–273, 275–276
Doll, L.S., 177–178
Donley, J., 47, 88, 98, 254
Dooling, D.J., 87
Dorosz, M., 125
Doussard-Roosevelt, J.A., 219, 236–237
Dudley, W.N., 3
Duffy, M., 4
Duke, L.W., 276
Duncan, J., 218

Ebbinghaus, H., 22–23, 28
Elias, J.W., x, 226–229
Elias, M.F., 228
Elias, P.A., 228
Ellis, H.C., 225
Erber, J.T., 4, 225, 229, 230
Erickson, R.C., 54–55, 184

Ericsson, K.A., 197
Erikson, E.H., 36, 268
Erikson, J.M., 268
Evankovich, K.D., 160, 183
Evans, G.W., 67, 201, 210
Every, O., 140
Eysenck, M., 225

Faraday, M., 25, 27–28
Farah, M.J., 218–219
Farkas, M.S., 219
Faulkner, D., 109, 116, 118
Feltovich, P.J., 88
Ferguson, 250
Ferris, S.H., 6, 54–55
Fisher, 95
Fisk, A.D., 238, 240
Fitzgerald, J.M., 259–260
Fivush, R., 40–41, 47, 50, 88
Flavell, J.H., 224
Fleiss, J.L., 131
Fleming, S., 140
Flicker, C., 54–55
Flores D'Arcais, G.B., 102
Fodor, J.A., 114, 140, 150
Foulke, E., 106
Fozard, J.L., ix, 184
Francis, D.E., 55
Freed, 157
Freeman, M., 268
Friedman, L., 183
Fry, E., 128
Furby, 144

Gabriel-Byrne, J., 237
Gallie, K., 241
Garfield, J.L., 140
Gaylord, S.A., 202
Geers, A.E., 116
Gelade, G., 220
Gentner, D., 247
Georgemiller, R., 68–69
Gershon, S., 54
Giambra, L., 238
Gibbs, J., 135
Giles, H., 103, 140
Gilewski, M.J., 4, 250

Gilligan, S., 226
Glaser, R., 88
Glisky, E.L., 159–162
Glover, J., 177
Gobert, J., 55, 61
Gold, D., 140
Gold, P., 275
Gollin, E.S., 15–16
Goodglass, H., 109
Goodman, G.S., 248
Gormican, S., 220
Gott, S.P., 4
Grady, J.G., 25
Graesser, A.C., 98
Graf, P., 156, 241
Graham, G., 178
Grams, A.E., 273
Granholm, E., 155
Green, G.M., 150
Greene, E., 254
Greenwald, A.G., 31
Grodzinsky, Y., 102
Grosjean, F., 102, 108–109, 112, 116
Growdon, 157
Gruendel, J., 41–44, 46–47, 88
Gruneberg, M.M., 3
Guider, R.L., 184

Habermas, J., 259–261, 265–266, 268
Hakim-Larson, J., 124
Hanesian, H., 177
Hanis, J.E., 238
Harker, J., 67
Harkins, S.W., 103, 156
Hart, K.C., 177
Hart, R.P., 156, 158
Hartley, J.T., 67, 274
Hasher, L., 68, 73, 149, 239–240
Hass, J.C., 140
Hassan, F., 68–69
Havighurst, R., 50
Haviland, J.M., 32–35
Haviland, S.E., 114
Hayashi, M.M., 140
Hayslip, B., x, 176, 178, 190, 194, 196, 225
Hazelrigg, M.D., 70
Hedrick, D.L., 140

Heindel, W., 155–156, 158–159
Heisey, J.G., 113
Hemsley, D.R., 161
Henwood, K., 103, 140
Herman, J.F., 15, 69–70, 210
Herman, T.G., 225, 229
Herrmann, D.J., 4, 9, 25, 249
Hertzog, C., viii, 4, 29–30, 202, 270, 272, 274–276
Hess, T., 41, 47
Hess, T.M., ix, 88–90, 123, 254
Hicks, B., 179
Hill, G.W., 8
Hill, R.D., 160, 182–186
Hirtle, S.C., 70
Hitch, G., 239
Hobart, C., 125
Hood, J., 68
Hoot, J.L., 178
Howard, D.V., ix, 113
Howieson, D., 54, 184
Hoyer, W.J., x, 98, 190, 197, 215, 217, 219, 237–238, 271
Hoyt, M.J., 140
Hudson, J., 40, 47
Huff, C., 157
Hulicka, I.M., 25
Hultsch, D.F., 4, 67, 69, 104, 108, 134, 216, 253, 270, 272–273, 275–276
Humphreys, G.W., 218–219
Hunt, E., 202
Hunt, R.R., 101
Hutchinson, K.M., 109
Hyams, N.M., 141
Hyland, D.T., 259–260

Ingram, 226
Isen, A.M., 225
Izard, C., 33

Jackson, C., 138
Jacobs, R., 186
James, W., 30–31, 236, 239–240
Jankovic, I.N., 70
Jastak, J., 127, 131
Jastak, S., 127, 131

Jaycock, K., 179
Jenkins, J.J., 11, 246
Jepson, K.L., ix, 150
Job, R., 67
Johnson, N.S., 253
Johnson, R.E., 129
Johnson, S., 270, 272, 276
Johnston, W.A., 219, 236
Jones, H.P., 249
Jonides, J., 70
Julesz, B., 219

Kahana, B., 184–185
Kahana, E., 184–185
Kahneman, D., 236, 240
Kane, R.L., 55
Kaplan, E., 54
Kapur, N., 54
Karol, R., 101
Kassian, S., 252
Kaszniak, A.W., 138, 140
Kausler, D., 67, 124, 228, 240–241
Keenan, J., 106
Kemper S., ix, 35, 134, 138–143, 145,
    149–150
Kempler, D., 138
Kennedy, J.E., 70
Kennelly, K., 176, 225
Kent, J., 249, 251
Kerschner, P.A., 177
King, P.M., 124, 135
Kinsbourne, M., 112
Kintsch, W.A., 102, 106, 114, 253
Kitchener, K.S., 124, 135
Kivnick, H.Q., 268
Klatzky, R.L., v
Klein, J.F., 116
Kliegl, R., 183
Knopf, M., 270, 274–275
Knowles, M.S., 174
Kobasa, S.C., 232
Koeske, R.D., 87
Kogan, N., 125
Kohlberg, L., 135
Kopelman, M.D., 155–158
Korkel, J., 274
Kowalski, D.J., 98
Kozlowski, L.T., 70

Kramer, D.A., 32–35, 54, 124–126
Krasic, K.C., 67–68, 202
Krauss, I.K., x, 5, 67, 201–203, 205–206,
    211, 270
Kuhn, D., 124
Kwentus, J.A., 156
Kynette, D., ix, 134, 139–140, 149–150

MacDonald, J., 4
MacDonald, M.L., 201, 210
MacKay, D.G., ix, 140
Madden, D.J., 109, 219, 238
Maloy, R.M., x
Mandler, J.M., 69, 253
Marcus, E.E., 175
Marcus, S.M., 102
Markus, H., 30–31
Marsh, G.R., 202
Marshall, V.S., 262
Marsiske, M., 190
Marslen-Wilson, W.D., 102, 108
Martens, S.K., 252
Martin, J., 4, 27
Martin, M., 4, 5
Martin, R.C., 103, 105
Martone, M., 159
Mattingly, I.G., 102, 105, 113
Maxwell, C., 27
McAndrews, M.P., 159
McCarthy, M., 6, 55
McCartney, K.A., 46
McClannahan, L.R., 201, 210
McClelland, J.L., 218–219
McCormick, D.J., 211
McCrae, R.R., 232
McDowd, J.M., 101, 104, 237
McGee, M.G., 203
McGee, N.D., 238
McKitrick, L.A., ix, 165, 167–169
McKoon, G., 14, 219
McNamara, T.P., 67
McNeill, D., 249
Meacham, J.A.; x, 265, 267
Metzger, R., 67–68
Meyer, B.J.F., 253
Miller, J., 82
Miller, J.L., 102
Miller, K., 67–68

Mitchell, D.B., 101, 158–159
Mittelman, D., 275
Modigliani, V., 162
Moffat, N.J., 159, 162–164, 169
Moore, J.W., 50
Moore, T.E., 68
Morris, P.E., 3, 238
Morris, R.G., 155–158
Morton, J., 109
Morton, K.R., 4, 271
Mross, E.F., 114
Muensterberg, H., 247
Murphy, L.J., x, 237
Murray, D.M., 247
Myer, B.J.F., 104
Myles-Worsley, M., 219

Nebes, R.D., 5, 238
Neely, J.H., 219
Neisser, U., 3, 18, 67, 253
Nelson, K., 40–51, 88, 92
Nelson, T.O., 273
Nersessian, N., 27
Neugarten, B.L., 50, 124
Newcombe, N., 203
Newmark, E.D., 34–35
Nezworski, T., 67–68
Niederehe, G., 4, 224, 226
Nissen, 157
Nolan, K.A., 102, 115, 118
Norman, S., ix, 134, 140
Norris, K.K.A., x, 211, 232
Novak, J., 177

Ober, B.A., 54
Obler, L.K., 138
O'Brien, K., 138
Ochalek, K., 252
Offermann, L.R., 174
Ohta, R.J., 67–68, 211
Okun, M.A., 174
Oliver, C., 67
Olsho, L.W., 103
O'Rourke, T., 249, 251
Osborne, D.P., 54
Osterhout, L., 114–115

Palij, M., 70
Palmer, J.C., 247
Papaniclaou, A.C., 55
Parasuramam, R., 236
Park, D.C., 3, 8, 15–16
Parker, R.E., 69
Parsons, T., 175
Payne, M., 159
Pennington, N., 124
Penrod, S.D., 249, 251–252
Percy, K., 174–175
Perlmutter, M., x, 25, 67–68, 250, 270–271
Peron, E., 67
Perrotta, P., 267
Perry, W.G., 124
Peterson, D.A., 174–176
Petrinovich, L., 7
Pezdek, K., 67–69, 201
Piaget, J., 124, 224
Pigott, M., 252
Pillemer, D.B., 259–261
Pinker, S., 105
Plude, D.J., x, 219, 236–238, 241–242
Pollina, L.K., 17
Poon, L.W., ix, 3, 6, 104–105, 107, 124, 182, 184, 231, 270–271
Posner, M.I., 219, 230–231, 236
Powlishta, K., 11
Prather, P., 115
Prescott, C., 273
Pressley, M., 273
Presson, C.C., 70
Presti, D.E., 219
Prill, K., 237
Prince, A., 105
Prinzmetal, W., 219
Puckett, J.M., 17
Puglisi, J.T., 8, 15–16
Pye, C., 141

Quahagen, M., 202
Quinlan, P.T., 219

Rabbitt, P., 9, 274
Rabinowitz, J.C., 156, 162
Rae, D., 55

Randt, C.T., 54
Rankin, J.L., 101
Rash, S., 138, 140–141, 150
Rashid, S., 249
Raskind, C.L., 274
Ratcliff, R., 114, 219
Ratner, H.H., 275
Reason, J., 26–27, 238–239
Rebok, G.W., 174
Reder, L.M., 122
Reese, H.W., 17, 51
Regnier, V.A., 5, 201
Reinhartz, G., 184
Reisberg, B., 54
Reiser, B.J., 88
Rice, G.E., 4, 104, 253
Rich, S.A., 160
Richards, B., 68
Richards, F.A., 124
Richardson, J.T.E., 18
Riddoch, M.J., 219
Riegel, K.F., 124, 260
Rieger, C., 113
Riley, K.P., x, 182–187
Risley, T.R., 201, 210
Roberts, P.M., 140
Rodriquez, I.A., 225
Rogan, J.D., 237
Rogoff, B., 6
Rogoff, R., 67–69
Ronning, R., 177
Roodin, P.A., 98, 197
Rose, T.L., 6, 184, 225
Ross, B.L., viii, 39, 42, 44, 46, 48, 51,
    97–98
Ross, L., 224
Rothenberg, P.S., 266
Rothkopf, E.Z., 177
Rowles, G.D., 184
Robin, D.C., 3–5, 231, 259–260
Rumelhart, D.E., 218–219
Ryan, E.B., 103, 118, 140
Rybash, J.M., x, 98, 197

Saffran, E.R., 141
Sagar, 157
Salama, M., 55, 61

Salmaso, P., 67
Salmon, D.P., 155–156, 158–159
Salthouse, T.A., 101, 124, 216,
    237–238, 274
Sax, D.S., 159
Schacter, D.L., 156, 158–164,
    218
Schaie, K.W., 51, 135, 174, 190–191,
    193, 202–203, 263, 274, 276
Schank, R.C., 46–50, 52
Scheidt, R.J., 191
Schell, D.A., 124, 126, 253, 275
Scheuder, R., 102
Shlechter, T.M., 25
Schneider, W., 240, 270, 274
Schonfield, D., 238
Schuck, J.R., 55
Schulenberg, J.E., 4
Schulz, R., 226
Schwartz, M.F., 141
Schwartzman, A., 140
Scogin, F., 6, 182–184
Scott, M.L., 55
Sehulster, J.B., 272
Shapiro, L.P., 102
Sharps, M.J., 15–16
Shaw, R.J., 113
Sherman, R., 67
Sheikh, J.I., 160, 183
Shiffrin, R.M., 239–240
Shimamura, A.P., 158
Shock, N., 70, 72, 74
Shrout, P.E., 131
Shults, C.W., 159
Siegler, I.C., 174
Simeone, C., 182
Simon, E., 240
Simon, H.A., 88, 197
Simons, M.A., 219
Sinnott, J.D., v, viii, 3, 5, 67, 71, 74,
    124, 206
Slauson, T., 138
Smiley, S.S., 129
Smith, A.D., 6, 8, 101, 240
Smith, C., 201
Smith, D.A., 98
Smith, S., 158
Smyth, M.M., 70
Snyder, D.R., 230–231

Sorensen, J., 116
Sowarka, D., 183
Spilich, F.J., 87
Sprott, R., 138
Squire, L.R., 156, 158–159, 169
Stampp, M.S., 160
Stasz, C., 48
Stead, C., 34–35
Steinberg, E., 4, 273
Stern, H.L., 241
Stern, W., 246–247
Sternberg, R.J., 190, 197
Stevens, A.B., 4, 168
Stine, E.A.L., ix, 8, 101, 104–108,
    115–116, 118
Stine, L., 239
Storandt, M., 182–183
Stuve, T., 249, 251
Sulin, R.A., 87
Sweeney J.D., 252
Swinney, D., 114–115
Sykes, R.N., 3

Taine, H., 22
Tanenhaus, M.K., 125
Tanke, E., 183
Taub, H.A., 253
Taylor, J.R., 156
Taylor, S., 47–48
Tenney, Y.J., 9
Thomas, R.L., 225
Thompson, D.M., ix
Thompson, D., 177–178
Thompson, L.W., 4, 250
Thorndike, E.L., 173
Thorndyke, P., 48
Thurstone, L.L., 91
Thurstone, T.G., 91
Till, R., 114
Tilse, C.S., 4, 271
Titus, W., 67
Tomarken, A.J., 223
Tomer, A., 182, 184–185
Tomoda, C., 138
Toner, H., 116
Trahan, D.E., 54
Treat, N.J., ix, 184
Treisman, A., 220

Trotter, S., 4, 273
Tulving, E., v, 162, 218, 240
Tun, P., 104
Tuokko, H., 241
Turner, T.J., 46
Tuten, C., 101
Tweney, R.D., 27–28, 36
Tyler, L., 102, 108–109, 112

Ulatowska, H.K., 140
Underwood, V.L., 4

Vandermaas, M., 47, 88, 98, 254
Van Dijk, T.A., 102, 106, 114, 252
Vanier, M., 103
Velton, E., 225
Ventis, D.G., x, 276
Vesonder, G.T., 87
Volans, P.J., 161
Voss, J.F., 87
Vygotsky, I., 261

Waddell, K.J., 6, 67–69
Wade, E., ix, 140
Wales, R., 116
Walicke, P.A., 159
Walker, V.G., 140, 149
Wallesch, G.W., 140
Walsh, D.A., 5, 67, 201–203, 205, 207,
    210, 212
Walton, M., 9
Watson, J.B., 224
Wayland, S.C., 109
Weaverdyck, S.E., 125–126
Weber, R.J., 201, 203, 207, 210, 212
Wechsler, D.A., 54–55, 61, 74, 142
Weinert, F.E., 270, 274–275
Weinsten, C.E., 4–5
Weisman, 178
Weldon, J.K., 201
Welford, A.T., 270
Welke, D.J., 3
Wellman, H.M., 29
Wells, C.E., 226
Wells, G.L., 247, 250, 252
Wessels, J., 109

West, R.L., viii, 3-7, 9, 11, 26, 56-57, 61-62, 167, 174, 182-186, 250, 273
Wetzler, S.E., 5
Whipple, G.M., 246
White, H., 13
White, S.H., 259-261
Whitehouse, P., 54
Willis, S.L., 184, 190-191, 193-194, 196
Wilson, B.A., 3, 7, 159, 231
Wingfield, A., ix, 8, 101-102, 104-105, 107-109, 113, 115-116, 118, 150, 239
Winkler, J., 47-48
Winograd, E., 6
Winterling, D., 61
Withnall, A., 173-174
Witken, H.A., 174
Wohlwill, J.F., 210
Woll, S.B., 98
Wood, P.K., 124

Woodruff, D.S., 33, 124-126
Woods, J.H., 177
Woods, R.T., 161
Worthley, J.S., ix, 4, 27, 140

Yarmey, A.D., 246, 248-249, 251-252
Yesavage, J.A., 6, 61, 160, 183-186, 225, 229
Yoder, C.Y., x, 226-227, 229
Youngjohn, J.R., 15, 56-57
Yuille, J.C., 252

Zacks, R.T., 66, 68, 73, 149, 239-240
Zajonc, R.B., 230
Zandri, E., 178
Zarit, S.N., 184-185, 276
Zelinski, E.M., 4, 67-69, 113, 250, 253
Zurif, W., 115

Subject Index

Acts, 92–97
  definition of, 92
Adult education
  computer applications for, 177–178
  effective instruction design for,
    175–177
  information organization for, 176–177
  learning capacity of elderly in,
    173–179
  presentation time, 175–176
  setting of, 174–176
Affective valence, 228–232
Age-Associated Memory Impairment
    (AAMI), 54, 59–63, 183–184,
    187
Aging, *see* Everyday memory aging
Alzheimer's-Type Dementia (AD), ix, 54,
    58–59, 62–63, 140, 155–170,
    183–183, 185, 241
  memory interventions in, 155–170
Analyses of variance (ANOVAs), 73,
    77–78, 80, 92, 96, 143, 194, 197
Autobiographical remembering, 259–268
  as emancipatory interest, 266–268
  as expression of technical interest,
    259–261
  as practical interest, 261–266, 268
    cooperative action, 261–266, 268
    interpersonal, 261–266

Backward digit span, 142–145
Benton error, 75
Benton Visual Retention Test, 60–61,
    74–75

California Verbal Learning Test, 54
Cohort-sequential research design, 264
Computer-aided instruction (CAI),
    177–178
Computer-simulated everyday memory
    battery, 58–63
Conditional terms, 92–94, 97
Continuous Visual Memory Test, 54
Cross-sequential research design, 263

DAT, 156, 163
Denman Neuropsychology Memory
    Scale, 54
Descriptions, 92–93, 98
Diary data, 22–36
  accuracy of, 23–24, 28–29
  cognitive development in, 32–36
  everyday thinking in, 34
  in memory research, 24–32
  reflective, 32–34
  as source of autobiographical memory,
    28–31
  syntactic complexity, 35
Discourse cohesion
  loss of, 140
Divided Attention task, 57
Domain-specific knowledge
  training in, 161–162
Domain-specific object-level extraction,
    215, 217–219

Ebbinghaus forgetting function, 28
Elaborations, 92–93

Encoding
  kinesthetic, 77–79, 81
  verbal, 77–79
  visual, 77–79, 81
ETS Basic Reading Skills test, 190–197
Everyday cognition
  impact of Gf on, 194–197
Everyday content, encoding, and retrieval
  condition, 12–14
Everyday memory
  assessment by computerized battery,
    54–63
  research designs for, 3–8
Everyday memory aging
  affect in, 223–232
    mechanism of, 230–231
    valence paradigm of, 226–229
  clinical interaction programs in,
    184–187
  contextual models of, 271–272
  definition of, vii
  individual differences in, 270–276
  information processing models of,
    271
  methodological choices in practice,
    182–187
  selective attention in, 235–242
    automatic performance, 239–240,
      242
    task complexity of, 237–238
Everyday visual perception
  knowledge factors in, 215–220
  models of aging in, 218–219
Eyewitness memory
  accuracy of, 249–252
  aging research in, 246–255
  children's, 248–249
  detail recall, 252–253
  historical perspective of, 246–
    248
  schemas of, 253–254

First-Last Names test, 56–58, 60–62
Forward digit span, 142–145

General crystalized ability (Gc),
  190–197

General fluid ability (Gf), 190–197
Geriatric Depression Scale (GDS), 61,
  185

Hesitation phenomena, 140
High-frequency loss, 103
Human immuno-deficiency virus (HIV),
  63
Huntington's disease (HD), 159

Interpersonal relationships, 261–265,
  268
  different-aged, 263–264
  distant, 264
  same-aged, 262–263

Knowledge structures, 87–88
Krauss Card Tasks, 203–204

Laboratory component process experiments, 3, 7–8, 15–16
Language processing methodologies,
  105–119
  context and gating, 105, 108–113
  crossmodal priming and online process-
    ing, 105, 113–115
  parsing and recall, 106, 115–118
  proportional density and speed rate,
    105–108
Linguistic limitations, 149–150
Linton's forgetting function, 28–29
Longitudinal research design, 262–
  265

Mean number of clauses per utterance
  (MCU), 145–147
Memory
  explicit, 156–158, 169
  implicit, 158–160, 169
  improvement via an affect, 228–
    232
  interventions, 160–170
    external, 161–162
    internal, 160

repetition, 161
  retrieval practices, 162–170
  knowledge effects on, 87–88
Memory aging
  everyday perception in, 218–219
  knowledge use in, 217–218
  value of ecological validity in, 216
Memory Assessment Clinic (MAC)
  battery, 7, 10, 15
Memory Assessment Clinic Self-Report
  Scale (MAC-S), 61
Memory Self-Efficacy Questionnaire,
  273
Memory skills training programs,
  182–187
Memory strategies, 24–27
Misplaced Objects test, 57–58, 68
Mnemonic strategies, 160–170
Mood-dependent research, 225
Mood-inductive procedure, 225
Multivariate analysis of variance
  (MANOVA), 145

Name-Face Association, 56, 58,
  60–62
Narrative Recall test, 57
Naturalistic studies, 3–4, 9–10
New York University Memory Test,
  54
Nursing home settings, 201–212
  environmental knowledge in, 202–203,
  205–212
  environment use in, 201–203,
  205–212
  spatial skills in, 201–212

Optional acts, 92
Optional slot fillers, 92–93

Pearson product moment correlations,
  73–74
Perceptual processing
  age differences for spoken language,
  101–119
Phonemic regression, 103–104
Primal Mental Abilities, 91

Primary Mental Abilities Test, 204–205
Pronominal anaphors
  error in, 140
Proportion of clauses left branching (LB),
  145–149
Prosody, 116–118
Psychometric ability
  ETS performance and, 191–194
  interface with everyday cognition,
  190–197

Reaction Time test, 58, 60
Recognition of Faces – Delayed Non-
  matching, 58, 62
Recognition of Faces – Signal detection,
  58, 60
Recruitment, 103
Rivermead Behavior Memory Test
  (RSMT), 15, 185

Script content
  adult age differences in, 87–98
  empirical investigations of, 90–97
Script reports, 39–52
  commonality in, 40–45
  context of, 43–45
  instructions for, 42
  prompting, 43
  props, 43
  idiosyncracy in, 40–49, 51
  impact of experience on, 47–51
  specific, 50–51
Scripts
  adult age differences in, 87–98
  content and structure, 90–97
  definition of, 88
  influence on memory aging, 88–90
Selective attention, *see* Everyday
  memory aging
Selective Reminding test, 57–58, 60, 62
Self-report measures, 3–4, 9
Self-Reported Memory, 272–276
Semantic integration, 134–135
Short Inventory of Memory Experiences
  (SIME), 25
Simulations, 3–7, 10–15
Spaced retrieval method, 85, 163–170

Spatial memory
  aging of, 66–82
    paradigm of, 70–72, 81
    theoretical issues relating to, 67–68
  automatic tasks and, 68, 75
  effortful tasks and, 68, 75–76
  encoding of, 68–69, 77, 82
  variables influencing, 68–69
Spatial relations, 66
Spatial representation
  modes of, 66, 78–79, 81–82
Spoken language, 101–119
  age differences in, 138–150
  special characteristics of, 102–104
Spontaneous segmentation, 115–119
Spontaneous speech, 138–139
Symbolic inferences
  complex, 130–132, 135
  simple, 130–132, 134
Symbolic processing, 124–135

Syntactic complexity, 138–142, 148
  development of, 35

Task-relevant knowledge, 215
Telephone Dialing test, 57–58, 60
Test batteries, 3, 7, 15
Text-based inferences, 129–131
Text-based statements, 129–130, 132
Time-sequential research design, 265
Tip-of-the-tongue experiences (TOTs), 4,
  26–27

Wechsler Adult Intelligence Scale, 60, 74,
  110, 131, 142–144
Wechsler Memory Scale, 7, 54, 60–61
Working memory, 142–150
  limitations of, 148–149
  linguistic complexity in, 147–148
  syntactic complexity in, 142–147, 150